Appalachian Health and Well-Being

Appalachian Health and Well-Being

Edited by
Robert L. Ludke
and
Phillip J. Obermiller

Foreword by
Richard A. Couto

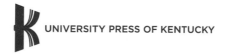

UNIVERSITY PRESS OF KENTUCKY

An earlier version of chapter 14 was published as "Identifying Appalachian Adults: An Empirical Study" by Robert L. Ludke, Phillip J. Obermiller, Eric W. Rademacher, and Shiloh K. Turner in *Appalachian Journal*. 2010;38(1). Copyright 2010, *Appalachian Journal*, Appalachian State University. Used by permission.

Scholarly publisher for the Commonwealth, serving Bellarmine University, Berea College, Centre College of Kentucky, Eastern Kentucky University, The Filson Historical Society, Georgetown College, Kentucky Historical Society, Kentucky State University, Morehead State University, Murray State University, Northern Kentucky University, Transylvania University, University of Kentucky, University of Louisville, and Western Kentucky University.

Editorial and Sales Offices: The University Press of Kentucky, 663 South Limestone Street, Lexington, Kentucky 40508-4008
www.kentuckypress.com

16 15 14 13 12   5 4 3 2 1

Library of Congress Cataloging-in-Publication Data

Appalachian health and well-being / edited by Robert L. Ludke and Phillip J. Obermiller ; foreword by Richard A. Couto.
    p. ; cm.
  Includes bibliographical references and index.
  ISBN 978-0-8131-3586-1 (hardcover : alk. paper) — ISBN 978-0-8131-3587-8 (ebook)
  I. Ludke, Robert L., 1945- II. Obermiller, Phillip J.
  [DNLM: 1. Rural Health—Appalachian Region. 2. Health Services Accessibility—Appalachian Region. 3. Health Status Disparities—Appalachian Region. 4. Health Status Indicators—Appalachian Region. 5. Residential Mobility—Appalachian Region. WA 390]
    362.109756'8—dc23   2011044469

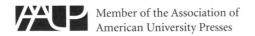 Member of the Association of American University Presses

To the health and well-being of Appalachians,
wherever they may live

Contents

Part III: Urban Appalachian Health

Illustrations

Foreword

As director of the Center for Health Services at Vanderbilt University from 1975 to 1988, I had the professionally and personally enriching experience of working with community leaders in rural, low-income communities in and around Tennessee. Our work, like the chapters of this book, addressed all the factors that promote health and well-being, including economic, political, psychological, environmental, and social ones. From these community leaders I learned to put health and health care in a socioeconomic and political context. I recall in particular Square Mormon, an African American farmer in predominantly black Fayette County in West Tennessee. He and his county were pioneers in the voter registration efforts of African Americans in the South. He understood his later work on health care, in his hometown of Rossville, as a seamless continuation of the "movement." "The people in Fayette County, when their eyes came open, they had really got sick for justice" (p. 72).[1]

Diagonally across the state, some 400 to 500 miles to the northeast in the Appalachian coalfields of Tennessee, eastern Kentucky, southern West Virginia, and southwestern Virginia, I was privileged to be part of other community leaders' efforts to develop health care services. They too were sick for justice—they wanted health care, jobs, and environmental quality, and they fought against ruinous extractive economies, scandalously inadequate tax systems, and the disparity between high levels of basic human needs and insufficient services.

More than thirty years mark the distance between that work and this book. Much has changed for the better. The chapters in this collection document measures of improved health status and ongoing innovations in the provision and coordination of services. There are also several constants from then to now, as this book shows. For instance, we still need to understand that health encompasses more than medical care and illness, and we still need to place these aspects in a broader context of their potential underlying determinants, which is the framework this volume uses. There is also a continuing connection between health and justice, or fairness. Readers will learn, if they do not already know, that Appalachia, as defined by the Appalachian Regional Commission, is not a homogeneous geographic or economic construct. Central Appalachia remains the poorest of the Appalachian subregions. The coalfields of eastern Kentucky, eastern Tennessee, southern West Virginia, and southwestern Virginia have higher rates of poverty and unemployment and lower rates of per capita income, labor force participation, and adults with a high school education compared with counties in other parts of Appalachia. Not surprisingly, Central Appalachia has the largest concentration of what the Appalachian Regional Commission refers to as "distressed counties," so called for their chronic poverty, unemployment, low educational attainment, and low per capita income.

Other subregions have seen both good and bad changes. Northern Appalachia has slipped from its position as the most prosperous subregion, signifying the decline of the country's "Rust Belt" areas. Southern Appalachia, part of the nation's "Sun Belt," has assumed the position as the most prosperous subregion. It has the most "attainment" counties, based on measures comparable to national averages of poverty, unemployment, educational attainment, and per capita income. Most of these are suburban counties around Atlanta, Georgia; Greenville and Spartanburg, South Carolina; and Winston-Salem, North Carolina.

Thus, economic inequality marks one difference between Appalachia and the rest of the country. Readers will learn, however, that there are differences in well-being, economics, and health among the subregions of Appalachia, among the Appalachian portions of the thirteen states that make up the region, between the Appalachian and non-Appalachian portions of these states, between metropolitan and rural counties, and even between Appalachian migrants and other residents of Cincinnati. In fact, there are greater variations in health and economics among the counties of Appalachia than between the region and the rest of the country.

The justice issue arises when we realize that differences in health status parallel the economic differences in Appalachia. For example, residents of Central Appalachian counties have the highest rate of premature mortality from heart disease and cancer among those aged 35 to 64 years. Also, people living in the distressed counties of Appalachia have the greatest risk for diabetes, perhaps because the prevalence of obesity (a risk factor for diabetes) is related to economic status, with distressed counties having more obese residents. Not surprisingly, people living in low-income counties report more life stressors and related mental health problems. This volume does not engage in reductionism and victim blaming; it does not attempt to pin responsibility for such conditions on some inherent shortcoming of these people—culture, idiosyncratic characteristics, or deficits in social capital. Central Appalachia has more severe health problems primarily because poor health is associated with low socioeconomic status and is thus a problem of justice.

The relatively new field of social epidemiology explains poverty and health status as social forms, not individual choices. Researchers in this field, invoking the work of Émile Durkheim, point to the social environments of groups that tend to remain different in the same way over time, such as the distressed counties of Appalachia. The social environment, including the construction of community bonds, influences what appear to be individual conditions, such as health and illness. Factors within the particular social environments of distressed counties or urban Appalachian neighborhoods do not determine which individuals will be poor or ill; they merely indicate that these residents run a greater risk for poverty and illness, absent an improvement in the social environment.[2]

These conditions of inequality invariably raise questions about justice, but they bedevil theories of justice as well. It is justice to treat all people the same, as espoused in the Declaration of Independence or the United Nations' Declaration of Universal Human Rights. It is also justice, however, to treat people with differences differently, such as providing handicapped parking spaces. Therefore, some inequalities may be tolerable. For instance, in practical terms, equality may not be possible with regard to distance from highly specialized trauma centers or genetics professionals (topics touched on in this book). Other unjust conditions may be intolerable, such as the differences in "allostatic load" within Appalachian counties. The combined and cumulative burden on the human body due to the "riskscape"—the social, psychological, and physical environmental contributors to health—puts some at greater risk for illness and premature mortality than others.

John Rawls famously used disparities in health status and their potential underlying determinants to formulate a theory of justice. Rawls's test to reconcile justice and inequality is simple: If you had no way of knowing whether you would have a physical handicap, would you choose to live in a world with or without handicapped parking spaces? Conversely, if you knew that certain rights were routinely denied or unavailable to people based on race, gender, and other factors, would you choose to have any of those factors? Justice requires us to remove those inequalities we would not choose to endure. When we do not know how we will fare (a veil of ignorance) in the distribution of assets and resources, our principles of justice are likely to be very different from those we would enact if we knew we would derive either advantages or disadvantages from that distribution. Choosing from behind a veil of ignorance and being averse to risk, we are likely to legitimate only those inequalities (e.g., handicapped parking spaces) that meet the needs of those who are less well off.[3]

This collection removes another veil of ignorance: the link between poverty and poor health. This enduring bond suggests that our practice of justice defies Rawls's premise that inequality is justified only when it addresses another form of inequality. Indeed, societies construct understandings of cultural and other differences that explain enduring inequalities as their defense against principles of justice and equality. The contributors to this volume do not invoke pejorative stereotypes or social science sophistry to explain and defend the health needs and disparities of the Appalachian region. Without these explanations, we are defenseless against claims for justice based on these disparities and their underlying determinants.

These are claims against justice, my friend Square informed me, but not the justice of Rawls, or "what would I pick for myself behind a veil of ignorance." Instead, we need another, less hypothetical theory of justice—the type Martha Nussbaum provides. Her premise differs from Rawls's, as does her effort to bring the real (not hypothetical) and differing conditions of people into her theory of justice. "The basic intuitive idea of my version of the capabilities approach [to justice] is that we begin with a conception of the dignity of the human being, and of a life that is worthy of that dignity—a life that has available in it 'truly human functioning.'" Nussbaum lists ten central human capabilities, including life, bodily health, bodily integrity (including safety), the ability to live with concern for and in relationship to the world of nature, and control over one's political and material environment. Nussbaum's concern is with an appropriate threshold level of these capabilities for all people in a society, and she assumes "a society that does not guarantee these to all its citizens, at some appropriate threshold level, falls short of being a fully just society" (pp. 74–75).[4]

Naturally, we can have intense debates over the appropriate threshold levels that measure the dignity of a human being in the United States. We can set these threshold levels low, as this volume shows has been done in Appalachia. Obviously, the lower the threshold, the more inevitably we compromise the standard of dignity for those human beings who do not meet these levels. Less obviously, the lower the threshold, the more we erode the human dignity of those who set or acquiesce to these levels.

These pages on the health and well-being of Appalachians reflect the values and practices of the United States. There is, of course, much to be proud of in these values and practices and in the progress we have made to express them more completely. However, these pages also tell us that some people in this country remain sick for justice.

> Richard A. Couto
> Distinguished Senior Scholar
> Union Institute and University

References

1. Couto RA. Prophets in health care. *Southern Exposure: Sick for Justice.* 1978;6(2):72–76.

2. Syme SL. Foreword. In: Berkman LF, Kawachi I, eds. *Social Epidemiology.* New York, NY: Oxford University Press; 2000:ix–xii.

3. Rawls J. *A Theory of Justice.* Cambridge, MA: Harvard University Press; 1971.

4. Nussbaum MA. *Frontiers of Justice: Disability, Nationality, and Species Membership.* Cambridge, MA: Belknap Press; 2006.

Introduction

The story of Appalachian health and health care is one of complexity and paradox. At various times and in different places throughout the region's history, health care has been the province of herbalists, granny women, missionaries, company doctors, nurse practitioners, labor unions, church groups, community-based organizations, private practitioners, and state and federal governments. At various times and places, the region has experienced a shortage of physicians, dentists, nurses, health educators, clinics, and hospitals. At times, the region has been a repository of underqualified and unqualified health practitioners, and it remains an area where a few unethical pharmacists and physicians trade in prescriptions for painkillers. The Appalachian region is also the place where many effective innovations and creative advances in health care have originated.

With nearly 25 million people living in a 205,000-square-mile area, Appalachia has been characterized as a place with pervasive health disparities and limited health care infrastructure and services.[a] It is a region with environmental, economic, and social conditions that contribute to poor health and substandard health care. Although knowledge about the health of Appalachians and its underlying determinants is growing, much is still unknown.

This volume takes a broad perspective by focusing on the health of all Appalachians, both residents of Appalachia and those who have migrated from the region. As some researchers have noted, "the facts about health in the mountains of Appalachia have been slow to emerge" (p. 1).[1] There are even fewer facts, mostly outdated, about the health of the millions of people who have migrated from Appalachia into urban areas and their descendants. Many of these migrants have settled in or near metropolitan areas across the nation, and they may be experiencing health disparities similar to those of their rural Appalachian counterparts.

Useful information about the health of Appalachians has yet to be compiled in a comprehensive and cohesive manner, limiting the education of students, health practitioners, and policy and decision makers. This situation has hindered the ability to translate what is known about the determinants of Appalachian health into effective health policy and health services delivery. It has also restricted the identification of gaps in our knowledge about Appalachian health and limited our understanding of the strategies needed to decrease the health disparities affecting rural and urban Appalachians.

This volume draws on a multidisciplinary group of researchers and clinicians, many of them nationally renowned for their work, to document what is known about the health of Appalachians, identify areas in need of further investigation, and assess the implications of this knowledge for policy development. This introduction sets the stage for these discussions by reviewing some of the earlier literature, examining some of the major developments in the history of health and health care in the region, defining some of the basic concepts related to the topic of Appalachian health, explaining some of the key methodologies used, and outlining the overall structure of the volume.

Historical Background

An exhaustive listing of historical resources relating to health in Appalachia is beyond the scope of this work. However, eight publications thematically similar to this volume illustrate the progress, or the lack thereof, made from the 1950s through the early 2000s.[b]

Report to the Council of the Southern Mountains on Health Care Services in the Southern Appalachian Region. Published in 1955, this report by the Rural Life Council at the Tuskegee Institute discusses health conditions; the availability of physicians, nurses, dentists, and institutional health care services such as hospitals and clinics; and the geographic distribution of these services in the region (then defined as 257 counties). In fewer than thirty pages, this highly quantitative analysis identifies the problems and some of the policy issues inherent in the health care systems of the southern mountains. What stands out is how difficult it was to collect health data at that time, forcing the researchers to be quite innovative. At one point, in the absence of any health indicators other than basic mortality data, the report uses "Rejection Rates of White Men Given Selective Service Examinations" as a proxy measure for Appalachian health status. Though aware of the medical, age, gender, and racial deficiencies of this data set, the researchers considered it the best metric available.

Although the report found the data on the relative health status of Appalachians to be inconclusive,[2] there was no ambiguity about the scarcity of health care. Doctors in the southern mountains were carrying heavier patient loads than their urban counterparts; they were older and were not being replaced by younger physicians. This situation, combined with the maldistribution of hospitals and clinics across the region, led the researchers to conclude: "The social conscience protests the lack of personnel and facilities to provide health care to relieve suffering and to prevent health impairment" (p. 25).[2]

Medical Services for Rural Areas. In this 1957 report, William Massie, chair of the Council of the Southern Mountains Health Committee, presents a case study of health issues in the coalfields of eastern Tennessee and the steps taken to address them. A health survey of residents in the Clear Fork Valley found that although self-reported morbidity rates were high, only one-third of respondents had seen a doctor, less than one-third had seen a dentist, and none reported a hospital visit in the previous year. Among children, "Scurvy and rickets were commonplace. . . . Pyorrhea was almost endemic. Decay of teeth far beyond normal was possibly related to high carbohydrate diet, frequent use of carbonated beverages and tobacco, and lack of prophylactic dental care" (p. 26).[3]

In cooperation with the state health department, the miners' union, state medical schools, and communities in the Clear Fork Valley, the Tennessee Health Foundation established a central clinic staffed with a public health nurse, a doctor, and a part-time dentist. Initial reluctance to use the clinic diminished in the face of quality care. Massie notes, "If the former medical care of patients with acute illnesses could be rated only as poor, the diagnosis and care of chronic or recurrent illnesses had been pitifully inadequate" (p. 26).[3] The clinic also succeeded because it was organized around the health needs and norms of the rural communities it served. For example, the wife of a local Baptist minister was hired to assist at the clinic. In Massie's words, "Her understanding of the local social and political structure proved particularly useful" (p. 26).[3]

Appalachia Medicine. Published from 1969 through 1973 by Appalachian Regional Hospitals, this quarterly journal covered a spectrum of topics, including health planning and education, physician recruitment, management of cardiovascular disease, health effects of air pollution, radiological techniques, treatment of gastrointestinal diseases, alcoholism treatment, and "decreasing the incidence of inappropriate prescriptions" (p. 78).[4] In addition to doctors and nurses, contributors included medical school faculty, hospital and clinic administrators, public health workers, community-based professionals, and local clergy. Some articles were devoted to educating health care providers about their patients' everyday lives—for example, "When Yesterday's People Become Today's Patients"[5] or "Life Style of the Coal Miner: America's Original Hard Hat."[6] Both of these articles relied heavily on Jack Weller's 1966 book *Yesterday's People*, then considered a key source on Appalachians. Since then, Weller has been criticized for promoting stereotypes.

Some articles described model programs, such as the Frontier Nursing Service and the Alice Lloyd College Outreach Reserves (ALCOR), which recruited student nurses to teach preventive medicine techniques in eastern Kentucky. The ALCOR educational effort was clearly a two-way street: "At the beginning of the summer the student nurses were asking the supervisor for Lysol, alcohol and other antiseptics, but toward the end of the experience they were only asking for soap and water" (p. 113).[7]

Rural and Appalachian Health. In 1971 the West Virginia University (WVU) School of Medicine hosted a conference on rural and Appalachian health, and two years later the conference proceedings were published.[8] This compilation of twelve essays and ten sets of comments is an indicator of both the status of Appalachian health care at the outset of the 1970s and the prevailing mind-set of the contributors. The focus is on health care systems rather than Appalachian health status, and information on the latter appears to be in short supply. The volume puts rural health care in an international perspective and calls for federal policies to address regional health problems.

Some contributors remained in the thrall of Weller, however, attributing Appalachian health problems to "social and cultural isolation" (p. 41),[9] "folk medicine and faith medicine" (p. 59),[10] and "individualism, traditionalism, religious fatalism, action-orientation, and stoicism" (p. 5).[11] In discussing environmental problems in West Virginia, one author invokes a cluster of rural north-central counties and concludes: "Except for the increased dangers of animal and insect bites and many types of rural accidents, [these counties] have fewer environmental problems than are apparent elsewhere. . . . Stream and air pollution is still minimal in these isolated counties" (p. 39).[9] This reticence is not surprising. Given its time and location, the conference was probably considered quite progressive for a state dominated by coal interests.

Apparently, the conference was also too progressive for many in the state's medical hierarchy. A fourth-year WVU medical student expressed his disappointment that so "few physicians and instructors from the West Virginia University Medical Center [are] attending this conference. Consider that only ten miles away there are about three hundred doctors who every day instruct us in what medicine is and what we should do with medicine; yet, when they do not seem to be interested in a thing like this conference, one really begins to question what it is all about" (p. 146).[12]

Streams of Idealism and Health Care Innovation. This 1982 monograph by Richard Couto discusses community mobilization around health care, principally in Appalachia. Its focus is on community-campus partnerships to establish health care centers run by local health councils. Here, health services are seen in the context of broader community development. In Couto's words, "it must be understood that a community is affected by a wide variety of social factors, and that health care cannot be singled out as a single factor to be addressed" (p. 101).[13] Over a ten-year span, federal support was garnered for rural clinics governed by community boards, nurse practitioners gained acceptance at the clinics, primary care was given due emphasis, and doctors from the National Health Service Corps contributed to a more even distribution of health care providers. College students and faculty involved in the project learned the fundamentals of community initiation and control of health care, positive community change beyond health care, and the key role of local leadership development.

At times, neither the power nor the assumptions deeply embedded in the health care system allowed for a successful outcome. In one instance Couto notes, "the bias of existing medical and political arrangements [was] invoked to render community claims of authority over the clinic illegitimate and unenforceable" (p. 109).[13] He is particularly critical of enumerating Appalachian cultural characteristics: "These stereotypes are applied too broadly and too inaccurately. In many instances the stereotypes serve the purposes of those who apply them, by explaining the inadequacies within the status quo in terms of inadequacies of people, rather than our institutions, where the fault may truly lie" (p. xvii).[13]

Health in Appalachia. The University of Kentucky's Appalachian Center sponsored a health-themed conference in 1988 and published the proceedings the following year.[14] In addition to twelve single-page summaries, *Health in Appalachia* includes twenty longer overviews, research reports, and demonstration projects. Overview topics include the political economy of Appalachian health and increasing access to health systems through finance reform. The research and analysis section is highly quantitative, with an emphasis on mental health issues. The discussion of demonstration projects includes those serving children and the elderly, advocating for networks and alliances, and promoting health education.

Many of the data analyzed in this publication come from eastern Kentucky or equally localized situations and are extrapolated to all of Appalachia. Nonetheless, there are many useful insights in this collection, salted with a few lingering stereotypes. Of particular interest is a roundtable of four rural physicians frankly discussing the realities of providing health care in eastern Kentucky. Their candor is refreshing when it is not alarming: "I found that in a lot of ways it's very easy to treat people who are less educated, because they don't question you as much" (p. 41).[15] Preceding a discussion of fatalism, another doctor comments, "I think there are stereotypes, and I think they stem from obvious sources. Some of them are still there, and some of them aren't. Some of them are nice, and I hope they don't change" (p. 41).[15]

Preventing Chronic Disease. In 2006 the National Center for Chronic Disease Prevention and Health Promotion published a special issue of this electronic journal focusing on health and health care delivery issues in Appalachia. Although these essays are useful and well-intentioned (and many are cited in this volume), for the most part, they lack a sense of environmental connectedness that Wendell Berry so eloquently evokes—for example, the interrelationships among agriculture, food, and health or the effects of extractive industries on drinking water and health.[16]

Encyclopedia of Appalachia. A more compelling resource is the section on health in the *Encyclopedia of Appalachia.* Also published in 2006, the section covers an eclectic set of topics, including a critical look at health systems in Appalachia, the effects of coal mining on workers' health, community-based health initiatives, and grassroots organizing for health care. Missing, however, is any mention of obesity, substance abuse, and many of the chronic diseases that disproportionately affect Appalachians.

Health Innovations

In addition to these research efforts, many collaborative and innovative health initiatives have originated in Appalachia. Community- and campus-based groups working together in the region have engaged in participatory health research, substance abuse cessation and treatment, clinical care, and advocacy for new health care policies and initiatives. A few examples of health care innovations in the region are offered here; others are presented as case studies in the chapters that follow.

The Frontier Nursing Service (FNS) was founded in 1925 in Leslie County, Kentucky, by Mary Breckinridge. Starting out as the Kentucky Committee for Mothers and Babies, the FNS pioneered the practice of nurse-midwifery in rural America. In addition to delivering home health care on horseback (and later in jeeps), the FNS eventually grew to include small clinics in rural areas, a hospital in Leslie County, and the Frontier Graduate School of Midwifery. Historian James C. Klotter notes that by 1965 "the Frontier Nursing Service had performed nearly 15,000 deliveries with an obstetrics-related death rate of 11.0 per 10,000 deliveries, versus the national average of 36.3" (p. 1643).[17]

Finding company-provided health care in the Appalachian coalfields inadequate, the United Mine Workers of America's Welfare and Retirement Fund built and staffed ten new hospitals in the coal mining areas of Kentucky, West Virginia, and Virginia in the 1950s. It also "established a new standard of care by combining group practice, preventive services, and appropriate referrals" (p. 1645)[18]; this was especially effective for black lung patients. When health professionals and community residents were brought together on the boards of clinics, they "pioneered in blending, very often in a stormy way, professional innovations with community-led health initiatives" (p. 1645).[18] Now known as Appalachian Regional Healthcare (ARH), the organization operates clinics, home health care agencies, pharmacies, and hospitals in Kentucky and West Virginia.

An example of community-based and -controlled health care is the Mud Creek Clinic. It was founded in Floyd County, Kentucky, in 1972 by

Eula Hall, who donated her home for use as a clinic. Burned to the ground by an arsonist in 1982, the clinic reopened in an outdoor setting the next day. "More than twenty years later, the [new] 5,200 square-foot clinic continued to serve more than seven thousand patients annually with a staff of more than twenty people" (p. 1662).[19] The clinic is an example of the determination of grassroots organizations to set up and sustain health care initiatives in rural Appalachia.

The Remote Area Medical Volunteer Corps (RAM), founded in 1985 by Stan Brock and based in Knoxville, Tennessee, is worldwide in scope but expends 60 percent of its effort in rural America, including Appalachia. RAM offers multiday clinics to provide medical, dental, and vision care primarily for the uninsured and underinsured. In addition to meeting the immediate health needs of people in places such as Wise, West Virginia, RAM clearly points to the need for a better system of providing health care across the region. RAM founder Brock is described as "impatient with those who suggest the people seeking help in Wise are somehow at fault and unworthy of care given poor health habits" (p. 4).[20] Brock himself says: "The rest of the population is not in the best of shape. . . . But in the case of the well-to-do and the well-insured, they can afford to take care of it" (p. 4).[20]

Definitions and Concepts

Despite the widespread acceptance of a unitary concept of "Appalachia," the region accommodates a wide variety of topographies, economies, ethnicities, population densities, social norms, and health risks. Consequently, several key concepts are used with particular care in this volume. They include a definition of the region as well as particular interpretations of Appalachian poverty, rurality, migrants, culture, community, and folk medicine.

Definition of Appalachia. Although there are many competing definitions of the region, this volume uses the 2009 definition of the Appalachian Regional Commission (ARC), which delineates Appalachia as encompassing 420 counties in thirteen states. This is a political definition that changes as counties are added or deleted, and it is used for purposes of regional planning and implementing economic development strategies. It is also useful for analyzing health data, which are most often aggregated at the

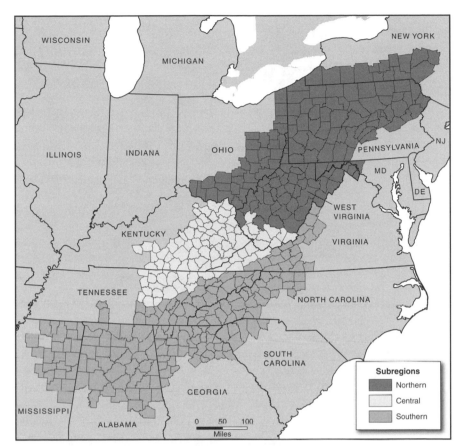

Map I.1. Subregions in Appalachia. (Map and data from Appalachian Regional Commission, October 2008.)

county and state levels. In those instances in which regionwide data are not available, health information from the Appalachian portions of states or special aggregations of Appalachian counties are adduced as case studies. Appalachia has historically been divided into three subregions (Northern, Central, and Southern) by the ARC (map I.1). In November 2009 the ARC expanded the number of subregions from three to five based on topography, demographics, and economics. Only the three original subregions are recognized in this volume because the Northern, Central, and Southern categories have been used to analyze nearly all health data to date.

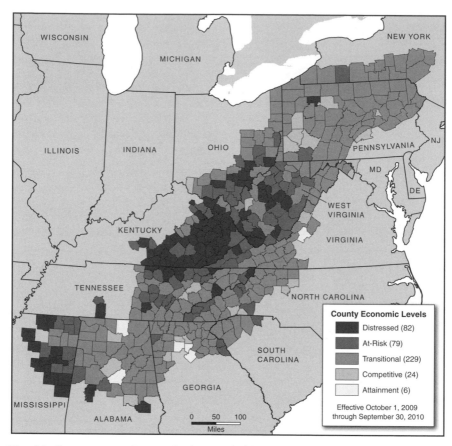

Map I.2. County economic status in the Appalachian region. (Map from Appalachian Regional Commission, October 2009. Data from U.S. Bureau of Labor Statistics, LAUS, 2005–2007; U.S. Bureau of Economic Analysis, REIS, 2006; and U.S. Census Bureau, 2000 Census, SF3.)

Poverty. Although economic deprivation is a serious problem in the region, poverty is neither universal nor evenly distributed in Appalachia. The ARC has devised a county typology involving five categories of economic status based on ranges of income, levels of unemployment, and rates of poverty: distressed, at-risk, transitional, competitive, and attainment.[c] As illustrated in map I.2, people of moderate economic circumstances are found in the Appalachian areas of every state, interspersed with pockets of relatively well-off people, especially in and near metropolitan areas.

Enclaves of people struggling economically are found throughout the region; however, areas of poverty are clustered in Central Appalachia and in Appalachian Mississippi.

Rurality. Appalachia is associated with a largely rural population in the public mind, despite the fact that the majority of Appalachians now live in metropolitan or urban counties. On average, Appalachia had more residents per square mile (114.1) than the United States as a whole (79.6) in 2000. But population density is not spread evenly across the region. Much of Appalachia's population is clustered in and around cities such as Pittsburgh, Charleston, Knoxville, Chattanooga, and Birmingham; many

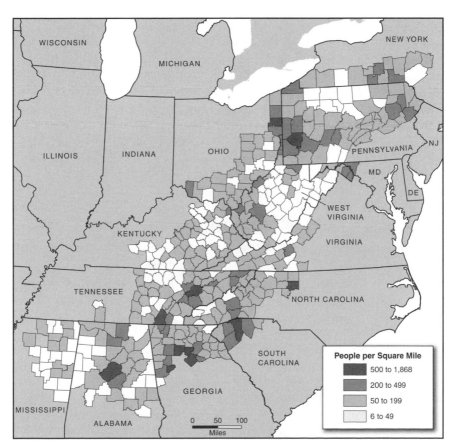

Map I.3. Population density in the Appalachian region. (Map from Appalachian Regional Commission, August 2010. Data from U.S. Census Bureau, 2009 Population Estimates.)

other Appalachians reside in the vicinity of major metropolitan areas adjacent to the region, such as Atlanta, Cincinnati, Greensboro, and Montgomery. Nevertheless, there are clusters of very lightly populated counties (fewer than 50 residents per square mile) in West Virginia and in the Appalachian areas of Pennsylvania, Ohio, Kentucky, Tennessee, Virginia, Alabama, and Mississippi (map I.3). These are among the most rural counties in the country.

Although direct access to hospitals, clinics, and physicians is attenuated by the topography of a region known for its valleys, rivers, and mountains, the residents of Appalachia's rural counties are by no means socially or culturally isolated from the rest of the country. Physical access to health services may be impeded by long distances or travel times, lack of personal or public transportation, or the cost of travel, but rural Appalachians participate in the national ethos through extended kinship networks, national organizations, travel, the Internet, cable and satellite television, newspapers, magazines, and telephones.

Migrant Urban Appalachians. In addition to the Appalachians living in and around the region's metropolitan areas, there are large numbers of migrants and their descendants living in cities outside the federally designated region. Often referred to as *urban Appalachians* because of their concentrations in large cities of the Northeast and Midwest, many left the region during the Great Migration of the twentieth century. Despite the passage of time, many Appalachian migrants and their descendants experience the same heterogeneity in socioeconomic status and health concerns as their counterparts who still live in the region.[21, 22]

Culture. Well-being lies above and beyond the concept of health.[23] When health is simply defined as the absence of disease, modern health care is often qualified to respond to health needs. But some people see their well-being in both physical and social terms, and they define illness more broadly than physician-diagnosed and -treated disease. An individual's well-being (happiness, satisfaction, independence, close familial and community ties, and diminished stress) may in fact require the avoidance of health care providers who are ineffective, incomprehensible, unaffordable, or otherwise detrimental to their patients' well-being.

Conversely, owing to a lack of reflection on their own assumptions and behaviors, health care providers frequently attribute underutilization or noncompliance to some aspect of a patient's "culture." In its extreme form, this mind-set can lead from passive stereotyping to active discrimination because people with unhealthy lifestyles are sometimes seen as "largely responsible for their own health status—have in fact chosen it. If so, then the justification for collective intervention, even in the provision of health care, becomes less clear" (p. 42).[24] Clearly, the notion of culture is a powerful concept in health care and requires careful consideration.

Where Appalachians are concerned, the concept of culture has often been vitiated by indiscriminate use of the term and vague referents. Even when Appalachian character traits or values are specified, they may be overly generalized or slanderously stereotypic. History, geography, geology, and the environment, along with social, political, and economic factors, are important considerations in Appalachian health outcomes, but they are too often conflated under the all-encompassing rubric of culture.

Appalachian culture is frequently adduced as a nebulous explanatory variable in the region's health status, but the science available to reinforce this position is scarce. To argue for a "mountain culture" in the coalfields or for a specific "rural culture" in Appalachian Ohio, for instance, one would have to specify the topic very carefully and document it thoroughly with relevant studies.[25] In those instances in which this research has been carried out, generalizing it to a wider area or to a larger population within the region remains problematic. In short, it is difficult to conceive of an accurate statement of "culture" for some 25 million people living in thirteen states, especially given the high annual turnover rate in the population through in- and out-migration.

This is not to say that local cultures do not exist. These cultures are present, particularly in rural Appalachia, just as they are in the field of medicine. In both cases, they are usually belief and behavior sets tied to specific areas in Appalachia or to specific locations within health care systems. Unfortunately, Weller's generalizations about Appalachians,[26] which even he came to doubt, still infect some contemporary thinking. These broad statements, usually summed up as definitive character traits and attributed to culture, are not used in this volume. In the words of medical psychologist Ellen Corin, "social and cultural variables are not reducible to a few discrete indices. Social and cultural environments have to be seen as systems of interacting variables and processes" (p. 119).[27] This approach to understanding the collective dimension of life in rural Appalachia is reinforced by anthropologists Elvin Hatch[28] and Susan Keefe[29, 30] in their studies of how Appalachians are continuously incorporating various aspects of modernity into their lives.

The challenge has been to find a balance between a bias toward cultural universality (there is no particularly "Appalachian" culture), on the one hand, and cultural exceptionalism (lists of specific cultural characteristics), on the other. This volume takes a pluralist stance that allows for both a biomedical and an ethnomedical approach to Appalachian health, without uncritically privileging either.

Community. The role of local communities in health care is another ambiguous concept. Community involvement is sometimes seen as a panacea and may be given a romantic (or at least an unrealistic) status in health care research and delivery. In some instances, community participation is used as a mere token, praised in theory but ignored in practice. At other times, the role of community is ignored owing to the belief that it lacks the scope and capacity to be of use in addressing health issues. Community-based organizations are dismissed as being oppressive, xenophobic, and parochial in their approach to health care.

None of these perspectives is accepted in this volume. Community involvement has worked too well and for too long to be easily dismissed in any discussion of health in Appalachia: "shared experiences in places, which form part of our identities, can be, and certainly are, mobilized to fight against collective threats and [for] collective goals" (p. 681).[31] Many in the region, however, understand the persistence and diligence required to mount successful participatory research or useful local health programs. Members of these local groups and community organizations are slow to romanticize the difficulties and barriers they have encountered.

The stance on community in this volume is based on two principles: (1) resolution of Appalachian health issues is best undertaken with full community participation, including decision making, and (2) community groups function best when they look beyond the local to make decisions in a wider context of social, economic, and scientific connections. Community-based participation is neither valorized nor rejected, but its central role in providing insight and effectiveness to health care systems serving Appalachians is recognized and accepted.

Folk Medicine. Home nostrums and folk remedies are frequently associated with Appalachian health behaviors in the popular mind. However, improvements in transportation and communication throughout the twentieth century sharply decreased Appalachians' knowledge of and reliance on folk diagnoses and remedies. Appalachians are now no more or less likely to use home remedies than other similar socioeconomic groups, and they appear to use over-the-counter medications for self-treatment at the same rate as other groups.[32] Today, substance abuse may be the most pronounced and deleterious self-medicating behavior among Appalachians.

In the past, specialized terms for certain physical conditions were used in parts of the region, and a few are still used today, especially by older Appalachians. With a little care, terms such as "high blood" or "nerves" need not interfere with effective communication and patient care. In analyzing research on this issue, anthropologist Anthony Cavender notes, "the language of health and illness in Southern Appalachia would not inhibit communication between health care provider and patient if the health care provider simply took the time to ask a few questions for clarification" (p. 182).[32]

Faith healing may be considered under the rubric of folk medicine and is also frequently associated with Appalachian health behaviors. Clinical observations of rural Appalachians indicate that most have fully integrated modern medicine with their trust in the healing powers of religious beliefs and practices. Like many other Americans, Appalachians continue to pray and engage in religious rites aimed at healing to complement the interventions of medical science.

The preceding concepts are presented here to avoid repetition in the individual chapters. Nonetheless, some background material is repeated in the chapters because an edited volume is rarely read cover to cover. Given that readers tend to select topics of interest, each chapter is meant to stand on its own to the extent possible.

The definitions and concepts presented here do not indicate that an orthodoxy has been imposed on the contributors to this volume. The attentive reader will find differing aggregations of subregions and various interpretations of particular health or social conditions. Most of these differences are driven by necessity (most data were collected when the region had fewer than 420 counties or fewer than five subregions) or by the specific timing or particular methodology of the research cited. In some instances, the same data are interpreted from different perspectives—for instance, the effects of substance abuse on lifestyle, mental health, and oral health. Just as there is heterogeneity across the region, this volume reflects the heterogeneity of Appalachian health research and analysis.

Minority Health

There are important Appalachian subpopulations (e.g., African Americans, Hispanics, Eastern Band Cherokee) and health cohorts (e.g., those with HIV/AIDS) that are not discussed in this volume. Although women's health is reasonably well represented here, many other subgroups in Appalachia are not. This is not an intentional omission; it is caused by an unfortunate lack of reliable regional data on these populations. Methodological strategies of random sampling do not routinely lead to reliable information on small groups. For example, African Americans constitute 8.2 percent of the Appalachian population, Hispanics 2.0 percent, and Native Americans 0.3 percent. These groups are largely urbanized, clustered in cities such as Knoxville, Chattanooga, Pittsburgh, Birmingham, and the suburbs of Atlanta. Relatively small numbers live in the rural counties of the region, where health disparities are most pronounced.[33]

The fact that these groups are hard to count does not mean they should be omitted from the region's health profile. Some of the research methodologies and policy suggestions in this volume directed at identifying Appalachians in urban areas can help rectify this lack of meaningful data on the region's minorities and smaller health cohorts.

A Note on Methodology

Some of the data presented in this volume were obtained through telephone surveys. Although telephone interviewing enables data to be collected from geographically dispersed persons at a relatively low cost and in a less time-consuming manner, the validity of the resulting data is dependent on a number of factors, including the quality of the questionnaire's design and administration, the manner in which the sample of potential interviewees is selected, and the representativeness of the final sample of individuals interviewed. This last factor is often a concern, given the number of persons without telephones and the difficulty of reaching respondents due to the increasing use of answering machines to screen calls, caller ID, privacy managers, and cell phones. Nationally, as well as in Appalachia, telephone availability in rural areas is becoming less of a problem. In fact, the proportion of homes with telephones in Appalachia increased from 71 percent in 1960 to 97 percent in 2000, with Appalachian families having similar access to phones as families living outside the region.[34] The growth in cell phone–only usage and the development of more sophisticated technologies for screening calls will continue to pose challenges for researchers trying to perform valid telephone surveys. Nevertheless, well-conducted telephone surveys can obtain representative samples of the population of interest and provide accurate data about the health and well-being of Appalachians.

Organization of This Book

Evans and Stoddart[23] argue that well-being and prosperity involve a dynamic interplay between the health and functioning of individuals and the health care system serving them. Although the ultimate objective of the health care system is to reduce and prevent disease, the system also interacts with genetic influences and the social and physical environments to determine the biological and behavioral responses of individuals. These responses not only have an impact on the onset or avoidance of disease as defined by the health care system; they also affect the health of individuals and their sense of well-being. Thus, to gain insight into the health status of rural and urban Appalachians, this volume examines their health and well-being from the perspective of potential underlying determinants—genetics, environments, lifestyles, and health care systems—as well as the various diseases and conditions that affect health and well-being: heart disease, diabetes, obesity, cancer, kidney disease, trauma, mental health, substance abuse, and oral health.[d]

Part I examines the genetic, environmental, behavioral, and systemic determinants of Appalachian health. Myers and Baugh discuss the genetic influences on health and the role of the family health history in ascertaining genetic risk. They provide evidence that dispels the lingering myth of frequent consanguineous marriages among Appalachians and argue for further studies on the prevalence and interaction of genetic risk factors, particularly given the socioeconomic and environmental living conditions of many Appalachians.

Appalachia is faced with a number of environmental issues related to the extraction of its abundant natural resources such as natural gas, coal, and timber. Hendryx examines the health threats associated with Appalachia's physical environment and their impact on the population's health. He recommends policies and programs to restore the physical environment for the promotion of public health.

Knight explores the notion of an Appalachian health lifestyle and discusses the underlying determinants and health effects of one particular lifestyle behavior: tobacco use. While arguing that no unique Appalachian health lifestyle has been found—and may never be found across a politically defined area—she concludes that more research is needed before the search is abandoned.

The central thesis of the chapter by Halverson and associates is that the underlying cause of poor health outcomes in the Appalachian region is the general absence of community-linked and community-responsive systems of health care. They enumerate four propositions for the effective resolution of health disparities among Appalachians and discuss them in detail.

Part II describes the current status of Appalachian health relative to specific diseases and conditions. McCracken and Firesheets address heart disease, the leading cause of death in the United States and in Appalachia, and point out the disparities in heart disease mortality and morbidity that exist between the region and the rest of the country.

Noting the prevalence of diabetes in Appalachia, Denham analyzes the health disparities linked to diabetes among residents of the region. She emphasizes the importance of diabetes self-management within the context of the family environment and presents several models for family-focused diabetes education.

Using data from national, state, and regional sources, Chubinski and Carrozza examine obesity, one of the major health issues facing Appalachian youth. Although a number of factors may contribute to obesity among Appalachians, the authors analyze the link between food scarcity and obesity in both rural and urban areas.

Focusing on the four leading anatomic sites of cancer and the two cancer sites for which screening tests exist, Fisher and colleagues describe the existing disparities in cancer incidence, prevalence, mortality, and screening behaviors, as well as cancer-causing behaviors and access to care. They present the Appalachian Community Cancer Network as a model for addressing these disparities.

Weaner and Schmidt examine chronic kidney disease, which is a silent killer of many Appalachians. Though arguing that the prevalence of kidney disease is difficult to assess in Appalachia, they present evidence of elevated risk factors for persons living in the region and discuss West Virginia's efforts to improve disease awareness and care.

Appalachians face unusual challenges related to occupational and recreational activities that expose them to a high risk of injury. Procter and colleagues discuss the problem of injury in Appalachia, including the role of trauma systems in caring for the injured and the inadequate development of these systems in rural areas.

Keefe and Curtin provide a detailed discourse on the mental health challenges in Appalachia from an ethnomedical perspective. They examine the prevalence of mental illness in Appalachia; the social, behavioral, economic, and ecological stressors affecting mental health; local knowledge about mental health and illness; coping strategies for dealing with adversity; help-seeking behavior; and mental health services in the region.

Substance abuse has become a major concern in Appalachia. Dunn, Behringer, and Bowers discuss the prevalence and health consequences, influencing factors, community response, and prevention and treatment of substance abuse in rural Appalachia. They argue for community-based programs to address the problem and describe a number of promising initiatives.

Often considered a sentinel marker of overall health status, oral health has become an area of critical importance. McNeil, Crout, and Marazita provide insight into the issues surrounding oral health in Appalachia; they also discuss the work being conducted by the Center for Oral Health Research in Appalachia.

Part III presents issues, techniques, and outcomes of health research conducted among Appalachian migrants and their descendants living in urban areas. The accurate identification of Appalachians is critical for determining the existence of health disparities affecting them as a distinct population subgroup. Ludke and colleagues analyze the results of several different approaches to identifying people of Appalachian heritage in the Greater Cincinnati area. Then Ludke, Obermiller, and Horner examine the health status and underlying health determinants of the urban Appalachian population in the Greater Cincinnati area. Their findings indicate that, relative to non-Appalachians, urban Appalachians are at greater risk for a number of health disparities.

Addressing the problem of health disparities in an effective and efficient manner requires community involvement in identifying critical issues and appropriate solutions. Brown presents examples of community-based participatory research methods applied by the urban Appalachian community in Cincinnati to investigate health issues of local concern.

This volume provides insight into the health of Appalachians, both rural and urban. It also identifies future research efforts and policy directions that can serve as the foundation for improving the well-being and prosperity of a population that continues to experience some of this nation's greatest health and economic disparities. As stated by Markus, Plaut, and Lackan, "When it comes to what gives rise to the good life and a global sense of well-being, place matters" (p. 614).[35] This point is illustrated by the mapping of the Gallup-Healthways Well-Being Index[e] across the entire United States.[36] Looking at this map, one is immediately drawn to the large cluster of congressional districts with some of the nation's lowest well-being—an area comprising most of the Appalachian region. If this work was replicated in urban areas such as Chicago, Detroit, and Cincinnati, akin to the work by Maloney and Auffrey[37] in identifying the social areas of Cincinnati, similar variations might be discovered, with those neighborhoods that are traditional Appalachian migration destinations having the lowest well-being. As argued by Evans and Stoddart,[24] well-being, or one's satisfaction with life, is strongly influenced by one's health and many of the underlying determinants of that health.

Notes

a. The National Institutes of Health defines health disparities as "differences in the incidence, prevalence, mortality, and burden of diseases and other adverse health conditions that exist among specific population groups in the United States."[38]

b. These materials include a sampling of publications from six decades, beginning in 1950. This cross section includes monographs, editions, serials, reference materials, and conference proceedings to reflect the broadest perspective on contemporary regional health available at the time. Both quantitative and qualitative research are represented, as are the perspectives of community-based observers and professional health care providers.

c. According to the ARC, "County economic status is determined by an index-based county economic classification system to identify and monitor the economic status of Appalachian counties. The system involves the creation of a national index of county economic status through a comparison of each county's averages for three economic indicators—three-year average unemployment rate, per capita market income, and poverty rate—with national averages. The resulting values are summed and averaged to create a composite index value for each county. Each county in the nation is then ranked, based on its composite index value, with higher values indicating higher levels of distress. Each Appalachian county is classified into one of five economic status designations, based on its position in the national ranking. Distressed counties are the most economically depressed counties. They rank in the worst 10 percent of the nation's counties. At-Risk counties are those at risk of becoming economically distressed. They rank between the worst 10 percent and 25 percent of the nation's counties. Transitional counties are those transitioning between strong and weak economies. They make up the largest economic status designation. Transitional counties rank between the worst 25 percent and the best 25 percent of the nation's counties. Competitive counties are those that are able to compete in the national economy but are not in the highest 10 percent of the nation's counties. Counties ranking between the best 10 percent and 25 percent of the nation's counties are classified competitive. Attainment counties are the economically strongest counties. Counties ranking in the best 10 percent of the nation's counties are classified attainment."[39]

d. Following Evans and Stoddart's terminology, this volume uses the phrase *health determinants,* but caution is advised. This is a very mechanistic approach to health conditions that may be affected by more variables (i.e., determinants) than are identified here. Moreover, there is no information on the relative proportions of the determinants' individual contributions to Appalachian health status. Readers may want to consider them more as contributing factors than definitive causes.

e. For the last three years, Gallup has called 1,000 randomly selected American adults each day and asked them about indicators of their quality of life. The Well-Being Index measures six domains of well-being, each of which is based on the scientific study of responses to the survey questions. The six domains are life evaluation, emotional health, physical health, healthy behavior, work environment, and basic access.[36]

References

1. Behringer B, Friedell GH. Appalachia: where place matters in health. *Prev Chronic Dis.* 2006;3:A113.

2. Jones LW, Shields M. Report to the Council of the Southern Mountains on health care services in the southern Appalachian region. Tuskegee Institute Rural Life Council; 1955.

3. Massie WA. *Medical Services for Rural Areas; the Tennessee Medical Foundation.* Cambridge, MA: Published for the Commonwealth Fund by Harvard University Press; 1957.

4. Kamienny F. Drug usage in the community through a vendor system. *Appalachia Medicine.* 1972;4:78–85.

5. Thomasina SM. When yesterday's people become today's patients. *Appalachia Medicine.* 1970;2:55–56.

6. Ross MH. Life style of the coal miner: America's original hard hat. *Appalachia Medicine.* 1971;3:5–11.

7. Markey L. Medical component of ALCOR: community outreach program for Appalachia. *Appalachia Medicine.* 1970;2:112–113.

8. Nolan RL, Schwartz JL, eds. *Rural and Appalachian Health.* Springfield, IL: Charles C. Thomas; 1973.

9. Schwartz JL. Rural health problems of isolated Appalachian counties. In: Nolan RL, Schwartz JL, eds. *Rural and Appalachian Health.* Springfield, IL: Charles C. Thomas; 1973:29–44.

10. Steinman GD. Health care barriers in Appalachia. In: Nolan RL, Schwartz JL, eds. *Rural and Appalachian Health.* Springfield, IL: Charles C. Thomas; 1973:56–64.

11. Loof DH. Rural Appalachians and their attitude toward health. In: Nolan RL, Schwartz JL, eds. *Rural and Appalachian Health.* Springfield, IL: Charles C. Thomas; 1973:3–28.

12. Fithian WTI. What it would take for me to practice in an isolated rural county. In: Nolan RL, Schwartz JL, eds. *Rural and Appalachian Health.* Springfield, IL: Charles C. Thomas; 1973:146–153.

13. Couto RA. *Streams of Idealism and Health Care Innovation: An Assessment of Service-Learning and Community Mobilization.* New York, NY: Teachers College Press; 1982.

14. University of Kentucky Appalachian Center. *Health in Appalachia: Proceedings from the 1988 Conference on Appalachia.* Lexington, KY: University of Kentucky Appalachian Center; 1989.

15. Florence J, Bates AA, Combs G, Benzoni T. The new country doctor. In: University of Kentucky Appalachian Center. *Health in Appalachia: Proceedings from the 1988 Conference on Appalachia.* Lexington, KY: University of Kentucky Appalachian Center; 1989:33–45.

16. Pollan M. Wendell Berry's wisdom. Available at: http://thenation.com/doc/20090921/pollan. Accessed September 21, 2010.

17. Klotter JC. Breckinridge, Mary. In: Abramson R, Haskell J, eds. *Encyclopedia of Appalachia.* Knoxville, TN: University of Tennessee Press; 2006:1642–1643.

18. Couto RA. Community-initiated health efforts. In: Abramson R, Haskell J, eds. *Encyclopedia of Appalachia.* Knoxville, TN: University of Tennessee Press; 2006:1645–1646.

19. Couto RA, Greene E. Mud Creek Clinic. In: Abramson R, Haskell J, eds. *Encyclopedia of Appalachia.* Knoxville, TN: University of Tennessee Press; 2006:1661–1662.

20. Berkes H. Rural medical camp tackles health care gaps: NPR. Available at: http://www.npr.org/templates/story/story.php?storyId=111066576. Accessed August 30, 2010.

21. Obermiller PJ. Migration. In: Straw RA, Blethen HT, eds. *High Mountains Rising: Appalachia in Time and Place.* Urbana, IL: University of Illinois Press; 2004:88–100.

22. Obermiller PJ, Howe SR. Moving mountains: Appalachian migration patterns, 1995–2000. In: Obermiller PJ, Maloney ME, eds. *Appalachia: Social Context Past and Present.* 5th ed. Dubuque, IA: Kendall/Hunt Publishing; 2007:85–99.

23. Evans RG, Stoddart GL. Producing health, consuming health care. *Soc Sci Med.* 1990;31:1347–1363.

24. Evans RG, Stoddart GL. Producing health, consuming health care. In: Evans RG, Barer ML, Marmor TR, eds. *Why Are Some People Healthy and Not Others: The Determinants of Health of Populations.* New York, NY: Aldine de Gruyter; 1994:27–64.

25. Huttlinger K, Schaller-Ayers J, Lawson T. Health care in Appalachia: a population-based approach. *Public Health Nurs.* 2004;21:103–110.

26. Weller JE. *Yesterday's People: Life in Contemporary Appalachia.* Lexington, KY: University of Kentucky Press; 1965.

27. Corin E. The social and cultural matrix of health and disease. In: Evans RG, Barer ML, Marmor TR, eds. *Why Are Some People Healthy and Not Others: The Determinants of Health of Populations.* New York, NY: Aldine de Gruyter; 1994:93–132.

28. Hatch E. Modernity with a mountain inflection. *Journal of Appalachian Studies.* 2008;14:145–159.

29. Keefe SE. Introduction. In: Keefe SE, ed. *Appalachian Cultural Competency: A Guide for Medical, Mental Health, and Social Service Professionals.* Knoxville, TN: University of Tennessee Press; 2005:2–26.

30. Keefe SE. Theorizing modernity in Appalachia. *Journal of Appalachian Studies.* 2008;14:160–173.

31. DeFilippis J, Fisher R, Shragge E. Neither romance nor regulation: reevaluating community. *International Journal of Urban and Regional Research.* 2006;30:673–689.

32. Cavender AP. *Folk Medicine in Southern Appalachia.* Chapel Hill, NC: University of North Carolina Press; 2003.

33. Hayden W. Appalachian diversity: African-American, Hispanic/Latino, and other populations. *Journal of Appalachian Studies.* 2004;10(3):293–305.

34. Black DA, Mather M, Sanders SG. *Standards of Living in Appalachia, 1960–2000.* Washington, DC: Population Reference Bureau; 2007.

35. Markus HR, Plaut VC, Lackan NA. Well-being in America: core features and regional patterns. In: Brim OG, Ryff CD, Kessler RC, eds. *How Healthy Are We?* Chicago, IL: University of Chicago Press; 2004:614–650.

36. Bloch M, Marsh B. Mapping the nation's well-being. Available at: http://www.nytimes.com/interactive/2011/03/06/weekinreview/20110306-happiness.html. Accessed May 26, 2011.

37. Maloney ME, Auffrey C, eds. *The Social Areas of Cincinnati: An Analysis of Social Needs.* 4th ed. Cincinnati, OH: University of Cincinnati School of Planning and University of Cincinnati Institute for Community Partnerships; 2004.

38. U.S. Department of Health and Human Services. *NIH Strategic Research Plan and Budget to Reduce and Ultimately Eliminate Health Disparities.* Vol. 1. *Fiscal Years 2002–2006.* Washington, DC: U.S. Department of Health and Human Services; 2002.

39. Appalachian Regional Commission. County economic status in Appalachia, FY 2009. Available at: http://www.arc.gov/research/MapsofAppalachia.asp?MAP_ID=49. Accessed September 30, 2010.

Part I

Appalachian Health Determinants

To better understand the background factors affecting the health of the region's population, this part examines some of the most misunderstood aspects of Appalachian health, including genetic predisposition, individual lifestyle behaviors, and the social and cultural dimensions of health. The system of providing health care to Appalachians is also scrutinized here, as well as the health effects of severe environmental pollution in some areas of Appalachia.

These chapters lay to rest the notion of inbreeding, stereotypically attributed to Appalachians; question whether there is really an overarching "Appalachian lifestyle"; and provide a nuanced look at health behaviors and beliefs in some parts of the region by avoiding a simplistic accounting of Appalachian cultural characteristics. Taken together, these chapters can put health care providers on a much firmer footing with their Appalachian patients who are seeking better health and a sense of overall well-being. The chapters on health systems and the environment will be of particular relevance to policy makers interested in addressing these large-scale issues.

1

Genetic Contributions to Health

Melanie F. Myers and Carol S. Baugh

Genetic factors are well-recognized contributors to the overall health of populations; however, their contribution to the incidence and prevalence of health conditions in the Appalachian population has not been systematically studied. This dearth of information may be due to the underrecognition of genetic conditions owing to the absence of systematic health surveillance systems in Appalachia; limited access to health care services and, specifically, to genetic specialists; lack of education among health professionals about genetic conditions; and limited investment in social capital, resulting in restricted resources and competing health and other priorities.[1,2] The economic and demographic diversity in Appalachia compounds the difficulty of ascertaining genetic contributions to health in the region, as well as among those who have migrated elsewhere.[3,4] Given the heterogeneity of Appalachia, there is likely to be a substantial amount of genetic diversity.

This chapter describes what has been published about the genetic influences on health in Appalachia. It begins with a brief overview of the health of Appalachians, followed by a review of the common inheritance patterns of genetic conditions. The main focus of this chapter is use of the family health history as a health promotion tool to capture shared environmental, behavioral, and genetic risk factors. Two components often included in a family history are ethnic origins and the prevalence of consanguinity—that is, individuals' relatedness through shared common ancestors. General challenges in assessing the genetic contribution to common chronic diseases are addressed at the end of the chapter, along with a discussion of the need for additional genetic studies and policy actions.

Health in Appalachia

Although there are limited data about genetic contributions to health in Appalachia, inferences can be drawn from information on mortality rates and disease prevalence. Health disparities have been well documented in rural Appalachia and are exacerbated by geographic, historical, and socioeconomic factors.[5,6] As a whole, the Appalachian region experiences higher mortality than the non-Appalachian United States with respect to heart disease, cancer, stroke, chronic obstructive pulmonary disease, and diabetes.[3,7] According to a 2004 Appalachian Regional Commission report,[3] high death rates due to heart disease are predominant in the Central and Southern subregions, whereas high death rates due to cancer are predominant in Central Appalachia alone. With the exception of white women aged 35 to 64 years, Appalachians have higher breast cancer death rates than non-Appalachians. Colorectal cancer death rates for white men and women are higher in the Southern subregion. The Appalachian region also has higher lung cancer death rates than elsewhere in the United States. High death rates from stroke are predominant in the Southern subregion, whereas high death rates among whites from chronic obstructive pulmonary disease are predominant in the Central subregion. High death rates due to diabetes are predominant in the Central and Northern Appalachian subregions. It is worth noting that heart disease, stroke, and cancer are all multifactorial conditions. Higher rates of obesity and smoking, lower rates of physical activity, and environmental exposure to coal mining, for example, undoubtedly contribute to the high death rates among Appalachians,[3] as do poor socioeconomic conditions such as poverty and the lack of health insurance.[5] Although efforts are under way to learn how genetic susceptibility influences the occurrence of common multifactorial diseases, this area of study is still nascent.

Inheritance and Genetic Conditions

To appreciate how genetics can contribute to health in individuals and populations, a general understanding of genes and chromosomes and the different categories of genetic conditions is essential. Genes, which are made up of DNA (deoxyribonucleic acid), are the basic units of inheritance.[8] Each person has two copies of a gene—one inherited from each parent.

Genes and DNA are further packaged into structures called chromosomes. Like genes, chromosomes come in pairs, with one chromosome in a pair inherited from each parent. Typically, each individual has forty-six chromosomes (twenty-three inherited from each biological parent). The first twenty-two pairs of chromosomes are called the autosomes and look the same in males and females. The sex chromosomes are the twenty-third pair. Females have two copies of the X chromosome, while males have one X and one Y chromosome.[8]

Mutations are changes in the DNA sequence that makes up a gene. These gene changes can be inherited and passed on from generation to generation (germline mutations), or they can be acquired during a person's lifetime (somatic mutations) as a result of environmental factors such as ultraviolet radiation or pollution. Somatic mutations are not passed on to the next generation.[8] Not all genetic changes or mutations cause disease or are harmful to health. Some genetic changes are neutral, and some can be protective. Mutations associated with disease can be inherited as single-gene disorders, or they can increase the risk of disease, as seen in multifactorial conditions.

Variations can also occur in the number of chromosomes or the amount of chromosomal material a person inherits. Inheriting too many or too few chromosomes, or inheriting only parts of chromosomes, can cause problems with growth, development, and function of the body's systems.[8]

Genetic conditions are often categorized into single-gene disorders, chromosomal disorders, and multifactorial or complex disorders.[9] Mitochondrial conditions are less common, but inherited DNA variations in mitochondria are useful in determining ancestry.

Single-Gene Disorders. Single-gene disorders are the result of disease-causing mutations within a single gene. Though individually rare, there are more than 6,000 known single-gene disorders that occur in about 1 out of every 200 births.[10] One common inheritance pattern involving single-gene disorders is autosomal recessive, whereby two mutations on the autosomal chromosomes are inherited (one in the copy of the gene from the mother, and one in the copy of the gene from the father). Examples of autosomal recessive conditions include cystic fibrosis, sickle cell anemia, and Tay-Sachs disease.

Single-gene disorders, particularly autosomal recessive disorders, may occur more often in certain ethnic groups or among children of related individuals. Children of related individuals have a higher risk of inheriting an autosomal recessive condition because they are more likely to inherit the same deleterious mutation from a common ancestor. Consanguinity involves mating between two individuals known to be related by blood. Inbreeding occurs if individuals from a small population tend to choose their mates from within the same population for social, geographic, or religious reasons. Parents may consider themselves unrelated but still share common ancestors.[11] Thus, ethnic origins and the amount of inbreeding or consanguinity within a population are key factors in determining the contribution of genetics to health conditions in that population.

Chromosomal Disorders. Chromosomal disorders are caused by extra or missing chromosomes or parts of chromosomes rather than errors in a single gene. The chance of having a child with a chromosome problem is not increased in consanguineous unions.[12] The chance of having a child with a chromosome problem increases as a woman gets older. Perhaps the best known chromosomal disorder is Down syndrome, which occurs when there is an extra copy of chromosome 21 (there are three copies of chromosome 21 instead of two copies).[13]

Multifactorial Disorders. Many common health problems run in families but are not inherited in the patterns characteristic of single-gene disorders. Multifactorial or complex conditions are caused by a combination of genetic, environmental, and behavioral factors and are much more common than single-gene or chromosomal disorders. With multifactorial conditions, an underlying genetic susceptibility is not sufficient to cause disease. The presence of many different genes in addition to environmental factors, such as exposure to hazardous chemicals, and a poor diet may all be required for a multifactorial or complex condition to occur.[14] In addition to shared genetics, it is not unusual for family members to share similar environmental risks such as diet, alcohol, or tobacco use (including smokeless tobacco).

Conditions inherited in a multifactorial manner are more likely to contribute to the overall health of a population than are single-gene or chromosomal disorders. Examples of multifactorial conditions include coronary heart disease, diabetes mellitus, cancer, schizophrenia, obesity, asthma, spina bifida, and nonspecific developmental delay.[15] Inbreeding can also affect the occurrence of multifactorial conditions, since individuals who share common ancestors may inherit the same predisposing factors associated with complex conditions. Traits such as height, eye color, and skin color are also inherited in a multifactorial manner.

Ascertaining Genetic Risk through Family Health History

Although efforts are under way to elucidate the interactive effects of genes and the environment in causing disease, family history is currently the most effective and readily available genomic tool that captures shared environmental, behavioral, and genetic contributors to disease. A family health history includes biological relationships and medical data,[16] and it can help identify individuals and families at increased risk for disease and risk factors for diseases such as obesity, high cholesterol, and hypertension. A family health history can be used to determine inheritance patterns, calculate risks, decide on medical management and testing strategies, distinguish genetic from other risk factors, and identify medical screening needs and health promotion recommendations for healthy individuals. The family health history can also be used as an educational tool for individuals and family members.[16] Increased awareness of family history can help promote health and prevent disease if those at risk adopt healthier lifestyles and undergo screening tests. These tests are important to detect disease early, when it is most treatable, and to detect treatable risk factors to prevent disease.

A family health history can identify risk factors for chronic diseases, but it is underutilized by clinicians and consumers.[17–20] Educating consumers about the benefits of family histories can empower individuals, allowing them to play a more active role in their own health care and consequently improve their health and prevent disease.[18]

Health-related studies in Appalachian communities suggest that individuals are aware that a family health history can identify risk factors for disease and that those with a particular family history should undergo screening for familial diseases. Appalachian women participating in focus groups in West Virginia recognized that a family history of cancer is an indication for more frequent cancer screenings.[21] In addition, surveys of Appalachians attending churches in the Ohio Valley region of western

West Virginia found a strong association between having a family history of colon cancer and having a colonoscopy.[22] How family history relates to the intention to undergo genetic testing (for conditions for which such testing is available) among Appalachians is unclear. In a social survey of adults using random-digit dialing in Kentucky, Kelly and coauthors[23] reported that a family history of cancer is not associated with an intent to undergo genetic testing for inherited cancer susceptibility syndromes, but greater worry about hereditary cancer is associated with greater intentions. Appalachian respondents reported greater worry than non-Appalachian respondents.[23]

Wallace and associates[24] asked urban Appalachian women how they intended to use the family histories they recorded during two educational sessions. Seventy-eight percent of the ninety-two women said they intended to share their family histories with their health care providers.[24] Those with a high risk of cardiovascular disease were more likely to share their family histories with providers than those at average risk.[25] Other intended uses of the family history included eating healthier (70 percent), becoming more active (54 percent), getting a checkup (40 percent), and trying to stop smoking (38 percent). Although actual behavior change was not recorded as part of this demonstration project, the results suggest that urban Appalachian women may be more likely to take steps to improve their health after learning about and recording their family health histories.[24] Family history is a readily accessible genomic tool that can lead to improved health and fewer acute or chronic diseases through early detection or risk reduction.

Ethnicity

Ethnicity or ancestral origin is an important component of a family health history at both the individual and the population level because, as previously mentioned, some genetic conditions occur more often in certain ethnic groups. For example, Tay-Sachs disease, Niemann-Pick disease, Gaucher disease, and Bloom syndrome are known to occur more often in individuals of Ashkenazi Jewish descent. Sickle cell anemia and other hemoglobinopathies are more common among individuals of African American ancestry, whereas familial Mediterranean fever, ß-thalassemia, and glucose-6-phosphate dehydrogenase (G6PD) deficiency often affect individuals of Mediterranean ancestry. Phenylketonuria and cystic fibro-sis are more common among people of English and Scottish ancestry, and α-thalassemia occurs more often in individuals from Southeast Asian, Cambodian, Chinese, Filipino, Laotian, and Vietnamese backgrounds.[26] When a new population is established by a small number of individuals from a larger population, there is a loss of genetic variation. Any genetic variations present in the "founder" population are likely to become more common in the new population. In addition, genetic changes that occur by chance are more likely to impact the health of a small population than a large population.

Since certain ethnic groups are at increased risk for specific genetic conditions, ethnic origin is important in understanding whether individu-als from Appalachia are at increased risk for genetic conditions. Although most Americans perceive Appalachia as a homogeneous region inhabited primarily by Caucasians, this is a common misrepresentation. While schol-ars may debate the percentages of the various ethnic groups that make up Appalachia, they agree that the region, from first European contact to the present, has always been diverse.

As Caucasians moved into the Appalachian Mountains in the 1700s, they encountered an already diverse region made up of a variety of Native American tribes, clans, and family groups. What is not commonly appreci-ated is the assortment of European and other populations that entered the area. Three hundred years ago, Scots-Irish, German, and English Europe-ans, as well as Africans, began to venture into Appalachia. Each group in-termarried with the existing culture (in this case, various Native American groups), creating an assortment of subcultures and genetic admixtures. The same story played out again with the arrival of southern and eastern Europeans, followed by those from Latin America, Mexico, Asia, and the Middle East. Because of the assortment of ethnicities in the Appalachian area, there are no clear increased risks for genetic diseases based on com-mon ancestry. Rather, any risks are specific to the many countries of origin of the Appalachian people.[27, 28]

The Melungeons are an ethnic group of mixed ancestry associat-ed with certain areas of Appalachia, most notably northeastern Tennes-see, southwestern Virginia, and southeastern Kentucky. Often considered a "mysterious" people who defy placement in a defined racial category, the

Melungeons have been characterized by anthropologists and others as "tri-racial isolates" with a mixture of European, black, and Native American ancestry.[29] Theories of the origins of the Melungeons are varied,[30] and descriptions of their physical characteristics have been inconsistent. Today, identification as Melungeon or as being of Melungeon ancestry seems to be based on self-reports and identification with certain surnames and geographic regions.[31]

Genetic research among individuals claiming Melungeon ancestry has focused primarily on trying to discover their ancestral origins through gene frequencies and DNA analysis. Pollitzer and Brown[32] suggest that blood type gene frequencies among the 177 Melungeons they studied are most similar to that of Europeans, with some Native American or African admixture. Guthrie[33] used the same sample to compare worldwide gene frequency distributions in five major blood group systems. He suggests the Melungeons' ancestors came from the Mediterranean region and coastal Europe, although he admits their ancestry could be English and African American, based on the same data. As evidence of a Mediterranean origin, Hirschman[30] describes several single-gene disorders that occur more often among both Melungeons and individuals of Mediterranean descent. These include Behcet's syndrome, Machado-Joseph disease, familial Mediterranean fever, sarcoidosis, and thalassemia. Furthermore, Hirschman suggests that selective mating within Melungeon bloodlines perpetuated these genetic conditions.[30] However, the lack of surveillance and data on the incidence and prevalence of these genetic conditions among Melungeons makes it difficult to appreciate their impact in this population.

Winkler[31] summarized the research conducted to determine the Melungeons' ethnicity through the analysis of mitochondrial DNA and concludes that DNA studies among 120 individuals self-identifying as Melungeon suggest they are "primarily of European descent, with some Native American and African-American ancestry. Some Melungeons have genetic sequences matching the Siddis of northern India, others reflect a Turkish or Syrian ancestry, some possess all of these genetic sequences, and others reflect only the 'generic' European genes" (p. 240).[31] It appears that the Melungeons, like the rest of Appalachians, have no uniform genetic background. Instead, they are a mixed ethnic population with varying degrees of admixture.

Consanguinity

The degree of consanguinity and inbreeding within a community is another important clue in assessing inherited disease risk, particularly autosomal recessive conditions. As noted earlier, individuals who are related or from the same small population may be more likely to inherit the same autosomal recessive mutation from a shared ancestor.[16] Communities may be more likely to experience inbreeding if opportunities for out-migration or in-migration are limited.

Consanguineous unions have been and remain a commonly accepted practice in many cultures. In parts of Asia, Africa, and the Middle East, 20 to 60 percent of marriages are between cousins.[11, 12] Attitudes toward consanguineous marriage often reflect long-standing religious or cultural beliefs. Historically, marriages between cousins have been beneficial economically because they keep land, property, or money in the family. In many cultures, marrying a cousin or other relative is considered socially beneficial because it can lead to more stable families.[34] In the United States, the rate of consanguinity is estimated to be less than 1 percent (www.consang .net). For marriages between first cousins, the absolute risk for birth disorders among offspring, including stillbirth, neonatal death, congenital malformations, and known autosomal recessive conditions, is between 3 and 5 percent, slightly higher than the overall background rate of 2 to 3 percent for offspring of unrelated couples.[11, 12] Unions between third cousins or more distant relatives are not thought to be associated with increased genetic risk.[11]

It is a common stereotype that marriages among members of rural communities in Appalachia are likely to be consanguineous. Accordingly, one would expect autosomal recessive genetic conditions to occur at an increased frequency in Appalachia. Although there are no data on the prevalence of consanguinity or autosomal recessive conditions in Appalachia, there are reports of consanguinity in specific counties or communities in Central Appalachia.[32, 35–39] The available literature does not substantiate an increased rate of genetic conditions in the region due to consanguinity.

From a historical perspective, rates of consanguinity and inbreeding across rural America may have been higher due to transportation barriers that existed in the eighteenth and nineteenth centuries. A 1951 publication examining intermarriage in a rural community in Kentucky through household surveys suggests that because the community was isolated and experienced very little immigration from the outside, most people in the community were related by blood.[36] In this community, an estimated 29 percent of 107 marriages were between third cousins or closer relatives; however, only 7 marriages were between first cousins. This study also suggests that class structure impacted the number of marriages between relatives. Those who considered themselves upper class *would not* marry outside their class and thus were forced to marry relatives. Similarly, those who were lower class *could not* marry outside their class and thus were also forced to marry relatives. Although the science behind the article is not well described, it is reasonable to conclude that class structure might influence the choice of a spouse, particularly in geographically remote communities.

A 1970 publication reports the frequency of consanguinity in more than 1,500 coal miners living in central and southern West Virginia who were being evaluated for respiratory diseases at one of two hospitals.[37] Among Caucasian respondents, reported rates of consanguinity were 1.5 percent among the surveyed generation and 1.1 percent among the respondents' parents. Rates of first-cousin marriages were 0.1 percent among respondents and 0.4 percent among the previous generation. No African American respondents reported marriages between first or second cousins. The authors concluded that rates of consanguinity in the surveyed population were no higher than those in the rest of the United States.

Studies about rates of consanguinity and inbreeding are best summarized by Tincher, who states that compared with populations elsewhere or at earlier periods in American history, "Appalachian inbreeding values do not seem extreme enough to justify labeling intermarriage as something unique or particularly common to the region" (p. 42).[38] Similarly, there is no evidence of an increased risk of single-gene disorders endemic to the Appalachian region. Although not systematically reported, there may very well be small kinship clusters where a particular genetic condition is more common. However, the same is true of other regions of the country and other parts of the world.[2] Documenting the geographic locations and incidence of genetic conditions in these small pockets is challenging due to the lack of systematic surveillance systems and the lack of access to genetics specialists and other health care providers. It is both expected and observed that out-migration trends in rural communities result in the disappearance of genetic isolates and a decrease in consanguineous pairings.[32, 39] Although not specific to Appalachia, a recent genetic study supports this conclusion, noting that increases in mobility, urbanization, and population admixture during the twentieth century have resulted in increasing genetic variation and more marginal inbreeding coefficients.[40]

Genetic Susceptibility to Disease

An underlying genetic susceptibility likely contributes to the incidence of multifactorial diseases in Appalachia and elsewhere. Studies have been conducted that look for associations between genetic variations and disease outcomes or traits using 100,000 to 1 million genetic markers across the human genome.[41] Such genome-wide analyses are increasingly identifying genetic variants associated with common chronic diseases. Although it is expected that this genomic research will eventually lead to personalized medical and pharmaceutical interventions, the clinical utility of knowing an individual's genotype for these variants has not yet been realized.[42–46] Most of the genetic variants associated with common diseases increase risk only slightly, and the impact of multiple genetic variants and the role of the environment are unclear.[42, 44, 47] The lack of predictive power and outcome data limits the clinical utility of genetic tests for genetic markers associated with disease susceptibility. The American Society of Human Genetics has stated that most health disparities are probably only modestly affected by genetics and are influenced more strongly by environmental factors such as diet, education, socioeconomic status, environmental pollution, and inequities in access to and provision of health care services.[48]

In spite of the limited predictive power of genetic variants identified by genome-wide analyses, efforts to encourage Appalachian communities to participate in new and ongoing large-scale studies of genetic and environmental factors that contribute to complex diseases could yield promising results. Individuals with genetic variations that predispose them toward a disease are statistically more likely to be affected. Similarly, those with genetic variants that protect them from a disease are statistically less likely to be affected.[14] Studies in geographic areas where certain diseases are more common may yield a greater understanding of the genetic and environmental risk factors for those diseases. Although genetic variations influence an individual's susceptibility to environmental influences, there are no data suggesting that Appalachians are more likely than other populations to be genetically susceptible to disease. To determine whether Appalachians are indeed more genetically susceptible to chronic diseases than other populations, the prevalence and interaction of genetic risk factors in Appalachian populations must be compared with those in non-Appalachian populations. For example, the Center for Oral Health Research in Appalachia is seeking to determine the genetic, microbial, individual, familial, and community factors that contribute to poor oral health in Appalachia. To do this, the center is obtaining DNA samples, collecting interview and survey data, performing a clinical oral health assessment, and conducting a microbiological assessment. This approach may lead to more effective intervention and prevention strategies in Appalachia. However, without a comparison group undergoing the same protocol, it is impossible to determine whether genetic susceptibility to poor oral health among Appalachians differs from that among other groups.[49]

The relationship between environmental pollutants and one's genetic makeup is complex. Direct measures of environmental pollutants and the duration of exposure to such pollutants are difficult to ascertain, as are individual-level health factors such as diet, smoking, alcohol use, and exercise. Appreciating biological pathways and the interactions of multiple genetic risk factors and multiple environmental risk factors requires complex models. In spite of these challenges, additional studies are needed in Appalachia to determine the interaction between one's genetic makeup and environmental exposures such as coal mining. As described later in this chapter, engaging Appalachians in such research will be critical to its success.

Access to Genetics Specialists

Lack of access to primary care providers is more acute in rural and low-income areas of Appalachia than in urban and high-income areas.[50, 51] Given the limited access to primary care physicians in the region, access to genetics specialists is even more limited. The two most common genetics specialists are masters-trained genetics counselors and physician-trained clinical geneticists. Map 1.1 presents the number of genetics counselors and clinical geneticists in Appalachia or within fifty miles of Appalachia,

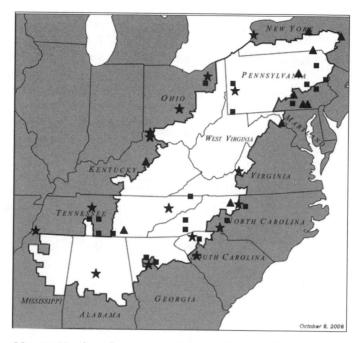

Map 1.1. Number of genetics specialists in the Appalachian Region
(★ 5 or more / ▲ 2–4 / ■ 1).

based on data from the National Society of Genetic Counselors (www.nsgc
.org) and the American College of Medical Genetics (www.acmg.net). Only
20 of 420 Appalachian counties had a genetics specialist listed as of May 1,
2009. Although the number of genetics outreach programs serving other
counties in Appalachia cannot be ascertained, map 1.1 suggests that access
to genetics specialists is limited. The lack of genetics specialists in Appalachia
may contribute to the underrecognition of genetic disorders in the region.

Further Research

The limited information about the contribution of genetic factors to the
incidence and prevalence of health conditions among Appalachians implies the need for additional research.

Just as Appalachia is geographically and economically diverse, the
people of Appalachia are genetically heterogeneous. Although health

disparities exist in areas of Appalachia, inbreeding is not a valid explanation for these disparities. Nongenetic socioeconomic factors such as poverty, environmental pollution, lack of health insurance, and patient and provider beliefs and behaviors are the most likely contributors to these health disparities. However, the contribution of genetic susceptibility and gene-environment interactions to complex health conditions is an important area of research to help elucidate the causes and biological pathways of disease. Given many Appalachians' emphasis on family,[52, 53] the family health history is a promising tool that can be incorporated into community participatory research efforts to promote health, prevent disease, and avoid the exacerbation of existing health disparities. Additional studies are needed to better understand local perspectives on the causes of these health disparities and the barriers to overcoming them. This work should provide insight into how the family health history can be used in Appalachia to educate families about their risk for disease, empower them to play a more active role in their own health care, and consequently improve their health and prevent disease.

Understanding providers' beliefs and practices, particularly regarding the family health history as a health promotion tool, is another potential area of research. Providers' behaviors and beliefs may contribute to health disparities in the Appalachian region. For instance, focus groups involving primary care providers in Tennessee suggested that providers may not routinely perform cancer screenings because of lack of time, because patients visit only for acute health problems as opposed to routine annual examinations, and because of conflicting professional guidelines about cancer screening.[54]

Although having a positive relationship with a health care provider is a motivating factor in seeking health care based on one's family health history,[24, 55] it is not known how willing providers will be to change medical management recommendations or suggest behavioral changes based on patient-generated information in the family health history. Also, it is not clear how often and how thoroughly providers in Appalachia collect family history information and how confident they are in interpreting that information. Therefore, research is needed to examine how providers in primary health care settings in Appalachia routinely and accurately assess risk based on the family health history and whether such assessments lead to behavioral changes or changes in medical management.

Awareness of individuals' and providers' understanding of genetics, genetic conditions, and how genetics contributes to disease is the first step in engaging Appalachian communities in studies related to genetics and health. Additional steps include encouraging Appalachian communities to participate in research efforts to identify genes that predispose to common chronic diseases, such as the Appalachian Cardiovascular Research Network's use of multidisciplinary approaches to identify genes related to cardiovascular disease.[56] In addition, more research is needed on gene-environment interactions in Appalachia, such as the interaction between genetics and exposure to coal mining. Such studies are important in elucidating biological pathways for disease and for developing both risk awareness and health promotion strategies. This requires research into the factors that discourage and facilitate community engagement in studies to identify genetic predisposition variants and gene-environment interactions.

Genomic research should not be conducted in isolation. Rather, it is only one piece of health information that needs to be incorporated with social and contextual variables. Given that most conditions occurring at an increased prevalence in Appalachia (and throughout industrialized nations) are multifactorial in nature, assessing the community's understanding of the different environmental, genetic, and behavioral causes of disease is critical to approaching health disparities in a culturally competent manner. From a public health standpoint, access to services, surveillance, and provider and consumer knowledge of single-gene and multifactorial conditions in Appalachia are all critical issues that need to be addressed and will help determine medical and educational needs as well as essential policy changes.

Policy Recommendations

Lengerich and colleagues[57] outline three broad recommendations for assessing and preventing disease in Appalachia that are applicable to multifactorial conditions with a genetic component:

1. Institute a regional approach to public health surveillance to support the collection and analysis of health-related data. These health surveillance efforts in Appalachia should include family history and other genomic information and should provide regional health

outcome data. Standard data-collection methods and practices need to be developed to incorporate genomic information into these health surveillance systems.

2. Implement community-based participatory interventions to reduce chronic disease among heterogeneous Appalachian communities. A community-academic partnership among researchers, community members, and health care providers is advised so that interventions to address the underlying determinants of health can be identified and implemented. These stakeholders need to be educated about family health history and the role of genetics in common complex disorders if they are to adequately address community health needs and consider the influence of individual hereditary.

3. Employ evidence-based approaches for public health practitioners that have been developed or evaluated with the Appalachian population in mind. Health care professionals and researchers in Appalachia need to be trained from an evidence-based medicine perspective that includes genetics as an underlying health determinant.

In addition to these three recommendations, policies need to be developed and implemented that address the limited availability of genetics specialists in Appalachia. This may include the incorporation of genetics into the training of rural primary care physicians and other health care professionals.

Progress on these policy recommendations will lead to improved health in Appalachia and a better understanding of the genetic contribution to disease in this region. In addition, a comprehensive approach to improving health that incorporates genomic information into surveillance efforts, includes community-based partnerships and education, and uses evidence-based approaches can serve as a model for health promotion and disease prevention efforts across the United States.

References

1. Blakeney AB. Health care in Appalachia. In: Edwards GT, Asbury JA, Cox RL, eds. *A Handbook to Appalachia.* 1st ed. Knoxville, TN: University of Tennessee Press; 2006:101–118.

2. Couto RA, Simpson NK, Harris G, National Cancer Institute, Division of

Resources Centers and Community Activities. *Sowing Seeds in the Mountains: Community-Based Coalitions for Cancer Prevention and Control.* Washington, DC: Appalachia Leadership Initiative on Cancer, Division of Cancer Prevention and Control, National Cancer Institute; 1994.

3. Halverson JA, Ma L, Harner EJ. An analysis of disparities in health status and access to health care in the Appalachian region. Washington, DC: Appalachian Regional Commission; 2004.

4. McLaughlin DK, Lichter DT, Matthews SA. Demographic diversity and economic change in Appalachia. Washington, DC: Appalachian Regional Commission; 1999. Available at: http://www.arc.gov/images/reports/demographic/demographics.pdf.

5. Mary Babb Randolph Cancer Center/Office for Social Environmental and Health Research. Underlying socioeconomic factors influencing health disparities in the Appalachian region. Final Report Contract No. CO-15198. Morgantown, WV: Department of Community Medicine, Robert C. Byrd Health Sciences Center, West Virginia University; 2008.

6. Gatz JL, Rowles GD, Tyas SL. Health disparities in rural Appalachia. In: Glasgow N, Johnson NE, Morton LW, eds. *Critical Issues in Rural Health.* 1st ed. Ames, IA: Blackwell Publishing; 2004.

7. Wilcox LS. Kitchen girl. *Prev Chronic Dis.* 2006;3(4):A111.

8. U.S. National Library of Medicine. Genetics home reference: your guide to understanding genetic conditions. Available at: http://ghr.nlm.nih.gov/handbook/basics. Accessed August 3, 2009.

9. National Institutes of Health, National Human Genome Research Institute. Frequently asked questions about genetic disorders. Available at: http://www.genome.gov/19016930. Accessed August 3, 2009.

10. U.S. Department of Energy Office of Science. Human Genome Project information: genetic disease information. Available at: http://www.ornl.gov/sci/techresources/Human_Genome/medicine/assist.shtml. Accessed May 13, 2009.

11. Nussbaum RL, McInnes RR, Willard HF, Thompson MW, Hamosh A. *Thompson & Thompson Genetics in Medicine.* 7th ed. Philadelphia, PA: Saunders/Elsevier; 2007.

12. Bennett RL, Motulsky AG, Bittles A, et al. Genetic counseling and screening of consanguineous couples and their offspring: recommendations of the National Society of Genetic Counselors. *J Genet Couns.* 2002;8(2):97–119.

13. March of Dimes. Pregnancy and newborn health education center. Available at: http://www.marchofdimes.com/pnhec/4439_4137.asp. Accessed August 3, 2009.

14. Twyman R. Polygenic and multifactorial diseases. Available at: http://genome.wellcome.ac.uk/doc_WTD020852.html. Accessed August 3, 2009.

15. Genetics through a primary care lens: a web-based resource for faculty

development. Available at: http://staff.washington.edu/sbtrini/index.shtml. Accessed May 13, 2009.

16. Bennett RL, Hudgins L, Smith CO, Motulsky AG. Inconsistencies in genetic counseling and screening for consanguineous couples and their offspring: the need for practice guidelines. *Genet Med.* 1999;1:286–292.

17. Acheson LS, Wiesner GL, Zyzanski SJ, Goodwin MA, Stange KC. Family history-taking in community family practice: implications for genetic screening. *Genet Med.* 2000;2:180–185.

18. Guttmacher AE, Collins FS, Carmona RH. The family history—more important than ever. *N Engl J Med.* 2004;351:2333–2336.

19. Yoon PW, Scheuner MT, Peterson-Oehlke KL, Gwinn M, Faucett A, Khoury MJ. Can family history be used as a tool for public health and preventive medicine? *Genet Med.* 2002;4:304–310.

20. Yoon PW, Scheuner MT, Khoury MJ. Research priorities for evaluating family history in the prevention of common chronic diseases. *Am J Prev Med.* 2003;24:128–135.

21. Lyttle NL, Stadelman K. Assessing awareness and knowledge of breast and cervical cancer among Appalachian women. *Prev Chronic Dis.* 2006;3:A125.

22. Tessaro I, Mangone C, Parkar I, Pawar V. Knowledge, barriers, and predictors of colorectal cancer screening in an Appalachian church population. *Prev Chronic Dis.* 2006;3:A123.

23. Kelly KM, Andrews JE, Case DO, Allard SL, Johnson JD. Information seeking and intentions to have genetic testing for hereditary cancers in rural and Appalachian Kentuckians. *J Rural Health.* 2007;23:166–172.

24. Wallace JP, Baugh C, Cornett S, et al. A family history demonstration project among women in an urban Appalachian community. *Prog Community Health Partnersh.* 2009;3:155–163.

25. Au MG, Cornett SJ, Nick TG, et al. Familial risk for chronic disease and intent to share family history with a health care provider among urban Appalachian women, southwestern Ohio, 2007. *Prev Chronic Dis.* 2010;7:A07.

26. Lashley FR. *Clinical Genetics in Nursing Practice.* 3rd ed. New York, NY: Springer; 2005.

27. Billings DB, Blee KM. *The Road to Poverty: The Making of Wealth and Hardship in Appalachia.* Cambridge, UK: Cambridge University Press; 2000.

28. Williams JA. *Appalachia: A History.* Chapel Hill, NC: University of North Carolina Press; 2002.

29. Winkler W. A brief overview of the Melungeons. Available at: http://www.melungeons.com/articles/jan2003.htm. Accessed August 3, 2009.

30. Hirschman EC. *Melungeons: The Last Lost Tribe in America.* 1st ed. Macon, GA: Mercer University Press; 2005.

31. Winkler W. *Walking toward the Sunset: The Melungeons of Appalachia.* 1st ed. Macon, GA: Mercer University Press; 2004.

32. Pollitzer WS, Brown WH. Survey of demography, anthropometry, and genetics in the Melungeons of Tennessee: an isolate of hybrid origin in process of dissolution. *Hum Biol.* 1969;41:388–400.

33. Guthrie JL. Melungeons: comparison of gene frequency distributions to those of worldwide populations. *Tennessee Anthropologist.* 1990;15(1):13–22.

34. Bittles AH. Consanguineous marriage and childhood health. *Dev Med Child Neurol.* 2003;45:571–576.

35. Cadle RG, Dawson T, Hall BD. The prevalence of genetic disorders, birth defects and syndromes in central and eastern Kentucky. *J Ky Med Assoc.* 1996;94:237–241.

36. Brown JS. Social class, intermarriage, and church membership in a Kentucky community. *Am J Soc.* 1951;57:232–242.

37. Juberg RC. Consanguineous marriages in West Virginia. *WV Med J.* 1970;66(2):42–43.

38. Tincher RB. Night comes to the chromosomes: inbreeding and population genetics in southern Appalachia. *Central Issues in Anthropology.* 1980;2(1):27–50.

39. Kirkland JR, Jantz RL. Inbreeding, marital movement, and genetic isolation of a rural Appalachian population. *Ann Hum Biol.* 1977;4:211–218.

40. Nalls MA, Simon-Sanchez J, Gibbs JR, et al. Measures of autozygosity in decline: globalization, urbanization, and its implications for medical genetics. *PLoS Genet.* 2009;5:e1000415.

41. Attia J, Ioannidis JP, Thakkinstian A, et al. How to use an article about genetic association: C: What are the results and will they help me in caring for my patients? *JAMA.* 2009;301:304–308.

42. Couzin J, Kaiser J. Genome-wide association: closing the net on common disease genes. *Science.* 2007;316:820–822.

43. Feero WG, Guttmacher AE, Collins FS. The genome gets personal—almost. *JAMA.* 2008;299:1351–1352.

44. Hunter DJ, Khoury MJ, Drazen JM. Letting the genome out of the bottle—will we get our wish? *N Engl J Med.* 2008;358:105–107.

45. Lango H, Weedon MN. What will whole genome searches for susceptibility genes for common complex disease offer to clinical practice? *J Intern Med.* 2008;263:16–27.

46. Offit K. Genomic profiles for disease risk: predictive or premature? *JAMA.* 2008;299:1353–1355.

47. Shriner D, Vaughan LK, Padilla MA, Tiwari HK. Problems with genome-wide association studies. *Science.* 2007;316:1840–1842.

48. The American Society of Human Genetics. Ancestry testing statement.

Available at: http://www.ashg.org/pdf/ASHGAncestryTestingStatement_FINAL.pdf. Accessed August 3, 2009.

49. Polk DE, Weyant RJ, Crout RJ, et al. Study protocol of the Center for Oral Health Research in Appalachia (COHRA) etiology study. *BMC Oral Health.* 2008;8:18.

50. Baldwin FD. Access to care: overcoming the rural physician shortage. *Appalachia Magazine,* May–August 1999. Available at: http://www.arc.gov/magazine/articles.asp?ARTICLE_ID=98&F_ISSUE_ID=13&F_CATEGORY_ID=.

51. Stensland J, Mueller C, Sutton J. An analysis of the financial conditions of health care institutions in the Appalachian region and their economic impacts. Washington, DC: Appalachian Regional Commission; 2002. Available at: http://www.arc.gov/researchreports.asp?F_CATEGORY=13. Accessed March 5, 2007.

52. Coyne CA, Demian-Popescu C, Friend D. Social and cultural factors influencing health in southern West Virginia: a qualitative study. *Prev Chronic Dis.* 2006;3:A124.

53. Denham SA, Meyer MG, Toborg MA, Mande MJ. Providing health education to Appalachia populations. *Holist Nurs Pract.* 2004;18:293–301.

54. Shell R, Tudiver F. Barriers to cancer screening by rural Appalachian primary care providers. *J Rural Health.* 2004;20:368–373.

55. Cree RA, Lynch J, Au MG, Myers MF. Decisions to seek healthcare based on family health history among urban Appalachian women. *J Genet Couns.* 2009;18:534–550.

56. West Virginia Idea Network of Biomedical Research Excellence. Appalachian Cardiovascular Research Network (ACoRN). Available at: http://www.wv-inbre.net/about.asp. Accessed August 3, 2009.

57. Lengerich EJ, Bohland JR, Brown PK, et al. Images of Appalachia. *Prev Chronic Dis.* 2006;3:A112.

2

Health and the Physical Environment

Michael S. Hendryx

Appalachia is known for its mountains and rivers, its forests, hills, and streams. It is known for its music and its heritage. It also includes large cities (Birmingham, Chattanooga, Pittsburgh), major industries, and, perhaps most centrally, coal. The complex interplay of historical, geographic, geologic, social, economic, and anthropogenic forces affects the health of the Appalachian population in profound ways. This chapter explores these influences, documents their impacts, and recommends policies and programs to restore the Appalachian physical environment for the promotion of public health. Because Appalachia suffers from major health disparities relative to the nation,[1-3] and because Appalachia is interconnected with citizens in the rest of the nation, such health promotion will benefit not only the region but also the entire country.

The Environmental Riskscape

Appalachia is the mountainous area in the eastern United States extending from southern New York to northeastern Mississippi. The region designated Appalachia currently includes 420 counties, although the data used in this chapter are based on the 410 counties so designated in 2007.[4] The topography of the region consists of three parallel belts running northeast to southwest; they are (from east to west) the Blue Ridge, the Ridge and Valley (which is actually hilly in most areas but has served as the major transit route within the region), and the Appalachian Plateau.[5] Throughout the region, east-west passages are rare and were difficult to navigate before modern transportation routes were constructed, especially in the South. Farmlands and valleys are small, offering limited opportunities for agriculture and the development of urban centers. Much of the area is covered by second-growth broadleaf forest that constitutes one of the most diverse temperate ecosystems in the world.

The Appalachian region is also divided into Northern, Central, and Southern subregions.[6] Historically, the Northern subregion has fared the best economically, but more recently it has been overtaken by economic growth in the Southern subregion. Poverty levels have remained persistently high in the Central subregion. As coal mining became more mechanized over time, employment in that industry began to fall, and the coal mining areas of eastern Kentucky and southern West Virginia have experienced disadvantageous socioeconomic conditions that persist to the present time.

Although this chapter focuses on the Appalachian physical environment and its relation to the population's health, poor health outcomes result from the combined effects of the total environmental "riskscape": genetic, social, psychological, behavioral, and physical environmental contributions. Models of the environmental riskscape conceptualize health as the consequence of both chemical and nonchemical stressors that impair the body's capacity to regulate, repair, and improve physical function.[7] The combined and cumulative burden the body experiences from this set of contributions is termed "allostatic load."[8] The more the body is biologically challenged by combined forces such as smoking, environmental toxicants, chronic stress, and poor diet, the more difficult it becomes to maintain a healthy system. The body's defenses and its regulatory capacity to respond to biological challenge eventually break down. Allostatic burdens begin in childhood, when poverty and chronic stress increase subsequent risks for physical illness, emotional distress, and risky behaviors, including substance abuse and overeating.[9–11]

The concept of allostatic load indicates that in many cases, illness does not result simply from exposure to a particular environmental agent; it requires exposure to that agent in the face of additional risk factors, be they genetic, psychological, behavioral, or social in nature. Likewise, positive health outcomes may result even in the presence of environmental exposure when other strengths or resiliencies are present in the riskscape. In Appalachia, the physical environment cannot be evaluated in isolation from these other impacts; rather, their interactive, synergistic effects must be considered jointly.

Table 2.1. Behavioral, Socioeconomic, and Health Care Disparities in Appalachia Compared with the Rest of the Nation

	Appalachia	Rest of Nation
Smoking rate (%), 2003	25.6*	21.8
Obesity rate (%), 2003	24.8*	23.7
Mean per capita income, 2000–2002	$20,962*	$23,602
Poverty rate (%), 2000–2002	15.5*	13.3
Unemployment rate (%), 2000–2003	6.2*	5.2
Percentage with high school education, 2000	71.2*	78.3
Percentage with college education, 2000	13.1*	17.0
Percentage without health insurance, 2000	13.8*	14.9
Primary care physicians per 1,000 population, 2001	1.34	1.31
Specialist physicians per 1,000 population, 2001	0.37	0.34

Note: Based on an analysis of county-level data from the 2006 Area Resource File and Behavioral Risk Factor Surveillance System data from the Centers for Disease Control and Prevention. Appalachian counties are those designated as such by the Appalachian Regional Commission as of 2007.
* Appalachia is significantly different from the rest of the nation ($p < .0001$).

People in Appalachia experience higher riskscape exposures across a spectrum of behavioral, socioeconomic, and environmental threats.[1,3] For example, smoking and obesity rates are higher in Appalachia compared with national averages (table 2.1). Many Appalachians also experience chronic socioeconomic disadvantages: lower income levels, higher poverty rates, higher unemployment rates, and lower rates of educational attainment (table 2.1). Socioeconomic disadvantage is one of the most powerful predictors of poor health outcomes in a population.[12–14] For example, Woolf and colleagues[13] demonstrated that a college education is eight times more powerful than combined advances in public health and medical science in preventing premature mortality.

In contrast to common perceptions, however, the region as a whole does not suffer from a shortage of medical professionals compared with the rest of the country (table 2.1). Federally designated health professional shortage areas are no greater in Appalachia than in the rest of the nation when it comes to primary care providers, dentists, and mental health professionals. This may be because shortages also exist in other geographic areas, such as the Mississippi Delta, or in remote rural areas outside Appalachia, or it may be due to the variability within Appalachia, with some parts of the region having shortages while others do not. Given that population-wide health problems are certainly more severe in Appalachia than elsewhere, the comparable supply of providers casts doubt on the common presumption that a greater number of providers equals better health; instead, it reinforces the idea that socioeconomic and behavioral impacts are the primary drivers of public health.

Higher average allostatic load is concentrated among persons with lower socioeconomic status (SES)[15]; by extension, the allostatic load is higher, on average, among the Appalachian population. Persons of low SES cannot afford highly nutritional diets. They experience chronic stress from economic concerns. They sometimes turn to buffering mechanisms intended to reduce stress that may have negative health consequences, including smoking, substance abuse, and overeating. Low SES populations are more likely to live in areas that are exposed to greater environmental pollution from industry, traffic, or resource extraction.[16]

Environmental Issues

No place in the country is immune from the threats to human health posed by the anthropogenic physical environment. In some ways, the threats to Appalachia, with its large rural and mountainous areas, are less severe. The region does not experience the large-scale exposure to pesticides and fertilizers that major agricultural areas may face. Rural communities are less exposed to the harmful automobile emissions concentrated in urban areas. Nevertheless, the region is faced with a number of serious environmental health threats.

Coal Plants. About half the electricity generated in the United States comes from coal.[17] According to data from the Environmental Protection Agency (EPA), there were 688 coal-fired power plants in the United States in 2007, including 95 in Appalachia.[18] Others were in development, and there were others located outside the region's borders but nearby and upwind. In Appalachia, 28 percent of all power plants are coal fired, compared with 15 percent of power plants in the rest of the nation. Coal is the dirtiest fossil fuel, releasing more carbon dioxide, sulfur dioxide, nitrous oxide, mercury, arsenic, lead, and other toxic elements and compounds per unit of energy than any other source. Coal plants are responsible for 87 percent of utility-related nitrous oxide, 94 percent of utility-related sulfur dioxide, and 98 percent of utility-related mercury emissions.[19] Pollution from coal combustion contributes to both acute and chronic morbidity and mortality,[20, 21] and it causes about 24,000 premature deaths among Americans every year.[22] In addition, it is responsible for millions of lost workdays and thousands of hospital admissions and emergency room visits annually.[22]

Air quality levels in Appalachia are among the worst in the nation. If a county fails to meet air pollutant criteria for ozone, carbon monoxide, nitrogen dioxide, sulfur dioxide, lead, or particulate matter, the EPA designates it a "nonattainment area." Between 2004 and 2006, 23 percent of Appalachian counties had one or more nonattainment episodes, compared with 16 percent of non-Appalachian counties.[23]

In addition to air pollution, fly ash, the residue left after coal is burned, is an environmental threat. Fly ash is a dry powder, but it is often mixed with water for easier transport, storage, and treatment. The dangers of fly ash are perhaps best illustrated by the catastrophic failure of the fly ash impoundment pond outside Harriman, Tennessee, in 2008. When this unlined, earthen-dam containment pond failed, it released more than 5.4 million cubic yards of sludge containing high levels of lead, thallium, iron, manganese, arsenic, cadmium, and other toxic elements.[24, 25] The actual spill exceeded the officially documented volume of the entire pond, burying homes, overrunning roads, bringing down power lines, and resulting in a massive fish kill. Fortunately, no humans were injured or killed during the spill. The exact contents of the sludge and its health implications are not yet understood, but this pond represents only one of 300 to 500 similar ponds nationwide.[26]

Coal Mining. It is not only the burning of coal but also the activities involved in extracting, processing, and transporting it that are environmentally damaging and pose health risks to the residents of Appalachia. These risks affect not only coal miners but all community residents. Contaminants from mining activities are conveyed to the air, water, and soil; from there, human contact is possible. Coal mining takes place in nine of the thirteen Appalachian states: Alabama, Kentucky, Maryland, Mississippi, Ohio, Pennsylvania, Tennessee, Virginia, and West Virginia. The

Appalachian coalfields constitute one of the three major coal regions in the country (the other two are the interior and western regions). In 2007, more than 377 million tons of coal were mined from Appalachia, representing about a third of the nation's total production.[27] Within Appalachia, West Virginia, eastern Kentucky, and Pennsylvania produce the most coal. More than 153 million tons of coal were extracted from West Virginia in 2007, making it the second highest coal-producing state in the nation after Wyoming.[27]

Coal itself contains many impurities, some of which are toxic or carcinogenic. The West Virginia Geological and Economic Survey tracks at least fifty-nine elemental impurities present in coal, including arsenic, beryllium, mercury, lead, cadmium, chromium, selenium, nickel, thallium, uranium, and zinc.[28] Arsenic, for example, is present at levels of 71, 22, and 29 parts per million in Southern, Central, and Northern Appalachian coal, respectively.[29] Coal also contains numerous toxic organic substances, such as polycyclic aromatic hydrocarbons (PAHs), which can contaminate air and water supplies through mining and processing activities.

Appalachia contained 1,200 active coal mines as of 2007.[30] Of these, 692 (or 58 percent) were surface mines, including mountaintop removal mines. Surface mining, as a percentage of total mining, has been increasing throughout Appalachia and particularly in West Virginia. Surface mines in that state were responsible for 45 percent of production tons in 2007, up from 19 percent in 1980.[30] This is important because surface mining causes more environmental disturbance than underground mines. Levels of ambient air pollution are higher at surface mines than at underground mines.[31] Surface and groundwater disturbance is also a major concern around surface mining operations. Between 1985 and 2001 surface mining in Appalachia permanently buried 724 stream miles through mountaintop removal and subsequent valley fills, and it will ultimately impact more than 1.4 million acres.[32]

Levels of ambient particulate matter (designated PM_{10} and $PM_{2.5}$, referring to matter less than 10 and 2.5 micrometers in diameter, respectively), sulfur dioxide, and nitrous oxide are elevated in areas proximate to coal extraction, processing, and transportation activities.[31, 33] These pollutants are health hazards, although the direct public health consequences of breathing compromised air around mining activities are poorly understood.

Mine drainage is another potential health hazard. Rivers and streams cannot support their original population size or diversity of species once they have been subjected to mine drainage. Human health consequences are also a concern in relation to mine drainage, but again, surprisingly little empirical research has been conducted on this issue.

Coal is not simply removed from the ground and tossed into a power plant. It must first be processed and transported. West Virginia alone has 162 facilities where coal is transported, loaded, or processed.[34] Processing involves crushing or pulverizing coal into small pieces or even into a powder so that it can be blown into furnaces and burned more efficiently. This crushing activity generates tons of dust around processing facilities.[33]

Processing also involves washing coal to remove noncombustible material and reduce the content of sulfur and metals.[29] The washing process results in contaminated water called slurry. This slurry contains both coal impurities and the chemicals used in coal processing, which may themselves be toxicants. Proprietary cleaning formulas are used, and these poorly understood formulas contain a variety of surfactants, coagulants, and flocculants.[35] The types of chemicals used include various benzenes, acrylamides, and PAHs. Billions of gallons of water are contaminated every year due to coal washing, and this water is treated in one of two primary ways. One method is to inject the wastewater underground into abandoned mining spaces, which may result in groundwater contamination. There are 649 current, suspected, and proposed underground injection sites in West Virginia.[36] The second method is to hold the water in earthen-dam impoundment ponds, which are often unlined. In West Virginia, there are about 137 impoundment ponds holding more than 140 billion gallons of slurry.[34] As noted earlier, the dams holding back the slurry can fail, with catastrophic consequences.[37]

Research has established clear connections between mining activity and water pollution.[38, 39] McAuley and Kozar[40] found an increased probability of contaminated groundwater proximate to Appalachian mining activity relative to nonmining areas. Wells in mining areas had higher levels of sulfate, aluminum, iron, manganese, and other constituents related to mine drainage. Shiber[41] reported elevated arsenic levels in domestic well water in Central Appalachia proximate to mining, although it is uncertain whether the arsenic resulted from mining or was naturally occurring. Stout and Papillo[42] reported levels of lead, arsenic, barium, beryllium, manganese, aluminum, iron, and zinc exceeding established EPA standards in one or more of fifteen sampled wells within two miles of a coal slurry impoundment in southern West Virginia.

Studies directly linking mining activity not only to water quality but also to human health are even more limited. Hitt and Hendryx[43] found that counties in West Virginia with higher levels of coal mining and processing were characterized by streams with poorer ecological integrity, as measured by benthic macroinvertebrate population size and diversity. Poorer stream integrity, in turn, was related to higher age-adjusted cancer mortality rates. Blakeney and Marshall,[44] reporting on a participatory action research program, concluded that a watershed in a Kentucky coal mining area was impaired due to mining and inadequate water treatment infrastructure and that human health was adversely impacted.

In general, it is well known that water contaminated with certain elements or compounds present in coal constitutes a serious health risk. Arsenic in water, for example, is clearly linked to lung and skin cancer.[45, 46] Environmental pollution from other elements and chemical compounds found in coal and coal processing are linked to a variety of serious and debilitating illnesses, including cardiovascular, respiratory, and kidney disease and some forms of cancer.[47–51]

The final phase of the precombustion coal cycle is transporting the coal from the mines to the processing plants and then to the power plants. This transportation takes place by truck, train, conveyor belt, and barge. Transportation has been identified as a source of ambient air pollution from coal mining,[31] caused by both the fossil fuels used to power the transportation vehicles and the dust coming off those vehicles.

Consistent with riskscape models, coal mining areas are associated with persistently low rates of educational attainment and high rates of poverty.[1, 52] These disadvantages overlap and interact with both air and water pollution from mining. Table 2.2 shows the same variables displayed in table 2.1, but with the Appalachian counties divided into those with and without coal mining. It can be seen that coal mining areas are significantly worse than nonmining areas in terms of smoking, poverty, unemployment, and college education.

Another difference between surface mining and underground mining

Table 2.2. Behavioral, Socioeconomic, and Health Care Disparities between Appalachian Counties with and without Coal Mining and Compared with the Rest of the Nation

	Appalachia, Coal Mining	Appalachia, No Mining	Rest of Nation
Smoking rate (%), 2003	27.2*	24.8	21.8
Obesity rate (%), 2003	24.8	24.8	23.7
Mean per capita income, 2000–2002	$20,841	$21,023	$23,602
Poverty rate (%), 2000–2002	17.3*	14.5	13.3
Unemployment rate (%), 2000–2003	6.8*	5.9	5.2
Percentage with high school education, 2000	70.6	71.5	78.3
Percentage with college education, 2000	11.9*	13.8	17.0
Percentage without health insurance, 2000	13.9	13.8	14.9
Primary care physicians per 1,000 population, 2001	1.36	1.32	1.31
Specialist physicians per 1,000 population, 2001	0.37	0.36	0.34

Note: Based on an analysis of county-level data from the 2006 Area Resource File and Behavioral Risk Factor Surveillance System data from the Centers for Disease Control and Prevention. Appalachian counties are those designated as such by the Appalachian Regional Commission as of 2007. Coal mining counties are those with any level of coal production from 1994 through 2006, based on statistics reported by the Energy Information Administration.
* Appalachian coal mining areas are significantly different from both nonmining areas and the rest of the nation (post hoc F test, $p < .05$ or better).

is that the former requires fewer employees to operate a mining site. Being able to extract large quantities of coal quickly with lower labor costs is one of the primary reasons that surface mining is on the rise. From a riskscape perspective, the decline in mining employment has important public health implications: less economic opportunity translates to increased stress, greater poverty, and weakened financial resources, resulting in negative health outcomes.

Other Environmental Health Issues. Although coal mining and coal combustion are two of the most serious environmental threats to the people of Appalachia, there are other potential hazards. Because of the region's topography and soil composition, large-scale agriculture is limited. However, to the extent that modern agricultural practices take place, they are characterized by the use of pesticides and fertilizers that can enter groundwater sources. Animal feedlots, such as chicken farms, are another potential source of pollutants. Four of the top five poultry states are located in the Appalachian region.[53] In the case of poultry, pollution occurs primarily through the production of large quantities of ammonia that enter water systems.

The EPA maintains records on a variety of industrial and other anthropogenic activities with potential impacts on environmental quality and health outcomes. These include a list of stationary sources of air pollution,[54] a toxics release inventory (TRI) database that maps the locations of sites that use or store more than 650 listed chemicals,[55] and a permit compliance system that tracks licensed chemical discharges into bodies of water.[56] The volume is staggering: in Appalachia there are 7,654 TRI sites, 4,043 air pollution point sources, and 20,585 permitted wastewater discharge sites. Compared with non-Appalachian counties, Appalachia has fewer TRI and air pollution sites but more water discharge sites per county. Research to understand the potential health consequences of this array of pollution sources has not been undertaken in a comprehensive or systematic way.

Logging is another major economic activity in Appalachia.[57] Although the environmental impacts of logging are not as detrimental to population-wide health as coal mining and coal combustion are, the industry is dangerous from an occupational perspective. Logging is recognized as one of the top occupational causes of death and injury,[57–60] as is coal mining, especially underground mining.[60] In 2007 there were 89 fatalities in the logging industry, equating to 90.8 fatalities per 100,000 full-time-equivalent workers, which makes logging the deadliest occupation in the country.[60] There are also several thousand nonfatal logging accidents every year.[59, 61]

Although topography may suggest that the risk for traffic-related injury or death is higher in Appalachia, this does not appear to be the case when Appalachia is compared with the rest of the nation. For example, death rates attributable to motor vehicle accidents among men and women aged 35 to 64 are no different in Appalachia than in the non-Appalachian

United States.[62] Because alcohol is often implicated in traffic fatalities, the relatively lower rates of alcohol consumption characteristic of the Appalachian population may play a part in keeping these rates down.[63] Other potential topography risks include landslides onto roadways, injuries related to outdoor activities such as hunting or backpacking, and road subsidence from mining.[64] Finally, a transportation threat linked to the region's coal dependence is the use of narrow, winding mountain roads by coal trucks. These vehicles are poorly regulated, and the truckers sometimes drive with overloaded trucks or at unsafe speeds because their compensation is based on how much they carry and how quickly they transport their loads.

Health Consequences

The Appalachian population experiences higher rates of chronic illnesses compared with the nation as a whole. These illnesses include diabetes, heart disease, and some types of cancer, including lung, colorectal, and cervical.[1,2] As a result, age-adjusted mortality rates are higher in Appalachia than in the rest of the nation (figure 2.1). To some extent, conclusions drawn about the causes of Appalachian health disparities may be based on assumption rather than fact. For example, a study that documented higher cancer mortality in Appalachia concluded that "elevated lung cancer death rates . . . are attributable to a high prevalence of smoking."[2] The role of smoking is

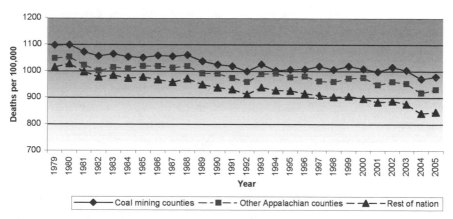

Figure 2.1. Total age-adjusted mortality per 100,000 by county group, 1979–2005. *Source:* Hendryx M, Ahern MM. Mortality in Appalachian coal mining regions: the value of statistical life lost. *Public Health Reports* 2009;24:541–550.

critical, but it is not the complete story. Environmental contributions to Appalachian health differentials have been largely overlooked. As a powerful case in point, one potentially important environmental contribution to poor population health is pollution from the extraction, processing, and transportation of coal.

Research on population health in the coal mining areas of Appalachia has documented substantial health disparities. This evidence includes higher age-adjusted mortality rates in mining areas from lung cancer and from cardiovascular, respiratory, and kidney disease.[65, 66] According to data from the Centers for Disease Control and Prevention, total age-adjusted mortality rates have been higher in coal mining areas compared with the rest of Appalachia and the rest of the nation every year since at least 1979 (figure 2.1). There is also evidence of higher self-reported rates of chronic illnesses and increased hospitalizations for conditions that are sensitive to potential environmental contaminants from the coal mining industry.[63, 67, 68] These health effects have been found in both women and men, suggesting that they are not simply the result of occupational exposure. These effects also become stronger as levels of mining increase, suggesting a dose-response effect. Furthermore, these adverse health consequences are only partially accounted for by standard risk variables such as poverty, education, race, and smoking, suggesting an independent environmental contribution.

The evidence indicates that (1) coal contains substances harmful to human health; (2) these substances and others used in the industry are released during extraction, processing, and transportation activities; and (3) human health in mining areas is impaired in ways consistent with an exposure hypothesis. Research is still needed to establish a direct connection between mining and health consequences; this can be done by (1) investigating air and water quality in mining areas, (2) relating air and water quality to human exposures through such indicators as blood tests for metals and inflammatory biomarkers and through pulmonary function tests, and (3) relating objective exposure measures to objective (e.g., diagnosed cardiovascular disease) and subjective (e.g., self-reported health status) health outcomes.

Returning once more to the riskscape model, it should be recognized that the costs associated with premature mortality among the residents of coal mining counties exceed the economic benefits from the mining industry. This statement is based on an analysis of the direct, indirect, and induced earnings impact of the Appalachian mining industry,[69] estimated at slightly over $8 billion in 2005 dollars.[3] The cost of premature mortality is found by estimating the number of excess annual age-adjusted deaths in coal mining areas; this estimate ranges from 3,975 to 10,923 excess lives lost per year, depending on the years studied and the comparison group.[3] The value of each life lost is converted to dollars using widely accepted value of statistical life (VSL) techniques.[70] Corresponding VSL total cost estimates range from $18.6 billion to $84.5 billion, with a point estimate of $50 billion—substantially higher than mining's $8 billion economic benefit.[3]

Improving public health by improving the Appalachian physical environment requires attention to a set of issues rooted in the larger socioeconomic context of the region. Improving the physical environment means reducing the harmful effects of both the coal extraction and the coal combustion industries. This could be partially accomplished through tougher environmental standards for air and water quality around mining activity and better enforcement of existing regulations. But ultimately, reducing the polluting impact of coal and improving other features of the physical environment (e.g., roads, health-oriented restaurants and grocery stores, recreational amenities) involve reducing the dependence on coal altogether and developing economic alternatives that result in more jobs, sustainable jobs, and jobs that require a more highly educated workforce. Jobs and education will do more to improve the physical environment, and subsequently public health, than minor adjustments to health care delivery systems or environmental regulatory standards.

Further Research

There are a number of areas in which further research is needed to better understand how the physical environment impacts population health in Appalachia.

First, what are the relative and interactive contributions of environmental, behavioral, socioeconomic, and health services variables on health outcomes? The relative importance of environmental contaminants in the context of other health risks, or the extent to which environmental exposures interact with other risks, is not clear and requires further study.

Second, what is the air, soil, and water quality in mining areas? Evidence indicates that air and water quality is impaired by the mining industry, but the research is limited. Additional research should focus on careful assessments of the types and quantities of air and water pollutants discharged at EPA-monitored sites. In addition, independent, systematic assessments of air, water, and soil quality should be undertaken in proximity to the extraction, processing, and transportation activities of the mining industry.

Third, what are the routes that lead from industrial activity to human exposure and subsequent health problems resulting from that exposure? Each of these elements has been established for the mining industry: coal and chemicals contain toxicants and carcinogens, air and water quality is compromised, and population health is impaired in ways not completely explained through conventional behavioral, socioeconomic, or health services risks. However, the causal links between the elements are still poorly understood and require further investigation.

Fourth, what economic redevelopment models would be most effective for the region? As coal mining continues to decline in economic importance, alternative economic models must be developed and implemented. These models require evaluation via demonstration projects or other research designs to determine which ones have the greatest acceptance among Appalachians and the greatest impact on their health and well-being.

Fifth, what community strengths or resiliencies can be brought to bear to improve community health? Some components of the physical environment, such as forests and rivers, might be useful in promoting positive health behaviors. Research is needed to understand how the physical environment not only compromises the health of the region's residents but also enhances their physical and mental health and well-being.

Policy Recommendations

The first two recommendations deal directly with changes to the physical environment; the rest address more fundamental drivers of health disparities.

Environmental Protection. Persons who live in low SES areas are more likely to be exposed to greater environmental risks; they are also subject to poorer enforcement of existing regulations.[71] One immediate step is to enforce the regulations that are already on the books. In addition, new regulations—such as the Appalachian Restoration Act, which has been introduced in the U.S. Senate and would protect streams from mountaintop removal mining waste—would be positive steps toward protecting the Appalachian physical environment.

Renewable Energy Alternatives. Todd[72] outlines an ambitious, thoughtful plan for the economic revitalization of Appalachia that has ecosystem restoration as a cornerstone. Other successful examples of ecologic restoration as economic stimulus have been documented.[73] A component of Todd's plan for Appalachia includes developing alternative energy based on available resources in the region other than coal.

Economic Restructuring. To ensure a healthy population, people must have dependable, meaningful, and fairly compensated employment. Possibilities that take advantage of Appalachia's strengths include outdoor and heritage-oriented tourism, small-scale agriculture, fishery development, sustainable timber, and technology development. Microloans have been used to create economic opportunity in developing nations,[74] and some areas of Appalachia may be suitable for similar investments. These programs provide small, low-interest or no-interest loans to entrepreneurs to begin new, needed businesses in underdeveloped areas; such loans could be funded through a restructuring of the existing tax system (see below). One requirement for loan approval would be that the recipients use the money to create jobs in areas typically underrepresented in the targeted communities (i.e., that are not related to the coal industry) but that are expected to be good sources of economic diversification.

Educational Investments. Investments in public education from preschool through graduate school are essential. Education is key to both poverty reduction and public health improvement.[13, 75] Economic and educational investments should go hand in hand because educated people will leave if economic opportunities are not present, and economic opportunities that offer high-end wages require educated people. Investments might target reductions in class size, provision of cutting-edge educational technologies, higher teacher salaries, and college scholarships for students in the most impoverished areas.

Tax Restructuring. Coal severance taxes exist in some but not all of the coal mining states in Appalachia. For example, the coal severance tax in West Virginia, 5 percent of the price per ton, has not been increased since its inception in 1987; it provided West Virginia with about $300 million in 2006.[76] Approximately 93 percent of this revenue funds state programs; 7

percent goes to county and local governments statewide, but only about 5 percent goes to coalfield communities. A restructuring of this tax could occur in two ways. First, the coal severance tax could be raised (a raise from 5 percent to 6 percent would generate an additional $60 million, assuming the same quantity of coal and price per ton). These additional funds could be dedicated to coalfield communities to support education, provide microloans, and develop economic alternatives as coal reserves are depleted. Second, the current tax dollars could be redirected so that a larger percentage goes to local coalfield communities and less to the state. Perhaps the 93/7 percent split in West Virginia should be reversed. The state would have to sacrifice these dollars, but because this money would be used for economic and educational investments in the state's neediest areas, West Virginia could recover these funds in the form of reduced public expenditures for Medicaid and other social welfare programs. Other Appalachian states could increase or implement severance taxes directed toward education and economic diversification as well.

A healthier Appalachian population can be created. This population will be educated, employed in meaningful and sustainable enterprises, and free from exposures to environmental contaminants from mining and industry. These objectives must be pursued jointly.

References

1. Halverson JA, Ma L, Harner EJ. An analysis of disparities in health status and access to health care in the Appalachian region. Washington, DC: Appalachian Regional Commission; 2004.

2. Huang B, Wyatt SW, Tucker TC, Bottorff D, Lengerich E, Hall HI. Cancer death rates—Appalachia, 1994–1998. *MMWR Weekly.* 2002;51:527–529.

3. Hendryx M, Ahern MM. Mortality in Appalachian coal mining regions: the value of statistical life lost. *Public Health Rep.* 2009;124:541–550.

4. Appalachian Regional Commission. ARC. Available at: http://www.arc.gov/index.do. Accessed September 25, 2009.

5. U.S. Department of State. Appalachia and the Ozarks: an outline of American geography, chap. 7. Available at: http://usinfo.org/enus/life/geotravel/geography/geog07.html. Accessed June 23, 2009.

6. Appalachian Regional Commission. Subregions in Appalachia. Available at: http://www.arc.gov/index.do?nodeId=938. Accessed September 25, 2009.

7. Morello-Frosch R, Shenassa ED. The environmental "riskscape" and social inequality: implications for explaining maternal and child health disparities. *Environ Health Perspect.* 2006;114:1150–1153.

8. Gee GC, Payne-Sturges DC. Environmental health disparities: a framework integrating psychosocial and environmental concepts. *Environ Health Perspect.* 2004;112:1645–1653.

9. Evans GW. A multimethodological analysis of cumulative risk and allostatic load among rural children. *Dev Psychol.* 2003;39:924–933.

10. Evans GW, Schamberg MA. Childhood poverty, chronic stress, and adult working memory. *Proc Natl Acad Sci USA.* 2009;106:6545–6549.

11. Gunnar M, Quevedo K. The neurobiology of stress and development. *Annu Rev Psychol.* 2007;58:145–173.

12. Woolf SH, Johnson RE, Geiger HJ. The rising prevalence of severe poverty in America: a growing threat to public health. *Am J Prev Med.* 2006;31:332–341.

13. Woolf SH, Johnson RE, Phillips RL Jr, Philipsen M. Giving everyone the health of the educated: an examination of whether social change would save more lives than medical advances. *Am J Public Health.* 2007;97:679–683.

14. Marmot MG, Wilkinson RG. *Social Determinants of Health.* 2nd ed. Oxford, UK: Oxford University Press; 2006.

15. Szanton SL, Gill JM, Allen JK. Allostatic load: a mechanism of socioeconomic health disparities? *Biol Res Nurs.* 2005;7:7–15.

16. Adler NE, Newman K. Socioeconomic disparities in health: pathways and policies. *Health Aff (Millwood).* 2002;21:60–76.

17. Freme F. Annual coal report, 2005. Washington, DC: Energy Information Administration, U.S. Department of Energy; 2006.

18. Environmental Protection Agency. eGRID clean energy. Available at: http://www.epa.gov/cleanenergy/energy-resources/egrid/index.html. Accessed August 30, 2010.

19. Environmental Protection Agency. National air quality and emissions trend report. Appendix A. Washington, DC: Environmental Protection Agency; 2003.

20. Wellenius GA, Schwartz J, Mittleman MA. Particulate air pollution and hospital admissions for congestive heart failure in seven United States cities. *Am J Cardiol.* 2006;97:404–408.

21. Krewski D, Jerrett M, Burnett RT, et al. Extended follow-up and spatial analysis of the American Cancer Society study linking particulate air pollution and mortality. Boston, MA: Health Effects Institute; 2009:140.

22. Physicians for Social Responsibility. Coal-fired power plants: understanding the health costs of a dirty energy source. Washington, DC: Physicians for Social Responsibility; 2007.

23. Environmental Protection Agency. The Green Book nonattainment areas for criteria pollutants. Available at: http://www.epa.gov/air/oaqps/greenbk/. Accessed November 23, 2009.

24. Dewan S. At plant in coal ash spill, toxic deposits by the ton. *New York Times,* December 29, 2008.

25. Petteway L. EPA announces new action to prevent coal ash release. Available

at: http://yosemite.epa.gov/opa/adpress.nsf/d0f6618525a9efb85257359003fb69d/b2856087. Accessed March 26, 2009.

26. Dewan S. Tennessee ash flood larger than initial estimate. *New York Times,* December 26, 2008.

27. Freme F. Annual coal report, 2007. Washington, DC: Energy Information Administration, U.S. Department of Energy; 2009.

28. West Virginia Geological and Economic Survey. Trace elements in West Virginia coals, 2007. Available at: http://www.wvgs.wvnet.edu/www/datastat/te/index.htm. Accessed October 6, 2007.

29. Kolker A, Palmer CA, Bragg LJ, Bunnell JE. Arsenic in coal. Fact sheet 2005–3152. Reston, VA: U.S. Geological Survey; 2006.

30. Freme F. Coal industry annuals/annual coal reports, 2008. Available at: http://www.eia.doe.gov/cneaf/coal/page/acr/backissues.html. Accessed May 19, 2008.

31. Ghose MK. Generation and quantification of hazardous dusts from coal mining in the Indian context. *Environ Monit Assess.* 2007;130:35–45.

32. Environmental Protection Agency. Mountaintop mining/valley fills in Appalachia: final programmatic environmental impact statement. Philadelphia, PA: Environmental Protection Agency, Region 3; October 2005.

33. Ghose MK, Banerjee SK. Status of air pollution caused by coal washery projects in India. *Environ Monit Assess.* 1995;38(1):97–105.

34. Hendryx M, Fedorko E, Anesetti-Rothermel A. A geographical information system–based analysis of cancer mortality and population exposure to coal mining activities in West Virginia, United States of America. *Geospatial Health.* 2010;4:243–256.

35. What is underground coal slurry injection? Available at: http://www.sludgesafety.org/coal_slurry_inj.html. Accessed August 30, 2010.

36. West Virginia Department of Environmental Protection. Groundwater/UIC, 2009. Available at: http://www.wvdep.org/item.cfm?ssid=11&ss1id=165. Accessed March 18, 2009.

37. Goodell J. *Big Coal: The Dirty Secret behind America's Energy Future.* Boston, MA: Houghton Mifflin; 2006.

38. Palmer MA, Bernhardt ES, Schlesinger WH, et al. Mountaintop mining consequences. *Science.* 2010;327:148–149.

39. Hartman KJ, Kaller MD, Howell JW, Sweka JA. How much do valley fills influence headwater streams? *Hydrobiologia.* 2005;532:91–102.

40. McAuley SD, Kozar MD. Ground-water quality in unmined areas and near reclaimed surface coal mines in the Northern and Central Appalachian coal regions, Pennsylvania and West Virginia. Reston, VA: U.S. Department of the Interior, U.S. Geological Survey; 2006.

41. Shiber JG. Arsenic in domestic well water and health in Central Appalachia, USA. *Water Air Soil Poll.* 2005;160:327–341.

42. Stout BM, Papillo J. Well water quality in the vicinity of a coal slurry

impoundment near Williamson, West Virginia. Wheeling, WV: Wheeling Jesuit University; 2004.

43. Hitt N, Hendryx M. Exploring the dynamic relationship between health and the environment. New York, NY: American Museum of Natural History Symposium; April 2009.

44. Blakeney AB, Marshall A. Water quality, health, and human occupations. *Am J Occup Ther.* 2009;63:46–57.

45. Ferreccio C, Gonzalez C, Milosavjlevic V, Marshall G, Sancha AM, Smith AH. Lung cancer and arsenic concentrations in drinking water in Chile. *Epidemiology.* 2000;11:673–679.

46. Yu HS, Liao WT, Chai CY. Arsenic carcinogenesis in the skin. *J Biomed Sci.* 2006;13:657–666.

47. Boffetta P, Nyberg F. Contribution of environmental factors to cancer risk. *Br Med Bull.* 2003;68:71–94.

48. Cakmak S, Dales RE, Judek S. Respiratory health effects of air pollution gases: modification by education and income. *Arch Environ Occup Health.* 2006;61:5–10.

49. Mastin JP. Environmental cardiovascular disease. *Cardiovasc Toxicol.* 2005;5:91–94.

50. Hodgson S, Nieuwenhuijsen MJ, Elliott P, Jarup L. Kidney disease mortality and environmental exposure to mercury. *Am J Epidemiol.* 2007;165:72–77.

51. Rosenman KD, Moore-Fuller M, Reilly MJ. Kidney disease and silicosis. *Nephron.* 2000;85:14–19.

52. Hendryx M. Mortality rates in Appalachian coal mining counties: 24 years behind the nation. *Environmental Justice.* 2008;1:5–11.

53. U.S. Department of Agriculture. Poultry—production and value 2007 summary. Washington, DC: National Agricultural Statistics Service, U.S. Department of Agriculture; 2008:Pou 3–1 (08).

54. Environmental Protection Agency. Air releases (AIRS/AFS), 2008. Available at: http://www.epa.gov/enviro/html/airs/index.html. Accessed March 30, 2009.

55. Environmental Protection Agency. Toxics release inventory (TRI), 2008. Available at: http://www.epa.gov/enviro/html/tris/. Accessed March 30, 2009.

56. Environmental Protection Agency. Water discharge permits (PCS), 2008. Available at: http://www.epa.gov/enviro/html/pcs/. Accessed March 30, 2009.

57. Kennard D. Timber supply in the southern Appalachians. Available at: http://www.forestencyclopedia.net/p/p2349. Accessed September 23, 2009.

58. Jarvis S. Logging fatalities investigated by OSHA: 1996–1997. *Forest Operations Review.* 2002;Fall:9–10.

59. Bell JL, Helmkamp JC. Non-fatal injuries in the West Virginia logging industry: using workers' compensation claims to assess risk from 1995 through 2001. *Am J Ind Med.* 2003;44:502–509.

60. Bureau of Labor Statistics, U.S. Department of Labor. Injuries, illnesses,

and fatalities. Available at: http://www.bls.gov/iif/oshnotice10.htm. Accessed September 25, 2009.

61. Sygnatur EF. Logging is perilous work. Available at: http://www.bls.gov/iif/oshwc/cfar0027.txt. Accessed November 23, 2009.

62. Appalachian Regional Commission. Motor vehicle accident mortality in Appalachia. Available at: www.arc.gov/images/reports/healthdisparities/mortality_motorvehicle.pdf. Accessed September 23, 2009.

63. Hendryx M, Zullig KJ. Higher coronary heart disease and heart attack morbidity in Appalachian coal mining regions. *Prev Med.* 2009;49:355–359.

64. Geohazards in transportation in the Appalachian region. 9th Annual Technical Forum. Lexington, KY, August 2009. Available at: http://www.marshall.edu/cegas/geohazards/2009pdf/Geohazards_Program2009.pdf. Accessed November 23, 2009.

65. Hendryx M. Mortality from heart, respiratory, and kidney disease in coal mining areas of Appalachia. *Int Arch Occup Environ Health.* 2009;82:243–249.

66. Hendryx M, O'Donnell K, Horn K. Lung cancer mortality is elevated in coal-mining areas of Appalachia. *Lung Cancer.* 2008;62:1–7.

67. Hendryx M, Ahern MM. Relations between health indicators and residential proximity to coal mining in West Virginia. *Am J Public Health.* 2008;98:669–671.

68. Hendryx M, Ahern MM, Nurkiewicz TR. Hospitalization patterns associated with Appalachian coal mining. *J Toxicol Environ Health A.* 2007;70:2064–2070.

69. Thompson EC, Berger MC, Allen SN, Roenker JM. A study on the current economic impacts of the Appalachian coal industry and its future in the region. Lexington, KY: Center for Business and Economic Research, University of Kentucky; 2001.

70. Viscusi WK, Aldy JE. The value of a statistical life: a critical review of market estimates throughout the world. *J Risk Uncertainty.* 2003;27:5–76.

71. Konisky DM. Inequities in enforcement? Environmental justice and government performance. *J Policy Anal Manag.* 2009;28:102–121.

72. Todd J. A new shared economy for Appalachia: an economy built on environmental restoration, carbon sequestration, renewable energy and ecological design. Burlington, VT: Rubenstein School of Environment and Natural Resources, University of Vermont; 2008.

73. Hibbard M, Karle K. Ecosystem restoration as community economic development? An assessment of the possibilities. *Journal of the Community Development Society.* 2002;33:39–60.

74. Gbezo BE. Microcredit in West Africa: how small loans make a big impact on poverty. *World at Work.* 1999;31(31):13–15.

75. Duncan CM, Coles R. *Worlds Apart: Why Poverty Persists in Rural America.* New Haven, CT: Yale University Press; 1999.

76. West Virginia Coal Association. Coal facts 2007. Charleston, WV: West Virginia Coal Association; 2007.

3

The Quest for an Appalachian Health Lifestyle

Evelyn A. Knight

Is there a distinctive Appalachian health lifestyle? This chapter explores the concept of health lifestyles and how research on this concept has been applied to the Appalachian region. It concludes with recommendations for researchers and practitioners engaged in addressing health issues from a lifestyle perspective.

Although there is no universal definition of the term *lifestyle* as it is applied to health research, in the most general sense, it refers to the behaviors and life course choices individuals and groups of individuals make that have the potential to impact their health status. Based on extensive epidemiological study over the past sixty to seventy years, these behaviors and life course choices can be categorized as follows: (1) behaviors that promote improved health and lower the risks for certain diseases, such as engaging in physical activity, consuming a diet that conforms to recommended guidelines, and choosing not to use tobacco products; (2) behaviors that prevent specific health problems or identify them early, when they may be more easily treatable, such as getting immunizations or undergoing blood pressure checks or mammograms; and (3) protective behaviors that reduce the exposure to health threats, such as using a seat belt or avoiding toxic exposures in the workplace.[1]

A wide variety of factors, or determinants, influence individuals' health behavior choices. These include knowledge, attitudes, and beliefs regarding the behavior itself and the relationship between the behavior and one's own health; the social norms and supports that influence beliefs and behavior; the structural or environmental factors that influence one's perception of what is possible; and the elements in one's societal and physical environment that either support or hinder the behavior. The approach to the study of health behavior based on these determinants is known as the socioecological model, and it is broadly applied in research and in practice.[2]

Given the breadth of influences on a wide variety of health behaviors, asking whether there is an Appalachian health lifestyle implies that there are broad cultural and structural commonalities in the region that result in widespread (perhaps even unique) Appalachian lifestyle patterns that can be observed and understood in relation to those commonalities. This chapter explores the information available to support or refute this assumption by examining regionwide studies of lifestyle behaviors. Then, using the example of tobacco-related behavior research, the chapter explores what has been learned about Appalachian lifestyle patterns at a subregional level.

Studying Health Lifestyle

In the United States, lifestyle information is most often collected through self-reports from random samples of the population or through convenience samples of well-defined local groups, such as users of specific health facilities. These key research tools are useful for describing general population trends or specific situations, but one must exercise care when using them to draw conclusions about health disparities or unique lifestyle characteristics of a subset of the U.S. population, including Appalachia, that encompasses subregions with different histories and diverse populations.

Vital Statistics. Records of vital statistics—which capture "official" events in the lives of American citizens, including birth and death—are the most complete, valid, and reliable data available for studying the health of the U.S. population. Analyses of mortality data, which are compiled from death certificates by the states and then combined into national data sets, have played a major role in highlighting regional health disparities.[3] For example, cardiovascular disease is the major cause of death among adults over age 35 in every state and among all ethnic and racial groups. Yet rates of death from cardiovascular disease vary greatly across the country, even when differences in the age distribution of various populations are taken into account. Similar disparities can be observed nationally for cancer mortality rates. When looking for explanations of these differences, health lifestyle comes under scrutiny. For example, extensive epidemiological research has found that specific health behaviors (though not the only determinants of these disparities) contribute to high rates of death from cardiovascular disease. These include smoking, sedentary lifestyle, and diet, with smoking considered the greatest preventable cause of death among the competing lifestyle risks.[4]

Data on the health behaviors that contribute to death are not available from death certificates, so researchers must depend on other data sources to examine differences in the prevalence of contributing health behaviors among various population groups. The key sources for these data are the Behavioral Risk Factor Surveillance System (BRFSS) and the National Health Interview Survey (NHIS), both of which use sampling techniques to estimate the prevalence of health-related behaviors.

Behavioral Risk Factor Surveillance System. Established in 1984, the BRFSS uses an annual telephone survey carried out at the state level. Each state chooses the size of the sample and the specific modules to be used each year, but the core questions and basic data-collection methodology are guided by the Centers for Disease Control and Prevention and are consistent across all states, allowing a comparison of behavior rates and confidence intervals between states.[5] At the county level, however, the BRFSS data may not be reliable in some cases due to the relatively small sample sizes. This has resulted in various approaches to aggregating and smoothing the data to overcome the limitations of small-area analysis.[6] The BRFSS data are based on self-reports and are subject to the limitations of such data.

National Health Interview Survey. The NHIS is a telephone survey used to monitor the health of the U.S. population. Using a sampling design based on each decennial census, the NHIS provides health data that are representative of the national population. The primary geographic sampling units are counties, small groups of contiguous counties, and metropolitan statistical areas. The data are not considered precise at the state level on a yearly basis, but years may be combined to produce state-level estimates. In addition to questions about health status and access to health care, the NHIS includes lifestyle questions related to cigarette smoking, leisure-time physical activity, alcohol use, and sleep.[7,8]

Primary Data. Neither the BRFSS nor the NHIS includes extensive information about the determinants of the behaviors under study, with the exception of basic demographic and geographic indicators. Researchers looking for larger local samples or in-depth information about the determinants of specific behavior risks must collect primary data. Locality-based research is fraught with its own methodological challenges, especially issues related to external validity, and it is rarely longitudinal. Nonetheless, when taken cumulatively, health behavior studies in Appalachian communities may increase the understanding of regional health behaviors.

Is There an Appalachian Health Lifestyle?

To answer the question of whether there is a unique Appalachian health lifestyle and what it might be, researchers begin by comparing mortality and morbidity rates between Appalachian and non-Appalachian populations using vital statistics data. If there are no observed differences at this level of analysis, Appalachian lifestyle behaviors would be considered benign. However, health disparities between Appalachia and other regions are well documented, as other chapters in this volume attest. In a widely cited analysis, Burkett[9] observes that for each of the top ten causes of death in the United States, mortality rates in both urban and rural Appalachian counties (as defined in 1988) are higher than in the rest of the country. Given these disparities, the search for causes becomes an endeavor of great interest.

One approach has been to examine patterns of lifestyle behaviors in the region and compare them with patterns in other regions. Such analyses are unable to detect a range of environmental differences in the populations under study, however, and as such, they obscure the importance of context to health outcomes. Nonetheless, these studies can hint at the need to delve into environmental differences that may be contributing to the observed population-level disparities. Another approach has been to carry out in-depth studies of local populations within the region for a better understanding of observed disparities in light of both socioecological factors and lifestyle in general. Several important studies have taken the first approach and are used extensively to describe health lifestyle issues in Appalachia. Other studies have undertaken more limited analyses, but social and environmental factors related to place have been ignored, for the most part, in all the work reviewed here.

The most complete analysis of health lifestyle behaviors in the Appalachian region to date is a 1995 monograph produced for the West Virginia Department of Health and Human Resources.[10] This report analyzed 1993 BRFSS data from the 399 counties designated as Appalachian by the Appalachian Regional Commission (ARC) at that time. The lifestyle behaviors studied were seat belt nonuse, current smoking, heavy drinking, binge drinking, and drinking and driving. There were insufficient data to report on smokeless tobacco use and sedentary lifestyle.[a] The researchers made three sets of comparisons for each risk factor: (1) the aggregated rate for the thirteen states designated as Appalachian compared with the aggregated rate for the other thirty-six states,[b] (2) the aggregated rate for all the Appalachian counties compared with the aggregated rate for all non-Appalachian counties, and (3) state-by-state comparisons between the aggregated Appalachian county rate and the aggregated rate for the rest of the counties in the state.

To demonstrate differences in health risks between the ARC-designated Appalachian region and the rest of the country, the researchers compared the aggregated data from the thirteen states partially or wholly within the Appalachian region with data aggregated from the other thirty-six states in the data set. In this overall analysis, the researchers identified significantly higher rates of smoking and failing to wear a seat belt and significantly lower rates of heavy drinking, binge drinking, and drinking and driving in Appalachian states compared with the other states. Differences in obesity, overweight, and hypertension awareness were not significant. Although there were observable differences in certain risk factors, given the vast demographic differences in the states being compared, especially in terms of the urban-rural continuum, it would be difficult to conclude that this analysis revealed meaningful information about an Appalachian health lifestyle.

At the next level of analysis, the population in the Appalachian counties across the thirteen states exhibited a significantly higher risk of injury and illness from not wearing a seat belt and current smoking compared with populations in non-Appalachian counties nationwide, including non-Appalachian counties in the thirteen-state region. In contrast, the Appalachian population exhibited a lower risk of injury and illness from heavy drinking, binge drinking, and drinking and driving than did non-Appalachian residents. There were insufficient data to compare physical activity behaviors. Differences among demographic groups for each risk factor were also noted, with the individual characteristics of gender, education, and age moderating the observed differences. Although this analysis focused on the Appalachian region per se, by comparing the Appalachian counties with all other counties, differences attributable to sociodemographics, the rural-urban continuum, and other place-based factors were obscured. Additionally, the region was treated as a totality, even though its subregions differ in important factors that contribute to lifestyle choices.

For the third analysis, the researchers compared the Appalachian and non-Appalachian counties in each of the thirteen states to look for differences in these key lifestyle factors (after reweighting the data according to the demographic characteristics of the Appalachian and non-Appalachian counties). Notably, only in Kentucky, New York, and North Carolina were there significantly higher risk factors in the Appalachian versus non-Appalachian portions of the state. In Virginia, North Carolina, Kentucky, Maryland, and Tennessee, one or more risk factor levels were lower in the Appalachian counties than in the rest of the state. Table 3.1 summarizes these comparisons.

This analysis shows that, at the state level, there does not appear to be a consistent pattern of differences between Appalachian and non-Appalachian health lifestyles. Several behaviors are more prevalent and others are less prevalent in the Appalachian counties of certain states. This state-by-state analysis cannot determine whether there are geographic pockets where health behaviors and other socioecological differences converge to create a unique health lifestyle pattern.

A more recent study,[11] using data from the 1990s, aggregated county-level BRFSS data at the labor market area (LMA) level.[c] There are seventy-nine LMAs that contain at least one Appalachian-designated county. Rates of smoking and physical activity in these LMAs were compared with rates in all other LMAs in the country. This analysis concluded that smoking and physical inactivity rates in the Appalachian LMAs varied across the region but were generally higher than elsewhere. Specific cancer screening behaviors were also compared, with the Appalachian LMAs showing varying but somewhat lower rates than other LMAs. This study confirmed that there is no singular Appalachian health lifestyle across the ARC-defined region. Like other studies, it was unable to draw meaningful conclusions about observed patterns because comparing Appalachian LMAs to all other LMAs

Table 3.1. Risk Factor Prevalence in Appalachian and Non-Appalachian Regions of the ARC-Designated Appalachian States, 1993

Risk Factor	Northern Region				Central Region					Southern Region			
	NY	PA	MD	OH	WV*	KY	VA	TN	NC	SC	GA	AL	MS
Seat belt nonuse	—	—	—	—	—	←	—	—	←	—	—	—	—
Obesity	—	—	—	—	←	—	—	—	→	—	—	—	—
Overweight	—	—	→	—	←	←	—	—	→	—	—	—	—
Hypertension awareness	—	—	→	—	←	←	—	—	—	—	—	—	—
Current smoking	—	—	—	—	—	←	—	—	—	—	—	—	—
Heavy drinking	←	—	—	→	—	→	→	—	—	—	—	—	—
Binge drinking	←	—	—	—	→	→	→	—	—	—	—	—	—
Drinking and driving	—	—	—	—	—	—	→	→	—	—	—	—	—

Source: Adapted from Thoenen E. *Health Risks: The Appalachian Lifestyle.* Charleston, WV: West Virginia Department of Health and Human Resources, Health Statistics Center; 1995.

Key:

← = Significantly higher in Appalachian region of the state.

→ = Significantly lower in Appalachian region of the state.

— = No difference between Appalachian and non-Appalachian regions of the state.

* Because all of WV is Appalachian, it was compared with non-Appalachian KY.

would be expected to identify health behavior differences, given the differences in underlying socioeconomic factors.

Another lifestyle issue of concern in Appalachia is substance abuse. A comprehensive study of mental health and substance abuse across the region found that methamphetamine, marijuana, and cocaine usage rates are lower in the region than in other parts of the country, as are rates of alcohol abuse and alcohol dependence.[12] However, the nonmedical use of prescription-type psychotherapeutics is higher among adolescents in Appalachia than elsewhere, and admission rates for addiction to opiates and synthetics are higher, especially in coal mining areas, than in other parts of the country. Use of opiates is increasing faster in Appalachia than elsewhere, especially in its coal mining areas. Note that, once again, the region was compared with the nation generally, meaning that the influences of contextual factors were obscured.

These broad, regional studies are important for their contribution to an understanding of the prevalence of specific health behaviors in the region. These risk behaviors are associated with poor health outcomes and early death, and they create a burden for communities, families, and individuals. However, because these studies use the political definition of Appalachia to analyze socially and ecologically influenced behaviors, the results do not contribute to an understanding of observed variations in the distribution of these behaviors or to the discovery of pathways to promote and support change.

Two lifestyle behaviors that have received widespread attention from health researchers focusing on the Appalachian region are smoking and the utilization of cancer screening services. Of the two, smoking is less dependent on the availability of support from the health care system, so an exploration of the research on this specific behavior may provide insights into the Appalachian health lifestyle question.

Appalachian Tobacco Use

Smoking is the number-one cause of preventable morbidity and mortality in the United States, and it is the second leading risk factor for six of the eight leading causes of death globally.[13] Tobacco use contributes to increased rates of cardiovascular disease, chronic lung disease, several cancers (especially lung cancer), diabetes, and low birth weight, making smoking a serious health concern.

Thoenen[10] and Halverson and coauthors[11] concluded that smoking prevalence in the 1993 ARC-designated Appalachian region was higher than outside the region, with high rates concentrated in Central Appalachia. Research has also shown that smoking rates are higher in some[11, 14] or all[10] of the Appalachian states than in the non-Appalachian states. However, according to Thoenen,[10] only in Kentucky was the smoking rate higher in the Appalachian than in the non-Appalachian part the state (see table 3.1).

To explore smoking as an Appalachian lifestyle characteristic, data (from the 1993 BRFSS) were extracted from Thoenen's study, and smoking rates in the Appalachian regions of the thirteen states were compared. Regional comparisons at the state level indicated that Appalachian Kentucky had a higher smoking rate than the Appalachian areas of eight other states. Only in North Carolina's Appalachian region were smoking rates as high as those in Kentucky. Notably, these two states are the top two tobacco producers in the country, and loyalty to the crop was very high, especially in the 1990s. The smoking rate for the Appalachian counties of North Carolina was not significantly higher than that for the rest of the state. The fact that the rate of tobacco use was higher in Appalachian Kentucky than in the rest of the state suggests that only in that state was an "Appalachian factor" involved. However, more recent data suggest that this difference has now been equalized; smoking rates in both Appalachian and non-Appalachian Kentucky are now lower than in 1993, and they are no longer significantly different.[15] There is no regionwide report on smokeless tobacco use, but the prevalence of its use among men in a convenience sample of Appalachian Ohio residents was reported to be 33 percent—much higher than the 5.1 percent in the rest of the state.[16]

Clearly, there are subregions of Appalachia where smoking rates are high. However, within states that have high smoking rates, the level of smoking in the Appalachian areas does not exceed that in the rest of the state, pointing to causes independent of the Appalachian designation.

Individual Determinants of Smoking Behavior

In classic health behavior studies, researchers look for determinants of the relevant behavior across a variety of socioecological factors ranging from individual knowledge and beliefs to environmental influences. Studies of specific Appalachian populations of smokers have searched for individual characteristics (e.g., knowledge, beliefs, personality, mental health status) as well as characteristics of the individuals' social environment (e.g., individual perceptions of social support systems and social norms) to explain behaviors related to tobacco, including smoking and smoking cessation, smokeless tobacco use and quitting, and smoking during pregnancy.

Knowledge. Although it is well understood that knowledge alone does not determine lifestyle behavior choices, it is a contributor to decision making. In a study intended to describe the determinants of rural adult smoking patterns in Appalachian Ohio, interviews of a convenience sample of smokers found differences between them and other non-Appalachian populations.[16] The authors concluded that the relatively low income level and generally low education level among those in the sample, coupled with their being raised in the region, characterized the sample as "typical" of Appalachian Ohio, if not representative. Respondents recognized the relationship between smoking and the risk for lung cancer, but only half the sample understood the relationship between smoking and cardiovascular disease. Fewer knew about the effects of environmental tobacco smoke than about the effects of smoking itself. Knowledge was related to education level, but greater knowledge was not associated with increased age, as has been observed in other studies. In this sample, younger participants had greater knowledge than older ones.

In another study,[17] information from focus groups in a nonmetropolitan Appalachian county (state not named) showed that smokers were aware of the pharmacological effects of nicotine and recognized it as an addictive substance. Participants identified negative consequences of smoking related to finances, health, and aesthetics as influences on their decision making. However, they also rationalized tobacco use with the observation that many people who smoke live into old age and that smoking can help control dietary intake.

Another focus group analysis revealed that knowledge of the dangers of tobacco use is high among adolescents in the Appalachian sections of seven states.[18] These adolescents cited concerns about exposing children to secondhand smoke and illnesses related to tobacco as deterrents to smoking.

These studies reveal that selected populations in the Appalachian region understand the risks of smoking, especially the pulmonary risks, and are sensitive to social issues surrounding the behavior. Although knowledge is an important component in the decision-making process, a host of other influences contribute to the adoption and maintenance of smoking behaviors in Appalachia and elsewhere.

Beliefs. It has also been hypothesized that the continuing high prevalence of smoking in parts of Appalachia may be associated with individuals' beliefs about quitting. Macnee and McCabe[14] examined readiness to quit in a randomly selected adult population in an Appalachian county in Tennessee and found a higher percentage (40 percent) of smokers in the precontemplation stage (not planning to quit) compared with national samples. They reported that in their sample, the classification of smokers into five stages of change[19] was not associated with education, gender, income, rating of health, age at smoking onset, amount smoked, or presence of tobacco as part of social life or occupation. Those in the maintenance stage—that is, nonsmokers—were more likely to report attending church more than twelve times a month. Negative views of smoking did not differ across the stages of change in the Tennessee sample, whereas decreases in negative views across these stages were found in national samples. However, there were statistically significant differences in views about the pros of smoking across the stages of change, as anticipated from studies of non-Appalachian populations. These Tennessee smokers reported using specific types of strategies for changing their smoking behaviors at different rates than did smokers in non-Appalachian studies. A similar study conducted in Appalachian Ohio identified 20 percent of smokers in the contemplation stage,[16] which was higher than that reported in the Tennessee sample and similar to that in a national sample.

The main conclusion to be drawn from the extant research on the relationship between beliefs and smoking is that it is complex and appears to vary across populations. There seems to be no consistent pattern in the Appalachian research reviewed here, although some differences from non-Appalachian samples were observed.

Personality and Mental Health Status. Personality[20, 21] and mental health characteristics[22] have also been associated with smoking behaviors. These variables were included in three studies that examined smoking among pregnant women in different Appalachian settings. In one study,[23] personality traits of smokers identified in other studies—specifically, being less sociable, more anxious, more vulnerable to stress, and more easily de-pressed—were not observed among the sample of pregnant women at a community health center in West Virginia. Smokers were not more nega-tive, although nonsmokers were more positive. Overall, personality traits[d] of the women in the study were more negative than those of middle-class women in a similar study, whether they were smokers or not. The research-ers noted that low socioeconomic status is often related to high negative personality measures.

Researchers in a different West Virginia setting explored the relation-ship between smoking and pregnancy as a transitional life event and found a complex association between smoking and depression.[24] Smoking was understood as integral to the women's social and personal context. The re-searchers did not conclude that their findings were unique to Appalachian women.

Another study,[25] conducted in a community clinic in Southern Appa-lachia, found that smoking during pregnancy was not associated with fac-tors observed elsewhere, including education level, living with a smoker, history of depression, or use of other substances. Factors that contributed to women's continuing to smoke during pregnancy were higher levels of smoking prior to pregnancy, inadequate prenatal care, and low family in-come. Why predictors of smoking cessation during pregnancy that were found in other studies, including emotional factors such as depression, did not apply to this disadvantaged population is not clear. The researchers were careful to note that the factors that predict smoking and successful smoking cessation during pregnancy vary across populations, as demon-strated in these three studies.

Socioeconomic Status. When looking for differences in individual de-terminants of smoking behavior across different populations, it is impor-tant to note that, nationally and globally, an individual's socioeconomic status is considered the single greatest predictor of tobacco use. An analy-sis of eight cross-sectional national surveys confirmed that poverty status is an independent predictor of smoking status as well as smoking cessa-tion.[26] Americans living below the poverty line are 40 percent more likely to smoke than are those living at or above the poverty line.[27] This is cor-roborated by an analysis of 2004 NHIS data on smoking behavior, which found that smoking varies substantially across population groups. Smoking prevalence decreases with increasing education and is higher among adults living in poverty.[28] Globally, epidemiological studies have identified an association between smoking behavior and poverty at both the individual and community levels of analysis.[29] Given the high rates of poverty in some parts of the Appalachian region, one would expect to find high smoking rates as well. However, the association between individual poverty status or community socioeconomic status and tobacco use has not been studied from a regional perspective.

Poverty may influence smoking behaviors at the individual level through mechanisms associated with behavioral modeling related to social position, nicotine exposure related to smoking behaviors, and positive rewards of nicotine use related to stress, even though smoking itself may be a stressor.[30] In light of the clustering of high smoking rates and high poverty rates in Central Appalachia, understanding this association is important for addressing this health risk in the region.

Social and Environmental Determinants of Tobacco Use

Social Determinants. Individual knowledge, perceptions, and beliefs are subject to social influences and are often dependent on social context. Often the most immediate social influence on an individual's lifestyle decisions is his or her family context. In several studies carried out in Appalachia, smokers reported that family circumstances, especially having a smoker in the household, influenced their decisions to smoke or to quit. Conditions within the family contributed to the use of both tobacco and alcohol, even though awareness of the risks related to such use was high. Adolescents in thirty-four focus group discussions in the Appalachian regions of seven states reported that family influences on their decisions to use or abstain from tobacco were very important.[18] Early experimentation with tobacco often occurred within the context of the family home. Specific deterrents to tobacco use cited by the adolescents included secondhand smoke exposure among children, the smell of smoke in the home and on family members, and personal experiences with illnesses related to smoking, such as lung cancer.

In a study of tobacco cessation among adolescent girls in tobacco-growing regions of Appalachian Ohio, Tennessee, and Virginia,[31] researchers observed that community support for tobacco and the prevalence of adult smoking, especially parental smoking, influenced the girls' decisions and perceptions. They concluded that local beliefs and social norms are related to local and family contexts. However, these phenomena are not necessarily unique to Appalachia.

The characteristics of one's social and political environment, including the prevalence of smoking itself, may influence decisions to begin and continue tobacco use. Macnee and McCabe[14] noted that there are fewer tobacco-related laws and fewer antismoking programs in areas that are economically dependent on tobacco. Nonetheless, Denham and colleagues[31] found that tobacco use in tobacco-growing areas of Appalachia is similar to that in other regions.

Environmental Determinants. Rurality is associated with tobacco use, and portions of Appalachia are highly rural. Researchers comparing BRFSS self-reported smoking data for 1994–1996 and 2000–2001 found rural smoking rates to be highest in Kentucky, Ohio, and Indiana and lowest in Utah, California, and Nebraska.[32] Although changes in prevalence between the two periods were negligible overall, a pattern was noted in which rural smoking prevalence declined in states where baseline smoking rates were already low, increased in ten states where baseline rates were not low, and increased in three states where baseline rates were high. The greatest increases in rural smoking were observed among the young and those in the lowest income category ($25,000 a year or less). Differences in urban and rural smoking rates were explained statistically by lower levels of income and educational attainment in rural areas and by being white or Native American. When only those in depressed income and low education categories were included in the analysis, rural rates were still higher than urban rates. African Americans residing in rural areas had lower smoking rates than their urban counterparts, but this pattern was not observed in any other racial or ethnic group. McMillen and associates[33] reported that rural areas were less likely than urban areas to have smoking restrictions in place, but this difference was not attributable to variations in the populations' knowledge about the risks of environmental tobacco smoke. Differences in home and work-site restrictions could not be explained by region, education, age, gender, race, or smoking status factors. In contrast, rural-urban differences in restrictions on smoking in public places were accounted for by variations in these demographic variables but not by differences in knowledge and opinion after controlling for smoking status, gender, race, age, and education. The researchers concluded that the social climate in rural areas results in greater exposure to environmental smoke, which influences individuals' perceptions of social norms that impact decision making.

Implications of Tobacco Use Research

This overview of tobacco use and its determinants in Appalachia shows that the prevalence of tobacco use varies across the region, with particularly high rates occurring in parts of Central Appalachia. Even where rates are high, as in Kentucky, the current rates are not higher in the Appalachian portion of the state than in the rest of the state. The strong association between poverty as a place-based determinant of smoking and the association between rurality and high smoking rates among white populations converge in areas throughout Appalachia to produce high rates of smoking. Thus, the inference by some researchers that smoking behavior is determined by Appalachian cultural characteristics appears to be unfounded.[16–18, 31] Some of the research cited here recounts, uncritically, what might be considered stereotypical characterizations as explanations for its results. For example, to call the influence of parents' smoking on youths' behavior "familism" or to label rationalizations about smokers living to an old age as "fatalism" relies on Appalachian stereotypes to suggest that these determinants and attributions are particularly Appalachian when, in fact, they are widespread. Marshall[34] observes that American Indian and Hispanic populations also focus on family and home characteristics. Nonetheless, health professionals are acutely aware that where prevalence rates are high, it is important to understand the social context that supports smoking and the barriers to smoking cessation.

With some notable exceptions, the search for an Appalachian health lifestyle has focused on the relationship between individual characteristics and behavior. Population characteristics affect health outcomes independently of individual characteristics. Therefore, understanding the observed disparities across the region requires more complex approaches to studying social and environmental determinants and access to societal resources, ranging from living history and local cultures to political structures and economic systems. Both individual and community levels of prosperity impact health through levels of knowledge (education), prestige, money, influence, and power and by the conditions that cause social stress and its physical impacts.[35] The recently created Centers for Population Health and Health Disparities are promoting multilevel research that incorporates biological factors, individual demographic characteristics and risk factors, social and physical contexts, and institutional and policy factors (called fundamental causes) in complex models that may elucidate the causes of health disparities and how "environment gets under the skin" (p. 1613).[36] This is the challenge faced by researchers seeking to uncover the fundamental causes of health lifestyle risks in Appalachia. Recognizing that lifestyle is place based[37] means that planning for health promotion and disease prevention programs needs to include a careful assessment of the local population and the local social, economic, political, and physical environmental conditions.

Further Research

A key question raised by this chapter is whether the search for a unique Appalachian health lifestyle should be abandoned. That existing research has not been able to identify an Appalachian health lifestyle may be attributable to limitations of the study methods used rather than to the absence of the phenomenon. Given the importance of the particularities of history, socioeconomic status, and place in lifestyle choices, however, the existing research supports the conclusion that if there is an Appalachian health lifestyle, it will not be distributed across a politically defined region. Using both epidemiological and social science methods may help answer the following overarching questions.

Do lifestyle behaviors in Appalachian communities differ from those in non-Appalachian communities with similar sociodemographic characteristics? Previous epidemiological studies compared geographically defined Appalachian populations with the sum of non-Appalachian U.S. populations, an approach that obscures differences based on rurality and socioeconomic factors. More complex, multilevel analysis may identify regional differences that cannot be explained by poverty or rurality. This question also needs to be addressed at the individual level to determine whether persons of Appalachian heritage have different lifestyle behaviors than those of non-Appalachian heritage. This issue has been difficult to assess, but doing so is necessary to identify an Appalachian health lifestyle.

In populations in which there is an association between poverty and important health behaviors such as smoking, what socioecological factors are consistent across these communities that may impact the behavioral choice? The broad range of environmental factors influencing deleterious lifestyle choices in poor communities has yet to be clearly differentiated. This information could expand practitioners' knowledge of causal factors that may be amenable to modification and add to researchers' understanding of the socioecological model of health behavior. Qualitative, in-depth studies can establish the basis for larger studies that use the community rather than the individual as the unit of analysis, which are lacking in the literature.[38]

How do social and environmental factors influence individual lifestyle choices in poor communities? A local, participatory action research approach to answering this complex question would begin to map the wide range of influences on individual health lifestyle choices and bridge the gap between the worldviews of researchers and the worldviews of those whose environments are often characterized by limited community resources and limited civic engagement. This research should be conceptualized against the backdrop of the wide range of models of poverty[39, 40] and the role of place in health outcomes.[41]

How do adaptations to the stress of personal and community poverty impact selected lifestyle choices, especially tobacco use? An association between poverty and smoking has been observed worldwide; the use of tobacco for stress relief has also been documented. When individuals perceive that they have limited control over life or occupational stressors, they often choose passive coping mechanisms that reduce the stress response rather than active coping behaviors intended to mitigate the source of stress.[42] Further understanding of these coping mechanisms is needed not only for tobacco use but also for other unhealthy lifestyle behaviors.

How do different types of tobacco policies impact underserved communities or communities with large health disparities? As a corollary, how can support for effective policies be built in these communities?[38] The research reviewed in this chapter has shown that poor and rural communities are less likely to have environmental tobacco control policies in place and are less likely to support such policies. At the same time, it has been hypothesized that smoking is more harmful to residents of disadvantaged communities.[43] Greater understanding of how policies differentially impact communities is needed to develop effective and acceptable public policies that support these communities.

Policy Recommendations

The Ottawa Charter for Health Promotion,[44] created by delegates at an international conference in 1986, proposed standards for the creation of health promotion–related public policy and recognized the complexity of the influences on health:

> Health promotion policy combines diverse but complementary approaches including legislation, fiscal measures, taxation, and organizational change. It is coordinated action that leads to health, income, and social policies that foster greater equity. Joint action contributes to ensuring safer and healthier goods and services, healthier public services, and cleaner, more enjoyable environments. Health promotion policy requires the identification of obstacles to the adoption of healthy public policies in non-health sectors, and ways of removing them. The aim must be to make the healthier choice the easier choice for policy-makers as well.[44]

Community empowerment and self-determination are considered the heart of health promotion and the basis for the creation of health promotion policy. Given this framework, policy recommendations for Appalachian health promotion include (1) assurances that health promotion infrastructure is available to all communities as an integral aspect of a public health and wellness system,[45] and (2) assurances that rural communities are included in health promotion policy debates, understand the issues, and have a voice in establishing state-level policies that will impact their communities.[46]

Notes

a. Obesity, overweight, and hypertension awareness were also included in the report.

b. Wyoming did not implement the BRFSS that year.

c. LMAs are defined as districts drawn to contain populations of at least 100,000 and that cross state and county boundaries.

d. Measurements included Costa and McCrae's five-factor personality inventory, the self-esteem index of the Clinical Measurement Package, Crnic's social support scale, and Braiker and Kelly's index of marital/partner satisfaction.

References

1. U.S. Department of Health, Education, and Welfare. Healthy people: the surgeon general's report on health promotion and disease prevention. DHEW (PHS) Pub. No. 79–55071. Washington, DC: Public Health Service, Office of the Assistant Secretary; 1979.

2. McLeroy KR, Bibeau D, Steckler A, Glanz K. An ecological perspective on health promotion programs. *Health Educ Q.* 1988;15:351–377.

3. Mary Babb Randolph Cancer Center/Office for Social Environmental and Health Research. Underlying socioeconomic factors influencing health disparities in the Appalachian region. Final Report Contract No. CO-15198. Morgantown, WV: Department of Community Medicine, Robert C. Byrd Health Sciences Center, West Virginia University; 2008.

4. Mokdad AH, Marks JS, Stroup DF, Gerberding JL. Actual causes of death in the United States, 2000. *JAMA.* 2004;291:1238–1245.

5. BRFSS. Behavioral Risk Factor Surveillance System operational and user's guide, version 3.0. 2006. Available at: ftp://ftp.cdc.gov/pub/Data/Brfss/userguide .pdf. Accessed December 15, 2009.

6. Jia H, Muennig P, Borawski E. Comparison of small-area analysis techniques for estimating county-level outcomes. *Am J Prev Med.* 2004;26:453–460.

7. U.S. Department of Health and Human Services. 2008 National Health Interview Survey (NHIS): public use data release. Hyattsville, MD: National Center for Health Statistics; 2008. Available at: http://ftp.cdc.gov/pub/Health_Statistics/ NCHS/Dataset_Documentation/NHIS/2008/srvydesc.pdf. Accessed December 15, 2009.

8. Centers for Disease Control and Prevention. About the National Health Interview Survey. Available at: http://www.cdc.gov/nchs/nhis/about_nhis.htm. Accessed December 15, 2009.

9. Burkett G. Status of health in Appalachia. In: Couto R, Simpson N, Harris G, eds. *Sowing Seeds in the Mountains: Community-Based Coalitions for Cancer Prevention and Control.* NIH Publication No. 94–3779 ed. Washington, DC: National Institutes of Health; 1994:62–80.

10. Thoenen E. *Health Risks: The Appalachian Lifestyle.* Charleston, WV: West Virginia Department of Health and Human Resources, Health Statistics Center; 1995.

11. Halverson JA, Ma L, Harner EJ. An analysis of disparities in health status

and access to health care in the Appalachian region. Washington, DC: Appalachian Regional Commission; 2004.

12. Zhang Z, Infante A, Meit M, English N, Dunn M, Bowers KH. An analysis of mental health and substance abuse disparities and access to treatment services in the Appalachian region. Washington, DC: Appalachian Regional Commission; 2008. Available at: http://www.arc.gov/assets/research_reports/AnalysisofMental HealthandSubstanceAbuseDisparities.pdf. Accessed December 15, 2009.

13. World Health Organization. Tobacco key facts. Available at: http://www .who.int/topics/tobacco/facts/en/index.html. Accessed December 28, 2009.

14. Macnee CL, McCabe S. The transtheoretical model of behavior change and smokers in southern Appalachia. *Nurs Res.* 2004;53:243–250.

15. Gross DA. The association of lung cancer mortality with income and education in Kentucky counties. Presentation to the University of Kentucky Center for Excellence in Rural Health. Available at: http://www.ruralhealthweb.org/index .cfm?objectid=6926E330–3048–651A-FE9E7C4519EF4612. Accessed October 16, 2009.

16. Wewers ME, Ahijevych KL, Chen MS, Dresbach S, Kihm KE, Kuun PA. Tobacco use characteristics among rural Ohio Appalachians. *J Community Health.* 2000;25:377–388.

17. Ahijevych K, Kuun P, Christman S, Wood T, Browning K, Wewers ME. Beliefs about tobacco among Appalachian current and former users. *Appl Nurs Res.* 2003;16:93–102.

18. Meyer MG, Toborg MA, Denham SA, Mande MJ. Cultural perspectives concerning adolescent use of tobacco and alcohol in the Appalachian mountain region. *J Rural Health.* 2008;24:67–74.

19. Prochaska JO, Velicer WF, DiClemente CC, Fava J. Measuring processes of change: applications to the cessation of smoking. *J Consult Clin Psychol.* 1988;56:520–528.

20. Smith GM. Personality and smoking: a review of the empirical literature. In: Hunt W, ed. *Learning Mechanisms in Smoking.* Piscataway, NJ: Aldine Transaction; 1970:42–61.

21. Munafo MR, Zetteler JI, Clark TG. Personality and smoking status: a meta-analysis. *Nicotine Tob Res.* 2007;9:405–413.

22. Lasser K, Boyd JW, Woolhandler S, Himmelstein DU, McCormick D, Bor DH. Smoking and mental illness: a population-based prevalence study. *JAMA.* 2000;284:2606–2610.

23. Song H, Fish M. Demographic and psychosocial characteristics of smokers and nonsmokers in low-socioeconomic status rural Appalachian 2-parent families in southern West Virginia. *J Rural Health.* 2006;22:83–87.

24. Cottrell L, Gibson M, Harris C, et al. Examining smoking and cessation during pregnancy among an Appalachian sample: a preliminary view. *Subst Abuse Treat Prev Policy.* 2007;2:14.

25. Bailey BA. Factors predicting pregnancy smoking in southern Appalachia. *Am J Health Behav.* 2006;30:413–421.

26. Flint AJ, Novotny TE. Poverty status and cigarette smoking prevalence and cessation in the United States, 1983–1993: the independent risk of being poor. *Tobacco Control.* 1997;6:14–18.

27. Anderson R, Oto-Kent D, Porter J, Brown K, Quirk L, Johnson S. Smoking habits and prevention strategies in low socio-economic status populations. West Sacramento, CA: Health Education Council; 2004. Available at: http://www.healthedcouncil.org/breakfreealliance/pdf/preres.pdf. Accessed October 16, 2009.

28. Centers for Disease Control and Prevention. Cigarette smoking among adults—United States, 2004. *MMWR Morb Mortal Wkly Rep.* 2004;54(44): 1121–1124.

29. World Health Organization. WHO report on the global tobacco epidemic, 2008—the MPOWER package. Available at: http://www.who.int/tobacco/mpower/en/index.html. Accessed December 28, 2009.

30. Jarvis MJ, Wardle J. Social patterning of individual health behaviors: the case of cigarette smoking. In: Marmot MG, Wilkinson RG, eds. *Social Determinants of Health.* New York, NY: Oxford University Press; 1999:224–236.

31. Denham SA, Meyer MG, Toborg MA. Tobacco cessation in adolescent females in Appalachian communities. *Fam Community Health.* 2004;27:170–181.

32. Doescher MP, Jackson JE, Jerant A, Hart GL. Prevalence and trends in smoking: a national rural study. *J Rural Health.* 2006;22:112–118.

33. McMillen R, Breen J, Cosby AG. Rural-urban differences in the social climate surrounding environmental tobacco smoke: a report from the 2002 social climate survey of tobacco control. *J Rural Health.* 2004;20:7–16.

34. Marshall CA. American Indian and Hispanic populations have cultural values and issues similar to those of Appalachian populations. *Prev Chronic Dis.* 2007;4:A77.

35. Anderson LM, Scrimshaw SC, Fullilove MT, Fielding JE, Task Force on Community Preventive Services. The community guide's model for linking the social environment to health. *Am J Prev Med.* 2003;24:12–20.

36. Warnecke RB, Oh A, Breen N, et al. Approaching health disparities from a population perspective: the National Institutes of Health Centers for Population Health and Health Disparities. *Am J Public Health.* 2008;98:1608–1615.

37. Behringer B, Friedell GH. Appalachia: where place matters in health. *Prev Chronic Dis.* 2006;3:A113.

38. Fagan P, King G, Lawrence D, et al. Eliminating tobacco-related health disparities: directions for future research. *Am J Public Health.* 2004;94:211–217.

39. Walls DS. Models of poverty and planned change: a framework for synthesis. *J Sociol Soc Welfare.* 1976;5(3):316–325.

40. Bradshaw T. Theories of poverty and anti-poverty programs in community development. Working Paper No. 06–05. Columbia, MO: RUPRI Rural Poverty

Research Center; 2006. Available at: http://www.rupri.org/Forms/WP06–05.pdf. Accessed December 28, 2009.

41. Macintyre S, Ellaway A, Cummins S. Place effects on health: how can we conceptualise, operationalise and measure them? *Soc Sci Med.* 2002;55:125–139.

42. Knight EA. Perceived control, coping style, and stress arousal in a job setting. In: Humphrey JH, ed. *Human Stress: Current Selected Research.* Vol. 2. New York, NY: AMS Press; 1987:55–72.

43. Pampel FC, Rogers RG. Socioeconomic status, smoking, and health: a test of competing theories of cumulative advantage. *J Health Soc Behav.* 2004;45:306–321.

44. World Health Organization. Ottawa charter for health promotion, 1986. Geneva, Switzerland: World Health Organization; 1986. Available at: http://www .who.int/hpr/NPH/docs/ottawa_charter_hp.pdf. Accessed December 28, 2009.

45. Troutman A. Establishing the center for health equity at a local health department. Presentation at the annual meeting of the American Public Health Association, Washington, DC, November 5, 2007.

46. Mittelmark MB. Promoting social responsibility for health: health impact assessment and healthy public policy at the community level. *Health Promot Int.* 2001;16:269–274.

4

Health Care Systems

Joel A. Halverson, Gilbert H. Friedell,
Eleanor Sue Cantrell, and Bruce A. Behringer

Scholars are engaged in active discussion about the underlying causes of poor health outcomes in the Appalachian region. One view is that cultural factors and traditions maintained over generations lead to unhealthy lifestyles and the inappropriate use or underuse of health services.[1] A different perspective points to a structural basis; that is, the roots of Appalachia's health problems lie in systemic characteristics, particularly those related to power and how—and by whom—decisions are made. At the same time, this view recognizes that population and social factors play a role.[2] Poverty, lack of jobs, illiteracy, inadequate education, poor housing, lack of public transportation, and lack of social support contribute to poor health in the region.[3]

The central thesis of this chapter, however, is that the underlying cause of poor health outcomes is the general absence of community-linked and community-responsive systems of health care across the region. This lack of engagement stems from systemic factors (e.g., service-driven reimbursement that results in no accountability for outcomes) and the difficulty of achieving direct community involvement in health issues, leading to significant health disparities in parts of Appalachia.

This chapter reviews health disparities in Appalachia and presents selected factors that affect health outcomes in the region. The discussion of these disparities centers on four key propositions: integration, collaboration, community action, and attention to local conditions. In support of these propositions, four case studies of health improvement efforts in the region are presented.

Health Disparities

The Appalachian region experiences excess mortality from major causes of death and illness when compared with the rest of the United States, making the residents of the Appalachian region a health disparity population.[4] Most disquieting is the high premature mortality in the 35 to 64 age group.[4] Central Appalachia, for example, has the highest rates of premature mortality from heart disease and cancers in the nation. There is no single explanation for the health disparities in Appalachia. They are likely the result of numerous variables intersecting in time and place, but four chief factors should be considered: availability, utilization, social distance, and lack of managed care.

Availability. One often-cited explanation is that the chronic economic distress pervading much of rural Appalachia has led to the lower availability of health services. A study authorized by the Appalachian Regional Commission[5] tested this hypothesis and found slow regional growth in the supply of physicians, a concentration of doctors in higher income areas, a low availability of dental and mental health care, many small hospitals struggling to stay open, and less access in rural areas to drug and alcohol treatment. Differential availability and access to medical resources likely contribute to regional heterogeneity in health outcomes. As recently as 2004, 318 of the 420 Appalachian counties (109 whole counties and 209 partial counties) were classified by the federal Health Resources and Services Administration as health professional shortage areas.[6] Medical care resources are unevenly distributed within Appalachia, and although there are primary care facilities throughout the region, the few major metropolitan areas contain the largest concentrations of medical care facilities. Pittsburgh, Pennsylvania, and Birmingham, Alabama, are the region's largest cities and have the greatest concentration of health care facilities in Appalachia. Large parts of the region have few major health care facilities, although a number of major metropolitan areas such as New York City; Atlanta, Georgia; Washington, D.C.; Cincinnati, Columbus, and Cleveland, Ohio; and Baltimore, Maryland, are on the periphery of Appalachia and may serve some health care needs in parts of the region. The degree to which out-of-region urban services reach into high-need rural Appalachian regions is unknown and probably not uniform. Although the importance of travel distance to medical care facilities in shaping health outcomes is not well understood, it is plausible that a lack of locally available medical care contributes to health disparities in the region.

Utilization. A second factor generally related to regional health disparities is the existence of many "upstream" population characteristics. For instance, Appalachia as a whole has lower disposable family incomes and educational achievement, two variables known to influence the use of services.[7, 8] Upstream factors impact health through a number of pathways. Over the course of life, all people experience some level of adversity, be it financial, personal, occupational, or medical. Populations in many parts of Appalachia are subject to repeated adverse life events involving some combination of these hardships. Adverse events typically trigger metabolic, hormonal, and physiological changes, as well as changes in behavior and attitudes. Repeated or multiple simultaneously occurring adverse events over the life course contribute to the risk of developing various chronic diseases via psychosocial and physiological pathways. For persons who experience repeated adverse life events, these experiences may be written into the physiology and pathology of their bodies.[9]

Figure 4.1 illustrates the interaction between people and communities and health services and systems. The large arrow in the middle of the figure represents individuals moving from a healthy state along a continuum toward a chronic disease state. Societal factors affecting the development and progression of chronic disease—the "underlying considerations"—are noted above the arrow, or "upstream." Interventions are noted below the arrow, or "downstream." These factors are listed separately, but in reality, they are interrelated. Prevention services may be available (as indicated below the arrow), but unless they are utilized, they will have no effect. For example, the immunization of children requires a connection between an available service and its utilization. The behavior of individuals and systems determines whether intervention services are utilized during the course of disease. In turn, the health behavior of individuals is influenced by community health attitudes. The education and literacy of residents influence the formation of community attitudes and may determine the occupations of community members. Conversely, social and environmental backgrounds, including occupation and employment, undoubtedly have a significant effect on community health attitudes and individual behavior.

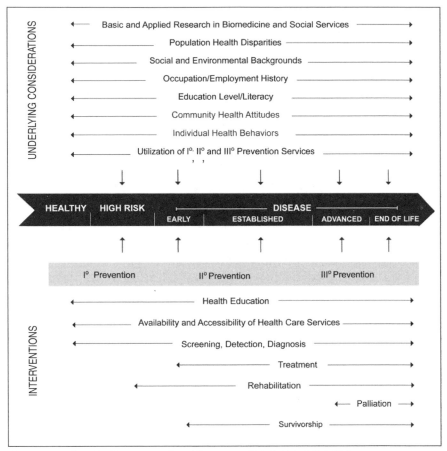

Figure 4.1. Chronic disease overview. (Courtesy of G. H. Friedell, MD.)

Utilization of downstream interventions depends in large measure on individual health behaviors conditioned by the upstream considerations noted. Figure 4.1 displays elements of clinical care as part of a continuum of optimal chronic disease care to achieve healthy outcomes. For individuals, moving through this continuum at an appropriate pace depends in part on community attitudes, perceptions and capabilities within the system, and the availability and utilization of community resources. Health care utilization is a function of many forces. The characteristics of individuals and their communities, as well as specific health services and systems factors, influence service delivery and use (see the explanation in figure 4.2 below). Simple availability of services does not equate to use, nor does the systematized organization and delivery of services ensure optimal utilization. Inequalities in availability, access, and quality of care or personal resources may lead to unequal care, unequal outcomes, and health disparities. In addition, because many health care providers working in Appalachia come from outside the region, their attitudes and expectations regarding health and their perceptions of unhealthy behaviors may present an upstream barrier to the provision of care.

Social Distance. A third factor related to regional health disparities is the social distance between some Appalachian populations and some health care providers. Educational and income differences are the most evident issues. Many mountain communities are served by health professionals from outside the region, often international medical school graduates. The use of medical terminology for those with limited health literacy is often cited as affecting communication, whether the providers are from Appalachia or from foreign countries. Providers' understanding and acceptance of local behaviors and preferences also affect the delivery and acceptance of health care. An important example is the effect of poor communication patterns on health care use and outcomes in the region.[10]

Although regional differences in health outcomes may reflect an underlying heterogeneity of local demographic, economic, infrastructural, and social factors, these disparities cannot be completely explained by the most often cited culprits: poverty, rurality, and lack of health insurance. Not all areas of the region with high poverty rates have comparably poor health outcomes.[4] Rural counties in Appalachia have generally poorer health outcomes compared with rural areas in some other parts of the country.[11]

Lack of Managed Care. The fourth factor is the low rate of managed care. The region retains a high reliance on standard indemnity insurance products. People usually contact the health system through primary care providers; others, due to the multiplicity of access barriers, are forced to use emergency care. In Appalachia, there are few examples of those primary care contacts taking place within vertically integrated systems that ensure the coordination found in other, often more urbanized, parts of the country. Managed care penetration rates are less than 15 percent in six

Southern Appalachian states. In four states—Maryland, New York, Pennsylvania, and Tennessee—the rates exceed 25 percent but are well below the national leaders in western states and Massachusetts.[12] The lack of managed care enrollment in Appalachia may be the product of fewer capital resources to finance plans, coupled with employer and consumer reluctance to utilize more restrictive insurance options. Low penetration rates for Medicare Part C plans result in less availability of the additional services that are now common among such plans.[13] Appalachians thus have fewer services such as disease management programs, lower community-wide adoption of care quality standards, an absence of care coordination, and few outreach and educational activities such as those included in managed care policies.

Addressing the Region's Health Disparities

Physical health can be seen as the result of the interaction of individual, extended family, and community action with available, accessible, and coordinated health care services and systems. In Appalachia, the relationship between personal and community economics and the region's health systems is often inconsistent. In some places, the lack of economic diversity makes it difficult to maintain locally resilient economies. This instability directly impacts the availability, economic viability, and continuity of regional health care services and the perceived investment opportunities they present. Lower per capita income means less money and greater personal economic concern about using disposable income for health services that are not covered by insurance. This is exacerbated by a reasonable mistrust of health systems that are characterized by uncoordinated services, duplication, and medical errors. Communities share stories of disconnected services that are often perceived as "high tech, low touch." Communication among health professionals, health systems, and patients and populations with low health literacy is inadequate.

Even when Appalachian patients and families are aware of and knowledgeable about healthy behaviors or appropriate uses of care, many encounter impediments when moving from knowledge to action. Risk factors are often the same for several of the leading causes of death. For instance, smoking, obesity, diet, and physical activity are influenced by one's environment and peers. Some Appalachians face the lack of risk reduction services, economic choices that require payment for such services, or the inability to successfully navigate the maze of services available for health improvement. These fundamental elements of a mature health system generally are not seen in the region or are found only in specific locales.

Addressing regional health disparities requires a complex task of assessment, definition, and intervention at both the community and health services levels. Effective resolution of the health disparities in Appalachia should be based on four propositions related to integration, collaboration, community action, and attention to local conditions.

Integration. There should be no division between local communities and health services and systems. Context is everything, particularly in Appalachia. Figure 4.2 presents a vision based on a health system model[14] in which structural relationships are constantly interacting with local behaviors and preferences to produce regional health outcomes. Currently, regional health disparities seem to be the outcome. Blaming Appalachians collectively for these disparities, or viewing them as victims, does not help identify effective ways to integrate socioeconomic conditions and local factors into a health system that is alert to individual health awareness, beliefs, and behaviors.

Collaboration. Some deeply rooted upstream socioeconomic factors persist and have a significant impact on the effective provision of health services and on downstream outcomes. Typically, outcomes have been

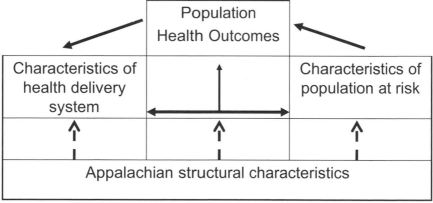

Figure 4.2. Appalachian health outcomes are the products of multiple factors. *Source:* Adapted with permission from Figure 1: Framework for the study of access to medical care. In: Lu Ann Aday and Ronald Anderson. *Development of Indices of Access to Medical Care.* Chicago, IL: Health Administration Press; 1975:7.

categorically measured to gauge progress (e.g., declines in infant mortality, cancer incidence and mortality, substance abuse overdoses and deaths), but a parallel assessment of upstream factors related to availability, accessibility, and utilization of patient care services is less frequent or comprehensive. As poor outcomes persist, a second proposition emerges: measures to assess upstream structural issues should be in the purview of communities but should be addressed by both communities and their health systems. In advancing this second proposition, it is important to ask a question: is it necessary to deal with all the upstream factors first, before addressing the health issues at the local or community level.[a] Although it would be highly desirable to do so, waiting is untenable when the need to improve the health of Appalachian communities is so great. The recipe for success lies in community engagement in defining a "healthy community" and determining the level of health care availability and quality desired. All relevant sectors of the community—including schools, businesses, civic organizations, religious communities, governmental entities, health professionals, and the media—should be engaged in assessing health interactions and community health outcomes. Health is understood differently when it is viewed as a community issue rather than a personal issue. Interactions and outcomes are impacted by quality education, a healthy workforce, economic vitality, and quality of life. The ability to afford, access, and retain vital health services for all citizens must be seen as a community goal and a shared responsibility. To the extent that certain upstream factors are barriers to accomplishing desired health ends, the local community has to deal with them. The will of an organized community can overcome many, if not all, such obstacles.

Community Action. The third proposition is that substantial health improvement is more likely not only when communities play an active role in defining health, but also when they involve residents and health care providers in community-wide initiatives that support changes in service delivery and individual health improvement. When communities are engaged in broad-based health improvement, they draw strength from community assent and personal involvement. Health services are more likely to accommodate change and play an active role when community-wide concern is evident. There are many examples of rural Appalachian communities becoming part of the solution for a broad variety of health problems.[15–17]

Awareness of Local Conditions. The fourth proposition is that Appalachia is not really a homogeneous region, although it is often characterized as one. Recent publications have pointed out variations among Appalachian subregions in demographic characteristics,[18] health risks and outcomes,[4] and cancer incidence and mortality rates,[19] including those for coal mining counties.[20] There is often sufficient variation between contiguous counties that one could argue for the existence of many different Appalachias. When viewed from a regional standpoint, descriptive characteristics commonly associated with parts of Appalachia, such as rurality, economic distress, and medical underservice, are accurate.[21] Although it is reasonable and necessary to have a common framework for addressing Appalachian health problems, the heterogeneity among Appalachian subpopulations indicates that flexibility is essential as local areas and communities adapt proposed solutions to fit community needs. Community-based participatory research is one effective means for communities to build on their local assets to link individuals, communities, and health services and systems to address local health disparities.

Model Cases for Reducing Health Risks and Improving Outcomes

Community involvement in assessing, planning, and reorganizing the provision of health care in Appalachia is illustrated in the following case studies. Each case demonstrates how elements of the four propositions enumerated earlier successfully redefine the relationship between the community and the health system and change upstream and downstream factors to address health disparity issues.

The Kentucky Cancer Program and Related Efforts. The Kentucky Cancer Program (KCP) comprises a statewide outreach program and a branch of the Cancer Information Service of the National Cancer Institute (NCI), as well as the Kentucky Cancer Registry.[22] Begun in 1984 as part of a statewide cancer control program, the registry achieved complete coverage of new cases in 1995 and became part of the NCI Surveillance, Epidemiology, and End Results (SEER) Program in 2000. With the development of the registry, it is now possible to accurately assess the incidence of cancer and changes in its incidence at any point in the past twenty years in different areas of the state. This includes Appalachian Kentucky, a fifty-four-county area in the southeastern part of the state with a rural, low-income, 98 percent white population of 1.1 million people.

According to Kentucky Cancer Registry data, the incidence of fatal lung cancer cases among Appalachian and non-Appalachian men in eastern Kentucky decreased between 1995–1999 and 2000–2006, but the rates remain some of the highest in the country. In contrast, there was a significant increase in the incidence of lung cancer among both Appalachian and non-Appalachian women. In a related manner, the rate of cigarette smoking has fallen in recent years among both Appalachian and non-Appalachian men, with no comparable drop among Kentucky women. The ongoing focus is on primary prevention (cigarette smoking cessation and prevention) in an effort to encourage individuals to modify their behavior. This has been difficult to get across to young people—the most important target population—when smoking is prevalent in their communities among parents, friends, teachers, and coaches. However, the city councils of three small eastern Kentucky cities, each a county seat (London, Campbellsville, and Prestonsburg), voted to make public places smoke free to improve the health of the community, despite protests from those who feared a loss of business if patrons could not smoke on the premises. This provides clear evidence of community support for smoking prevention and cessation (i.e., individual behavior change).

The KCP's outreach services include a fifteen- to twenty-member District Cancer Council (DCC) in each of the fifteen multicounty Area Development Districts in the state. At least once a year, each DCC reports cancer incidence and mortality data to the Kentucky Cancer Registry. Issues of particular importance to the residents of each area are emphasized, and the KCP cancer control specialist who staffs the DCC for each region facilitates the community's response to such concerns. Follow-up community activities of KCP regional coordinators have played major roles in efforts to reduce cervical and breast cancer. The incidence and mortality rates for both cervical cancer and invasive breast cancer dropped for Appalachian and non-Appalachian women in eastern Kentucky between 1995–1999 and 2001–2005. The quality of care for women with breast cancer appears to be equally good in Appalachian and non-Appalachian Kentucky, but the fact that the mortality rate in eastern Kentucky remains relatively high in spite of a lower incidence indicates that improving survival is most likely hindered by low levels of screening and early diagnosis.

In addition to the KCP's efforts, the state legislature has supported cervical and breast cancer screening, the Centers for Disease Control and Prevention and the NCI have supplied funding, and the Kentucky Department for Public Health provides services through local health departments in each county. These and other cancer control efforts have all contributed to increased screening, effective treatment of identified precancerous cervical lesions, the treatment of more breast cancer cases, and the consequent reduction in cervical cancer incidence and mortality in Appalachian Kentucky. Special efforts, such as the work of the NCI's Appalachia Leadership Initiative on Cancer to foster the development of community cancer coalitions (twenty-four in eastern Kentucky between 1991 and 1997), have heightened community awareness of cervical and breast cancer—the first step in increasing screening for these diseases. However, one major barrier may be low levels of educational attainment in this population, which may be correlated with low rates of screening. In addition, the availability and accessibility of screening services are continuing problems, especially in rural areas in the state. These problems have been compounded by the distance and travel times to screening and other facilities. As a consequence, even when services are available and accessible, they are not as well utilized as they could be.

In spite of these hindrances, screening for cervical and breast cancers has increased over the years. As a result, cancers are identified earlier and in more treatable stages, which is partly responsible for the drop in mortality. The number and quality of treatment centers in Appalachian Kentucky have also improved, especially in the field of radiation oncology. One example of improved breast cancer management is the approach of physicians and administrators at the 350-bed King's Daughters Hospital in Ashland, Kentucky. All patients with breast cancer who are seen by staff physicians are evaluated by a panel of surgeons, radiotherapists, medical oncologists, radiologists (who share mammograms and other reports), and pathologists (who discuss the pathological findings in available biopsies) before definitive treatment begins. The head nurse on the oncology service and the cancer registrar are also present at this evaluation, and the panel's conclusions are made available to the primary physician.

Improving Health Care in Hancock County, Tennessee. The 1990 census cited Hancock County, Tennessee, as the poorest county in the state and among the ten poorest counties in the nation. It had high unemployment, a per capita income less than half the national average, and one of the lowest educational attainment levels in the state. Jobs were limited to public employment, farming, and small manufacturing. Although county residents had a history of low teenage pregnancy and infant mortality rates, the overall mortality rates from chronic illnesses such as heart disease were high then and remain significantly high today.[23] More than two-thirds of all children were uninsured or were covered through TennCare, Tennessee's Medicaid program. The Hancock County Hospital closed in 1992, leaving the county with only one full-time and one part-time general-practice physician, an active volunteer rescue squad, and a small health department. As part of the Empowerment Zone initiative of the 1990s, Hancock County conducted a series of public meetings that resulted in the development of a long-term strategic plan. Key health issues were identified, and gaps in health care services were documented. Foremost among these issues was the absence of fundamental preventive services and primary care for children and the concomitant low utilization of such services.[b]

The strategic plan called for a partnership among multiple county agencies and external organizations to garner resources to address health issues. Consequently, a regional community health center system opened an office in the county to improve access to primary care, the county's emergency medical services participated in a federal demonstration project to test a telecommunications link between the rural community and a regional tertiary care center, and the Hancock County Health Council was formed through the Tennessee Department of Health, assuring a continuous assessment of county health needs and communication within the county and with external partners.

Moreover, a rural health outreach grant was awarded to the East Tennessee State University (ETSU) College of Nursing (located eighty-five miles away), the regional community health center, and the county health department. These organizations performed physical examinations for the public and obtained baseline data on the health of the county's children. These examinations identified multiple issues, particularly childhood risks for long-term chronic illnesses.

Based on these data, the first high school–based health clinic in the state was funded in 1995 by a federal Healthy Schools, Healthy Communities grant. Nurse practitioners from ETSU and local staff began delivering health services in the Hancock County schools, including primary care and prevention services, health education, individual and group student counseling, and classroom instruction. A behavioral health specialist addressed long-term child and family issues. Clinic personnel became child health advocates, working with parents, changing students' awareness of health issues, and seeking pediatric and adolescent care and support services from in- and out-of-county providers.

Thanks to a high degree of collaboration among multiple partners, a new critical access hospital opened in 2006. Local leaders used the Empowerment Zone's strategic plan to promote an understanding of the county's health needs assessment and to engender support for a plan to finance the new medical facility. County leaders invited regional health and hospital systems to explore ownership and management options for the hospital. One system was selected, and county health care providers negotiated with the hospital to ensure internal support for key health services and cooperation in addressing health status issues. The facility now provides emergency services for pediatric patients and serves as the keystone for a more integrated health system that is accessible to all, regardless of the ability to pay.

Hancock County provides an example of the level of community commitment and vision needed to improve health services, form a cohesive health system, and use partnerships to address local health issues. The continuum of care now available to the county's 1,700 children is exemplary. Primary prevention activities have become part of the Tennessee Coordinated School Health Program. Primary care is now supported through a school-based health clinic administered by the ETSU College of Nursing and a regional community health center, both funded by the Health Resources and Services Administration. Secondary and emergency care has been reestablished in the county. Specialty care and tertiary hospital services are assured by clinical arrangements developed through the new county hospital managed by Wellmont Health System. The school-based health clinic has reported some evidence of health status improvements among children, particularly in terms of childhood obesity and the early identification of potentially disabling conditions. High quality standards are in place for the delivery of care, and through the auspices of the County Health Council, organizational relationships and community involvement intended to improve the health of the county's children are maintained.

Combating Obesity and Cardiovascular Risks in West Virginia. West Virginia, the only state completely within the Appalachian region, has persistently had adverse outcomes from cardiovascular disease. In addition, West Virginians are among the most obese people in the nation. More than 60 percent of adults are overweight, and 30 percent are obese; the state ranks second in childhood obesity, with 20.9 percent of children aged 10 to 17 being overweight or obese. The Coronary Artery Risk Detection in Appalachian Communities (CARDIAC) project was started as a school-based public health risk factor screening program in 1998 through collaborative efforts by West Virginia University and Alderson-Broaddus College.[24] Initiated as an individualized, population-based strategy to address the high morbidity and mortality from heart disease in West Virginia, its mission has expanded to include all chronic illnesses associated with obesity, such as diabetes and, more recently, asthma.

Three key stakeholder groups were identified at the beginning of CARDIAC: individuals, schools and surrounding communities, and policy makers and legislators. The CARDIAC program has identified numerous children at risk of obesity and has helped develop a number of school-based interventions to teach children about nutrition, physical activity, and tobacco avoidance.

Since its inception, CARDIAC has grown from a small pilot project in three rural West Virginia counties to a multidimensional effort involving all fifty-five counties in the state, with voluntary participation open to all fifth graders in West Virginia. The screening consists of a short family history of premature coronary artery disease and diabetes, as well as symptoms of and treatment for asthma. Body mass index (BMI) is calculated, blood pressure is measured, and a fasting lipid profile is obtained.

One of the benefits of CARDIAC extends from its relationship to the Rural Health Education Partnership (RHEP), a component of an association between West Virginia's institutions of higher education and its rural communities. RHEP enables health science students from the state's three medical schools and nursing students from participating colleges to complete required rotations in local rural communities. These students participate in CARDIAC and learn disease prevention and health promotion techniques under the supervision of field faculty, school health nurses, and CARDIAC staff.

A community-based program aided by information derived from CARDIAC is Camp NEW You (NEW stands for nutrition, exercise, and weight management). This is a two-week summer residential program with yearlong follow-up for at-risk 11- to 14-year olds who are above the 85th percentile in BMI and are referred by their primary care providers. The first camp was held in 2008 on the campus of West Virginia University. The program expanded to Marshall University and may eventually extend to smaller colleges in the state.

Documenting the health status of West Virginia youth through the CARDIAC project was instrumental in passage of the Healthy Lifestyle Act of 2005 (HB 2816). This initiative formalized and expanded CARDIAC's BMI screening in schools, required increased physical education in elementary and middle schools, and mandated modest improvements in the school nutrition program.

Tackling a Growing Substance Abuse Problem in the Region. A study conducted by the Substance Abuse and Mental Health Services Administration mapped the use of nonmedical pain relievers by substate regions, and Appalachian counties frequently appeared in the regions of highest use.[25] Some states (Virginia, West Virginia, North Carolina) have published reports that included maps of overdose fatalities, showing a clear pattern: the highest mortality rates occurred in contiguous counties that form the Central Appalachian region. A report to the Appalachian Regional Commission indicated that, compared with national rates, Appalachia has higher rates of hospital discharge from co-occurring mental health and substance abuse diagnoses and higher admission rates for opiates and synthetics.[26] The study also found a high and growing use of heroin, opiates, and synthetics in coal-producing counties in the region.

Past experience in Appalachia involving the abuse of alcohol and codeine-containing analgesics did not prepare providers, individuals, mental health and substance abuse counselors, law enforcement, or the court system to deal with the abuse of highly addictive semisynthetic opiate prescription drugs. In fact, most of the agencies and professionals countering substance abuse did not perceive this new wave of drug abusers as being significantly different from the occasional abuser of the past. However, two different professionals in southwestern Virginia saw the nature of this new problem and its local effects from two entirely different perspectives.

The first individual, a primary care physician in a rural coal mining community, made several observations. First, he was seeing more substance abusing patients who were quickly becoming addicted and rapidly escalating their doses and methods of administration to achieve the maximal effect of the drug. Second, several patients presented with unusual skin lesions and multinodular infiltrates on chest X-rays. These were later determined to be related to immunological reactions to excipients in the tablets, which were crushed and then injected into the skin (accounting for the skin lesions) or directly into a vein (and deposited in the lungs). Ultimately, the physician enlisted others in the local health care system to help him conduct a "town hall" meeting. Approximately 700 individuals from the community attended, including those who had been directly affected by substance abuse. They identified the problem and began to formulate a response. As a result of this community effort, led in large part by one physician, more treatment options, Alcoholics Anonymous and Narcotics Anonymous groups, and even a residential treatment facility were developed over the next ten years.

The second individual, an attorney, recognized an increase in crime related to drug use. After practicing law for several years and acquiring a sense of the court system's caseload, he was struck by the increase in the absolute number and percentage of cases that were drug related, either directly or indirectly. He researched prior years' statistics for his own and several surrounding counties and observed that certain crimes were increasing, especially larceny and breaking and entering. Further research showed that the increase in crime paralleled the increase in prescription drug abuse. With the help of fellow attorneys, the court system, judges, and treatment and recovery professionals, a drug court was established, and more options for treatment in lieu of incarceration were made available.

In both instances, a tipping point was reached when an observant health or legal professional recognized a problem and was appropriately positioned to take the message to his respective health care system and community. Struggling with soaring foster care cases as more children were removed from homes with addicted parents, rising crime rates, and other social ills accompanying a burgeoning substance abuse problem, communities were eager to redefine substance abuse services and their position in the health care system through a dialogue to address the issue. Several years have passed, and the abuse of prescription drugs persists in these areas, but there are now more resources and treatment options available within the area, including more targeted, evidence-based prevention programs and recovery support.

Further Research

A number of research questions evolve from the ideas presented in this chapter, and answering them will increase our understanding of the region's health issues and aid in developing projects and plans to improve the health care system's capacity, functioning, and utilization.

Given the sparse distribution of medical care resources in Appalachia, what impact does travel distance to medical care facilities have on overall population health? Although some logical assumptions can be made regarding health care access and outcomes, it is not clear how or to what extent the distribution of medical care facilities influences health outcomes. A related and perhaps more critical question is, how does travel distance to medical care facilities influence attitudes about health care and careseeking behavior?

Given the generally poor economic conditions in parts of the region and a lack of infrastructure that contributes to upstream health factors, how do contextual factors interplay with the health care system? It is critical to identify contextual barriers to health improvement and ways to circumvent these barriers so that progress toward integrated health systems can be achieved.

Given the significant heterogeneity in both contextual circumstances and health status in different parts of Appalachia, what are the distinguishing characteristics of areas with favorable outcomes as opposed to those with less favorable outcomes? Clearly, there is an opportunity to learn lessons from communities that are relatively health prosperous and share that insight with communities that are less so.

Policy Recommendations

The ideas presented in this chapter lead to a number of policy suggestions. For instance, one of the key issues in Appalachia is the local recognition of health problems. In many cases, local populations may be unaware of their health status and health risks relative to other parts of the region and the country, but intuitively, they acknowledge poor health outcomes. Therefore, state and local officials should be urged to share and highlight health outcome deficiencies among local, regional, and national populations. From a health disparity standpoint, only when health problems are identified can they be effectively addressed. Although communities are often able (and best suited) to identify local health issues, regional and national statistics allow local community health issues to be related to broader regional and national health outcomes; they can also serve as a tool to muster support for health improvement efforts. Health policy at the state and national levels is greatly influenced by broad-scale health outcome measures, as opposed to locally defined health issues. It is critical that intersecting broad-scale and local health issues be articulated to local populations by local officials and community groups. In this way, local realities that affect health behavior and define pathways by which local health care systems are accessed can be addressed most effectively. In addition, national and state health policy to address health disparities must be flexible enough to account for diversity and differences among local and regional populations.

Policies to address identified gaps in local health outcomes need to focus on primary prevention in addition to secondary and tertiary clinical care. All too often, the health care system responds to financial incentives that emphasize emergent needs, with less attention to alleviating barriers to access that force residents to use health care as a last resort. The failure to address primary prevention, or the lack of a system of health care in Appalachia to do so, may largely explain the persistent adverse health outcomes in the region. The systemization of health care in the region should include a continuum of health services, from primary prevention to tertiary care, that eliminates gaps in health services and promotes a progression of care through all service domains.

Notes

a. *Community* is defined as a population within a geographic boundary. In urban areas, community is readily defined as the population in that city or town.

In contrast, in rural Appalachia, community is generally thought of as the population within county boundaries. However, within a county, there is a county seat community and perhaps other small towns with their own communities.

b. School-age children represent 25 percent of Hancock County's population of 7,000.[27]

References

1. Coyne CA, Demian-Popescu C, Friend D. Social and cultural factors influencing health in southern West Virginia: a qualitative study. *Prev Chronic Dis.* 2006;3:A124.

2. Eller RD. *Uneven Ground: Appalachia since 1945.* Lexington, KY: University Press of Kentucky; 2008.

3. Braveman P, Egerter S. Overcoming obstacles to health. Princeton, NJ: Robert Wood Johnson Foundation; 2008.

4. Halverson JA, Ma L, Harner EJ. An analysis of disparities in health status and access to health care in the Appalachian region. Washington, DC: Appalachian Regional Commission; 2004.

5. Stensland J, Mueller C, Sutton J. An analysis of the financial conditions of health care institutions in the Appalachian region and their economic impacts. Washington, DC: Appalachian Regional Commission; 2002. Available at: http://www.arc.gov/researchreports.asp?F_CATEGORY=13. Accessed March 5, 2007.

6. Bureau of Health Professions. Area resource file (ARF). Rockville, MD: U.S. Department of Health and Human Services, Health Resources and Services Administration, Bureau of Health Professions; 2005.

7. Culter D, Lleras-Muney A. Education and health: evaluating theories and evidence. Working Paper 12352. Cambridge, MA: National Bureau of Economic Research; June 2006. Available at: http://www.nber.org/papers/w12352/. Accessed March 5, 2007.

8. Flores G, Bauchner H, Feinstein AR, Nguyen US. The impact of ethnicity, family income, and parental education on children's health and use of health services. *Am J Public Health.* 1999;89:1066–1071.

9. Brunner E, Marmot M. Social organization, stress, and health. In: Marmot M, Wilkinson RG, eds. *Social Determinants of Health.* Oxford, UK: Oxford University Press; 1999.

10. Hutson SP, Dorgan KA, Phillips AN, Behringer B. The mountains hold things in: the use of community research review work groups to address cancer disparities in Appalachia. *Oncol Nurs Forum.* 2007;34:1133–1139.

11. Halverson J, Hendryx M. A rural socioeconomic risk and resiliency inventory and associated health outcomes. Morgantown, WV: West Virginia Rural Health Research Center; 2009.

12. Kaiser Family Foundation State Health Facts. Distribution of the non-elderly

uninsured by age, states (2006–2007), U.S. (2007). Available at: http://www.statehealthfacts.org/index.jsp. Accessed March 25, 2009.

13. Centers for Medicare and Medicaid Services. Medicare Advantage (Part C). Available at: http://www.medicare.gov/navigation/medicare-basics/medicare-benefits/part-c.aspx. Accessed February 18, 2011.

14. Aday LM, Anderson R. *Development of Indices of Access to Medical Care.* Ann Arbor, MI: Health Administration Press; 1975.

15. Rice TJ, Bernstein SB. The process of community intervention in an isolated Appalachian mountain hollow. *Med Care.* 1971;9:365–371.

16. Stewart GW. Social and cultural perspectives: community intervention and mental health. *Health Educ Quart.* 1993;20(Suppl 1):S99–S111.

17. Liburd LC, Giles HW, Mensah GA. Looking through a glass, darkly: eliminating health disparities. *Prev Chronic Dis.* 2006;3:A72.

18. Hopenhayn C, Bush H, Christian A, Shelton BJ. Comparative analysis of invasive cervical cancer incidence rates in three Appalachian states. *Prev Med.* 2005;41:859–864.

19. Wingo PA, Tucker TC, Jamison PM, et al. Cancer in Appalachia, 2001–2003. *Cancer.* 2008;112:181–192.

20. Hendryx M, Ahern MM. Relations between health indicators and residential proximity to coal mining in West Virginia. *Am J Public Health.* 2008;98:669–671.

21. Appalachian Regional Commission. ARC-designated distressed counties, fiscal year 2009. Available at: http://www.arc.gov/index.do?nodeId=3301. Accessed March 25, 2009.

22. University of Louisville. Kentucky Cancer Program. Available at: http://kycancerprogram.org/. Accessed May 25, 2011.

23. Tennessee Institute of Public Health. County profile health rankings, 2007. Available at: http://state.tn.us/tniph/countyprofiles.html. Accessed April 2, 2009.

24. West Virginia University, Department of Pediatrics. Coronary artery risk detection in Appalachian communities. Available at: http://cardiacwv.org/index.php. Accessed May 25, 2011.

25. Office of Applied Studies. The NSDUH report: nonmedical use of pain relievers in substate regions: 2004 to 2006. Rockville, MD: Substance Abuse and Mental Health Services Administration; June 19, 2008.

26. Zhang Z, Infante A, Meit M, English N, Dunn M, Bowers KH. An analysis of mental health and substance abuse disparities and access to treatment services in the Appalachian region. Washington, DC: Appalachian Regional Commission; 2008. Available at: http://www.arc.gov/assets/research_reports/AnalysisofMentalHealthandSubstanceAbuseDisparities.pdf. Accessed March 25, 2009.

27. U.S. Bureau of Census. Hancock County, Tennessee. Available at: http://factfinder.census.gov/servlet/acssafacts?_submenued=factsheet_o_sse=on. Accessed April 2, 2009.

Part II

Appalachian Health Status

This part discusses the nature, prevalence, interconnections, and implications of various health conditions in the region. The issue of health disparities both in the region as a whole and in the states with Appalachian counties underlies the following chapters. Although it is not known precisely why these disparities exist, the data clearly indicate that Appalachians are disproportionately affected by cardiovascular disease, diabetes, specific cancers, and obesity. Other less obvious but equally serious health concerns involve kidney disease, traumatic injuries, mental and oral health, and substance abuse.

These chapters go beyond documenting Appalachian health inequalities; they examine some of the more effective programs for dealing with them. Case studies highlight the key role of local communities in defining needs and promoting health care services. Each chapter also indicates where data crucial for program design and implementation are missing and how they might be obtained.

5

The Heart of Appalachia

Ann L. McCracken and E. Kelly Firesheets

Heart disease,[a] the leading cause of death of both men and women in the United States, costs an estimated $475 billion for health care services, medications, and lost productivity in 2009.[1] Among adults over 20 years of age, some 80 million Americans, or 38 percent of men and 34 percent of women, are currently living with one or more types of cardiovascular disease. This form of heart disease affects the heart itself or the blood vessel system, especially the veins and arteries leading to and from the heart. Nationally, more than 830,000 people die of cardiovascular-related conditions every year.[2]

Rates of heart disease are not equally distributed across the U.S. population. According to reports from the Centers for Disease Control and Prevention (CDC),[3] some of the highest rates of heart disease are in Appalachian areas, including southern Ohio, West Virginia, and eastern Kentucky. In 2008, 8.1 percent of West Virginians reported that they had been diagnosed with angina or coronary heart disease—the highest percentage in the country and nearly twice the national average of 4.3 percent.[4] Four of the five states with the highest heart disease death rates (West Virginia, Pennsylvania, Mississippi, and Alabama) contain Appalachian counties (only Oklahoma, which ranks second, does not).[5] Nearly 15 percent of hospitalizations in the 406 Appalachian-designated counties in 2000 were due to heart disease, exceeding hospitalizations due to chronic obstructive pulmonary disorders, all cancers, stroke, and diabetes combined. Eastern Kentucky, southern West Virginia, and western Virginia have particularly high rates of hospitalization for heart disease.[6]

Barnett and coauthors[7] point out that disease incidence is influenced by social, economic, behavioral, psychological, and physiological risk factors, while disease mortality is affected by the speed of diagnosis and the efficacy of medical care. Death certificate data from 1990 to 1997 reveal that heart disease was the leading cause of death among elderly men and women in Appalachia. Elderly white men living in Appalachia had higher death rates than those who lived outside the region.[6] These data are not surprising, given that heart disease is generally considered a disease of the elderly; more than 83 percent of people who die of coronary artery disease are aged 65 or older.[8, 9] However, young Appalachians are not immune to heart problems. In fact, nearly a third of hospitalizations for heart disease in Appalachia were for individuals between 35 and 64 years of age.[6]

These statistics have led many to believe that the risk factors for heart disease may be more prevalent among Appalachians than non-Appalachians. This chapter explores that proposition by presenting the known risk factors for heart disease and reviewing national and regional data on their prevalence among Appalachians. Additional evidence regarding the prevalence and relative effect of various risk factors is provided through a case study analysis of heart disease among Appalachians in the Greater Cincinnati metropolitan area. The chapter ends with research and policy recommendations that address the prevalence of heart disease among Appalachians.

Risk Factors for Heart Disease

To improve the heart health of individuals in Appalachia, it is important to understand the risk factors influencing their long-term health. Some of these factors, such as age, sex, and heredity, cannot be changed, while others can be manipulated. For example, in a case-controlled study of fifty-two countries, nine risk factors subject to change accounted for greater than 90 percent of the likelihood of having an initial acute heart attack. These factors are cigarette smoking, abnormal blood lipid levels, hypertension, diabetes, abdominal obesity, lack of physical exercise, low daily fruit and vegetable consumption, alcohol overconsumption, and low scores on a psychosocial index that included depression, locus of control, perceived stress, and life events.[10] Risk factors can be grouped using a variety of other frameworks as well. Practitioners and health researchers have identified health, lifestyle, and behavioral factors that increase the risk of developing

Table 5.1. Risk Factors for Heart Disease

Health Factors	Behavioral Factors	Contextual Factors
High cholesterol	Smoking	Poverty
High blood pressure	Overweight (body mass index > 25)	Geography
Diabetes	Physical inactivity Alcohol use Stress	Medical resources

heart disease.[11] Others examining the relationships between socioeconomic status and health outcomes group risk factors in two categories—compositional and contextual. Compositional factors focus on the individual, such as health, lifestyle, and behavior, whereas contextual factors are shared by all individuals in a similar environment.[6] Both types are relevant in Appalachia; however, contextual factors such as geography and poverty may be particularly salient for people living in some areas. For purposes of this discussion, the risk factors for heart disease are categorized as health factors, behavioral factors,[b] and contextual factors[c] (table 5.1).

Health Factors

High Cholesterol. Individuals with high total cholesterol levels are at greater risk of developing heart disease. Blood cholesterol at or below 200 mg/dL is considered desirable, whereas a level at or above 240 mg/dL doubles the risk of heart disease.[12] A health needs assessment of seven Appalachian counties undertaken by the Appalachian Rural Health Institute[13] determined that the prevalence of high cholesterol in these Appalachian counties was 37.6 percent, slightly higher than the national rate of 35.6 percent. Other studies confirm elevated rates of high cholesterol among Appalachians.[14, 15] The percentage of people who have high cholesterol levels has been increasing. From 1995 to 2007, nine of the thirteen states with Appalachian counties experienced gains greater than the national average gain of 9.5 percent. In North Carolina and Georgia, high cholesterol rates increased more than 15 percent. West Virginia had the highest percentage of people with high cholesterol (42.2 percent).[4]

Typically, high cholesterol is associated with older age. However, in a study of 1,338 fifth-grade students in fourteen West Virginia counties, overweight children had a 2.4 times greater risk of having high total lipids and a 5.3 times greater risk of having low levels of high-density lipoprotein (HDL)—or "good" cholesterol—than children at healthy body weights.[16] These data suggest that early intervention targeting children may be needed to lower rates of high cholesterol and, in turn, heart disease in the region.

High Blood Pressure. Hypertension, or high blood pressure, is a major risk factor for heart disease and other serious medical conditions.[17] Health data indicate that hypertension is prevalent among Appalachian populations.[18] According to a CDC report, the Appalachian region has the highest hospitalization rates for hypertension (between 782 and 955 per 100,000 people).[19]

Between 1997 and 2007, the number of persons diagnosed with hypertension rose faster in eight of the thirteen Appalachian states than in the rest of the nation, which had a 5.6 percent increase. Georgia had the greatest increase, from 19.7 percent in 1997 to 30.4 percent in 2007. Approximately 33 percent of residents in Tennessee, West Virginia, and Alabama had been diagnosed with hypertension in 2007, compared with about 28 percent in 1997.[4]

Diabetes. In addition to the physical problems generally associated with diabetes (hypoglycemia, ketoacidosis, and renal problems), individuals with type 1 and type 2 diabetes are at increased risk of developing heart disease.[20] While an estimated 8.3 percent of American adults have diabetes,[21] rates are much higher in Appalachia. For example, eight of the ten states with the highest rates of diabetes are Appalachian states, and West Virginia has the overall highest rate of diabetes in the United States (11.9 percent).[4]

Behavioral Factors

Tobacco Use. In 1997, 97 percent of the total U.S. burley tobacco production occurred in Appalachian states.[22] It is well known that smoking is one of the leading contributors to heart disease.[23] According to information from the Ohio Tobacco Prevention Foundation,[24] over 32 percent of adults in Appalachian Ohio use cigarettes, and 6.6 percent of Appalachian adults use some form of smokeless tobacco. In 1995 the West Virginia Department of Health and Human Resources found that the rate of adult smokers in 399 Appalachian counties was 24.2 percent—significantly higher than the 21.9 percent rate in the rest of the country.[25] Although the national rate decreased to 18.3 percent in 2008, two of the three states with the highest smoking rates were in Appalachia: West Virginia (26.5 percent) and Kentucky (25.2 percent).[4]

There are geographic and racial differences in smoking rates within Appalachia. Smoking rates among whites are highest in eastern Kentucky and central and southern West Virginia (25.4 to 36.6 percent). Rates among blacks are higher in Northern Appalachia (29.9 to 37.6 percent) than in Southern Appalachia (11.3 to 28.4 percent).[6]

Obesity and Overweight. Obesity is becoming a health issue across the United States and is related to heart problems in Appalachia. The three states with the highest obesity rates in Appalachian Mississippi (33.4 percent), Alabama (32.2 percent), and West Virginia (31.9 percent).[4] West Virginia (68.8 percent), Tennessee (68.0 percent), and Alabama (67.9 percent) have the highest rates of overweight and obese persons in the United States.[4] Among whites, the highest rates of obesity are found in northern Pennsylvania, southern New York, central West Virginia, and eastern Kentucky Appalachian counties.[6]

Physical Inactivity. Physical activity increases endurance, builds muscular strength, and helps control blood lipid abnormalities, diabetes, and obesity—all risk factors for heart disease.[26] In addition, exercising and modifying other unhealthy behaviors after having a heart attack results in a better quality of life and slightly increased survival rates.[27]

Nationally, approximately 35 percent of mortality from coronary artery disease is attributable to physical inactivity.[6] Three Appalachian states—Mississippi, West Virginia, and Kentucky—are among the top five states most likely to have residents who do not participate in physical activities.[4] Research suggests that persons who either live in rural areas or have lower incomes are less likely to meet physical activity recommendations.[28] Both these factors are likely to affect Appalachian heart health.[29]

Alcohol Use. When consumed in moderation, alcohol is beneficial for heart health.[30, 31] Moderate alcohol consumption (one to two drinks per day for men; one drink per day for women) can raise HDL (good) cholesterol; however, heavy drinking (in excess of these amounts) can raise the level of triglycerides in the blood and lead to high blood pressure, cardiomyopathy, and cardiac arrhythmia.[32]

Recent research suggests that alcohol consumption may be less common in Appalachia than in other regions of the country.[33] West Virginia has one of the lowest rates of heavy drinkers (2.1 percent). The only two states with Appalachian counties that exceed the national average (5.1 percent) are Ohio (5.8 percent) and Pennsylvania (5.5 percent).[4] However, Appalachian youth are more likely to report heavy alcohol use (2.9 percent) than their non-Appalachian peers, which may have implications for the future onset of heart disease.[34]

Stress. Stress includes an individual's behavioral, psychological, and physical reactions to physical, environmental, and social conditions.[35] Contextual factors such as poverty may contribute to prolonged stress; however, reactions to the effects of stress are highly dependent on the perceptions and experiences of the individual. In some cases, stress can lead to health conditions such as anxiety, depression, pain disorders, and ulcers.[36] Although the exact biological mechanisms that link stress to heart disease are unclear,[9] the negative effect on the cardiovascular system is well documented.[37] Stress is implicated in a number of heart problems, including heart attack, increased blood pressure, and irregular heartbeat. At the same time, research shows that medical interventions for heart disease are more effective when they are supplemented with psychological techniques that teach new coping mechanisms to reduce emotional stress.[38]

Contextual Factors

Socioeconomic Status. Strong evidence suggests a link between socioeconomic status and health, and there is a significant relationship between the incidence of heart disease and socioeconomic status.[39–41] In a study of disparities in heart disease, cancer, and stroke in the Appalachian region, poverty and lack of health insurance increased rates of premature mortality.[42]

Geography and Medical Resources. Regular medical care is critical in reducing the morbidity and mortality associated with heart disease. A number of factors influence the use of medical services, including insurance status, availability and quality of medical professionals, severity of the health problem, and proximity to health care resources.[6] Forty-two percent of Appalachians live in rural areas, with limited access to physicians, hospitals, and other medical facilities. Many rural residents have to travel relatively long distances to meet with a specialist.[6, 43]

Although the number of physicians in Appalachia increased between 1990 and 1999, they remain unevenly distributed. In 1999, 27 percent of Appalachian counties were designated health professional shortage areas; another 47 percent of the counties had shortages in parts of them. These shortage areas are clustered in central West Virginia, eastern Kentucky, northeastern Mississippi, and central Alabama.[6] In 1999 there were six counties in Appalachia with no physicians and eighty-one counties (20 percent) with no hospitals.[6] Also, Appalachian counties in central West Virginia, eastern Kentucky, northeastern Mississippi, and the mountain ridge from western Carolina to northwestern Virginia are less likely to have specialists.[44]

In addition, medical facilities that can greatly increase the chance of surviving a major cardiac event and improve the quality of life for people with heart disease tend to be located in the more prosperous and populated Appalachian counties.[6] In 2006 there were 635 short-term (less than thirty-day stay) hospitals, 126 hospitals with coronary intensive care units, 245 hospitals with cardiac rehabilitation units, and 1,380 cardiologists (in 2007) in Appalachian counties. These medical facilities were clustered in metropolitan areas such as Pittsburgh and Knoxville, while neighboring rural counties might lack such facilities and providers.[7, 45, 46] For example, Allegheny County, Pennsylvania (where Pittsburgh is located), had 238 cardiologists, 29 hospitals, 7 coronary intensive care units, and 12 cardiac rehabilitation units, while 76 rural counties had none of these resources.[47] Thus, individuals living in rural Appalachia must often travel across county or state lines to receive medical care.

A Case Study of Risk Factors and Heart Disease

The literature supports the need for additional study of the risk factors for heart disease among Appalachians. The Greater Cincinnati Community Health Status Survey (GCCHSS) provides an opportunity to explore the prevalence and relative effects of several of these risk factors. Conducted in 2005 to collect information about health and health-related behaviors, the GCCHSS included random-digit-dialed telephone interviews with adults aged 18 years or older in the Greater Cincinnati area, including twenty-two counties in Ohio, Indiana, and Kentucky. Four of the Ohio counties (Adams, Brown, Clermont, and Highland) are designated Appalachian counties. Of the 2,077 respondents, 468 were either first-generation (210) or second-generation (257) Appalachians, based on their own or their parents' county of birth. The first- and second-generation Appalachians constituted the Appalachian sample; all other survey respondents were designated non-Appalachian. The Appalachian sample was not weighted, given that it was a subsample of the regional sample. The risk factors included in the analysis were history of high cholesterol, history of hypertension, history of diabetes, current smoking, lack of moderate exercise, overweight, alcohol consumption, high stress, income less than 200 percent of the federal poverty level, not consistently insured, and no medical home.[d]

Nearly 15 percent of Appalachians reported that they had been diagnosed by a medical professional as having heart trouble or angina, which was significantly greater than the rate among non-Appalachians (10 percent). Because heart disease is typically more prevalent as age increases, some of the differences observed between Appalachians and non-Appalachians could be related to the fact that the Appalachian respondents, as a group, were slightly older (mean age of 47.4 years versus 44.6 years for non-Appalachians). However, the literature does not reveal a sharp increase in the prevalence of heart disease in these years. Thus, the age difference was statistically significant, but it was not substantial, and the results were not adjusted for age. The analysis focused on the following questions.

Are there differences in the prevalence of risk factors between Appalachians and non-Appalachians with heart disease? Appalachians with heart disease differ from non-Appalachians with heart disease (table 5.2). More than four out of five Appalachians had hypertension, and three out of four had high cholesterol. These rates were significantly higher than those seen among non-Appalachians. Appalachians were more likely than non-Appalachians to be living at less than 200 percent of the federal poverty level. They were also more likely to report getting little to no exercise but were less likely to report having had at least one drink of alcohol in the past thirty days.

Are there differences in the prevalence of risk factors between Appalachians with heart disease and Appalachians without heart disease? Compared with Appalachians without heart disease, those with heart disease experienced health risk factors (high cholesterol, hypertension, and diabetes) at

Table 5.2. Prevalence of Risk Factors for Appalachians and Non-Appalachians with Heart Disease

Risk Factor	% Appalachian (N = 69)	% Non-Appalachian (N=151)	Chi-Square P Value
High cholesterol	75.4	54.7	.004*
Hypertension	85.5	60.9	.000*
Diabetes	23.2	19.2	.497
Current smoking	27.5	20.5	.250
No moderate exercise	31.4	14.5	.003*
Overweight	65.2	74.0	.182
Alcohol consumption	27.5	50.7	.001*
High stress	50.7	54.7	.587
Less than 200% of federal poverty level	72.6	46.2	.001*
Not consistently insured	15.7	13.2	.623
No medical home	15.7	10.7	.288

Source: Greater Cincinnati Community Health Status Survey, 2005.
*Statistically significant at the $p < .05$ level based on chi-square test of proportions.

higher rates and were more likely to live in poverty and not get adequate exercise (table 5.3). However, they were more likely to have consistent insurance coverage and less likely to have had a drink of alcohol in the past thirty days. Although they were less likely to have these risk factors, approximately one out of three Appalachians without heart disease had high cholesterol, hypertension, and incomes less than 200 percent of the federal poverty level. Nearly seven out of ten were overweight, three out of ten were not consistently insured, and one out of four did not have a medical home.

Do Appalachians and non-Appalachians without heart disease differ with respect to risk factors associated with heart disease? A comparison of Appalachians without heart disease and non-Appalachians without heart disease revealed several significant differences (table 5.4). Appalachians without heart disease had higher rates of health risk factors (high cholesterol, high blood pressure, and diabetes), higher rates of behavioral risk factors (overweight), and lower rates of behavioral protective factors

Table 5.3. Prevalence of Risk Factors among Appalachians with and without Heart Disease

Risk Factor	% with Heart Disease (N = 69)	% without Heart Disease (N = 399)	Chi-Square P Value
High cholesterol	75.4	33.8	.000*
Hypertension	85.5	38.7	.000*
Diabetes	23.2	11.5	.008*
Current smoking	27.5	31.8	.477
No moderate exercise	31.4	10.8	.000*
Overweight	65.2	68.1	.637
Alcohol consumption	27.5	43.7	.012*
High stress	50.7	45.1	.388
Less than 200% of federal poverty level	72.6	35.7	.000*
Not consistently insured	15.7	29.4	.018*
No medical home	15.7	24.1	.122

Source: Greater Cincinnati Community Health Status Survey, 2005.
* Statistically significant at the $p < .05$ level based on chi-square test of proportions.

Table 5.4. Prevalence of Risk Factors among Appalachians and Non-Appalachians without Heart Disease

Risk Factor	% Appalachian (N = 399)	% Non-Appalachian (N = 1,354)	Chi-Square P Value
High cholesterol	33.8	23.1	.000*
Hypertension	38.7	24.0	.000*
Diabetes	11.5	7.4	.008*
Current smoking	31.8	30.7	.675
No moderate exercise	10.8	10.8	.997
Overweight	68.1	58.4	.001*
Alcohol consumption	43.7	59.3	.000*
High stress	45.1	51.0	.039*
Less than 200% of federal poverty level	35.7	26.8	.001*
Not consistently insured	29.4	17.8	.000*
No medical home	24.1	19.8	.061

Source: Greater Cincinnati Community Health Status Survey, 2005.
* Statistically significant at the $p < .05$ level based on chi-square test of proportions.

Table 5.5. Logistic Regression Results for Heart Disease Risk Factors (N = 374)

Predictor	Odds Ratio	P Value
High cholesterol	2.594	.0036*
Hypertension	3.689	.0004*
Diabetes	2.088	.0606
Current smoking	1.216	.5896
No moderate exercise	2.141	.0493*
Overweight	0.611	.1709
Alcohol consumption	0.531	.0901
High stress	1.023	.9458
Less than 200% of federal poverty level	2.329	.0119*
Not consistently insured	0.818	.6228
No medical home	1.381	.4613
Over age 65	1.532	.2732

Source: Greater Cincinnati Community Health Status Survey, 2005.
*Statistically significant at the $p < .05$ level.

(consuming alcohol in the past thirty days). Appalachians without heart disease were also more likely to be living in poverty and to lack consistent insurance coverage, but they were less likely to experience high stress.

Which risk factors are the most powerful predictors of heart disease among Appalachians? The results of a logistic regression analysis of the risk factors for heart disease among Appalachians are presented in table 5.5. Appalachians with hypertension were approximately 3.7 times more likely to have heart disease than those without hypertension. Appalachians with high cholesterol and those with incomes less than 200 percent of the federal poverty level were about 2.5 times more likely to have heart disease than those without high cholesterol or above the 200 percent level.

Results. The results of the case study indicate that first- and second-generation Appalachians in the Cincinnati tristate area are at increased risk for developing heart disease, and they experience many of the risk factors that contribute to heart disease. Prevalence rates for heart disease, as well as for the associated risk factors, were high among the Appalachian cohort. Even among the Appalachian respondents who did not have heart disease, there was a higher prevalence of high cholesterol, hypertension, and diabetes than in the general population.

A higher percentage of people without heart disease (in both the Appalachian and the non-Appalachian samples) were not consistently insured and had no medical home compared with those who had heart disease. Non-Appalachians with heart disease were less likely to be current smokers than were those without heart disease. Moreover, those who had been diagnosed with heart disease were less likely to have consumed alcohol in the past thirty days than those who had not been diagnosed with heart disease. This is consistent with other research that indicates that moderate alcohol consumption is related to health status[48] and specifically to cardiovascular health.[30]

Heart Health Promotion in Appalachia

The Healthy People 2010 goal was to reduce deaths from heart disease to 166 per 100,000 population.[49] The Appalachian rate of 651 deaths per 100,000 is four times that goal.[6] Reducing deaths from heart disease and increasing life expectancy must involve health promotion and the adoption of healthy lifestyles (primary prevention), early identification and treatment of disease (secondary prevention), and adequate treatment and rehabilitation of those with more advanced disease (tertiary prevention). Because Appalachians are at particular risk for heart disease, a few innovative programs have taken steps to address the problem.

The Coronary Artery Risk Detection in Appalachian Communities (CARDIAC) project in West Virginia screens schoolchildren for heart disease risk factors and refers those found to be at high risk for further testing, education, and treatment.[16, 50] In one CARDIAC project that included 1,338 West Virginia fifth graders, 17.5 percent were identified as being overweight and 27 percent were identified as obese. However, relatively few of these students (63 percent of the obese and 26 percent of the overweight children) had been identified by their pediatricians as being over the recommended weight. Because obese children are at greater risk for high cholesterol and high blood pressure, this raises obvious concerns about the early identification and treatment of health problems.[16]

A program targeting specific risk behaviors is the Be Active North Carolina–Appalachian Partnership, which focuses on increasing physical activity in Appalachian North Carolina. This initiative assesses physical activity needs and challenges, provides resources for exercise in schools, and encourages work sites and community agencies to promote regular exercise.[51]

Collaboration is a necessary ingredient in prevention and risk reduction interventions. CareSpark, which represents seventeen counties in northeastern Tennessee and southwestern Virginia, is one example of a coordinated effort to improve health in Central Appalachia. CareSpark develops the infrastructure to improve access to health information technology, coordinates health improvement efforts between providers and patients, and collects health data for public health interventions. This program has identified five priority health issues as its focus, three of which are related to cardiovascular health.[52]

Further Research

The disparities experienced by Appalachians in terms of heart disease and the associated risk factors emphasize the need for additional research to more fully understand the nature of this problem and to develop and implement effective prevention strategies. Suggested areas of research include the following.

Data Improvement. One consistent problem in the existing literature is the lack of comprehensive health data, particularly for rural Appalachians. Researchers could contribute to the overall health of the region by experimenting with new ways to collect health data in Appalachia and by exploring ways to share these data with the community.

Differences within Appalachia. Subregional differences in health status and risk factors make it clear that Appalachia does not have a homogeneous population. It follows that approaches to prevention and health care that work in one community may not be equally effective throughout the entire region. Researchers can help develop more targeted programs by exploring the differences among races, geographic locations, and economic classes in Appalachia.

Distribution of Resources. There continue to be discrepancies in the distribution of health care resources throughout the region. Geographic information systems and mapping analyses may be useful to explore the distribution of resources and their impact on the utilization of health services and on health status.

Epidemiological Analyses. Given the complex interactions among the heart disease risk factors, further research is needed to clarify the nature of heart disease and risk in Appalachia. Path analysis methodologies may be helpful in understanding the direct and indirect contributions of each risk factor to the development of heart disease. Although costly and time-consuming, research that utilizes longitudinal data panels may provide unique insight into the development of heart disease and its underlying causes.

Policy Recommendations

Increasing access to health care is critical in the effort to reduce cardiovascular disease among Appalachians. To increase access to health care in the Appalachian region, the following issues should be addressed.

Monitoring the Implementation of Health Care Reform. Although health care reform legislation has passed and there are numerous implications for Appalachians, many of the major reforms will not be implemented until 2014. Monitoring the implementation of this legislation is paramount to ensure that those who were meant to benefit do so.

Diminishing Geographic Barriers to Care. Increasing the number of health care professionals will not solve all the access issues in Appalachia. Medical care tends to be clustered in population centers, which are not readily accessible to everyone in the region. Even county hospitals may be too far away for some people, depending on the size and geography of the service area. Many people in Appalachia are forced to travel great distances for health care, which makes it very difficult for them to obtain regular care, let alone ongoing care for chronic conditions. Many Appalachians would benefit from the adoption of an approach that brings medical services to the people. For example, mobile clinics could travel between smaller communities or work sites, offering services on a regular basis. School-based health centers could provide medical care to students and their families. Employer-based clinics could offer preventive care and treatment for minor problems.

Eliminating Financial Barriers to Care. Poverty is an abiding problem in parts of Appalachia, and it is a huge challenge to health care access. Mining and other industries that have traditionally sustained Appalachia are losing momentum, and the region has been particularly hard hit in the recent recession.[53] In the short term, outreach programs may help connect individuals and families to benefits such as Medicaid and the Children's

Health Insurance Program (CHIP), allowing them to continue to receive care. In the long run, regional policy makers should explore options to expand the availability of health care coverage, particularly to individuals and small businesses. For example, pooled purchasing agreements or regional health insurance purchasing cooperatives may offer more options to small, geographically isolated businesses.[54]

Notes

a. *Heart disease* is a term used to describe a broad range of diseases that affect the heart and, in some cases, the blood vessels.[55] It is often used interchangeably with *cardiovascular disease,* which generally refers to conditions that involve narrowed or blocked blood vessels that can lead to a heart attack, chest pain (angina), or stroke.

b. Although behavioral factors are important contributors to heart health and disease, data on individual behaviors are difficult to obtain. Unlike mortality data, which are documented on legally required death certificates, there are few ways to collect data on people living with chronic disease and even fewer ways to gather information on the behaviors that contribute to chronic disease. One national survey, the Behavioral Risk Factor Surveillance System (BRFSS), attempts to do this. To ensure that there are an adequate number of responses to draw conclusions about a specific geographic area, county-level data for the Appalachian region may be aggregated into seventy-nine labor market areas (LMAs)—areas where people live and work.[6] Even these larger areas may lack the data needed to accurately report on subgroups (e.g., black men and women). The lack of precision in existing data makes it difficult to fully understand the role of behavioral risk factors in Appalachian heart health. However, it does provide insight into the specific challenges facing the region.

c. Several contextual factors have been identified as potential contributors to the risk of heart disease. These contextual factors are generally out of the individual's control. Some parts of Appalachia have relatively high levels of unemployment, low incomes, and low levels of educational attainment. These factors, along with geographic barriers, translate into decreased access to social, economic, and medical care resources and, ultimately, to more adverse health outcomes.[6]

d. Risk factors used in the analysis were defined as follows: *cholesterol:* history of high cholesterol; *hypertension:* history of hypertension; *diabetes:* history of type 1 or 2 diabetes; *smoking:* current smoker; *moderate exercise:* engages in moderate activities for at least ten minutes at a time in a usual week; *overweight:* body mass index greater than 25; *drinking:* consumed at least one drink of alcohol in the past thirty days; *high stress:* stress level is "a lot higher" than the respondent would like; *under 200 percent of the federal poverty level:* calculated using 2005 poverty guidelines; *not consistently insured:* respondent went without insurance at some point in the past year; *no medical home:* respondent does not have one particular place to receive medical care. More information about the GCCHSS, including survey data and definitions, can be found at www.healthfoundation.org/gcchss .html.

References

1. American Heart Association. Cardiovascular disease cost. Available at: http://www.americanheart.org/presenter.jhtml?identifier=4475. Accessed August 31, 2010.

2. American Heart Association. Heart disease and stroke statistics—2010 update. Dallas, TX: American Heart Association; 2010.

3. Centers for Disease Control and Prevention. Updated heart disease maps. Available at: http://www.cdc.gov/dhdsp/library/maps/heart_disease_map_all.htm. Accessed August 31, 2010.

4. Centers for Disease Control and Prevention. BRFSS prevalence and trend data. Available at: http://apps.nccd.cdc.gov/BRFSS/index.asp. Accessed February 17, 2010.

5. Hoyert DL, Heron MP, Murphy SL, Kung H. Deaths: final data for 2003. National Vital Statistics Reports 54(13). Hyattsville, MD: National Center for Health Statistics; 2006. Available at: http://www.cdc.gov/nchs/data/nvsr/nvsr54/nvsr54_13.pdf. Accessed September 12, 2010.

6. Halverson JA, Ma L, Harner EJ. An analysis of disparities in health status and access to health care in the Appalachian region. Washington, DC: Appalachian Regional Commission; 2004.

7. Barnett E, Elmes GA, et al. Heart disease in Appalachia: an atlas of county economic conditions, mortality, and medical care resources. Morgantown, WV: Prevention Resource Center, West Virginia University; 1998.

8. Stern S, Behar S, Gottlieb S. Aging and diseases of the heart. *Circulation.* 2003;108:e99–e101.

9. American Heart Association. Risk factors and coronary heart disease. Available at: http://www.americanheart.org/presenter.jhtml?identifier=4726. Accessed August 31, 2010.

10. Yusuf S, Hawken S, Ounpuu S, et al. Effect of potentially modifiable risk factors associated with myocardial infarction in 52 countries (the INTERHEART study): case-control study. *Lancet.* 2004;364:937–952.

11. Centers for Disease Control and Prevention. Heart disease prevention. Available at: http://www.cdc.gov/heartdisease/prevention.htm. Accessed August 31, 2010.

12. Centers for Disease Control and Prevention. Cholesterol fact sheet. Available at: http://www.cdc.gov/DHDSP/library/fs_cholesterol.htm. Accessed August 31, 2010.

13. Appalachian Rural Health Institute. Disease prevalence. Athens, OH: Appalachian Rural Health Institute; 2006.

14. Edwards JB, Shuman P, Glenn LL. Relationships among health risk factors and objective physical findings in well rural Appalachian women. *Fam Community Health.* 1996;8:4.

15. Ramsey PW, Glenn LL. Risk factors for heart disease in rural Appalachia. *Fam Community Health.* 1998;20:4.

16. Demerath E, Muratova V, Spangler E, Li J, Minor VE, Neal WA. School-based obesity screening in rural Appalachia. *Prev Med.* 2003;37:553–560.

17. American Heart Association. Why blood pressure matters. Available at: http://www.heart.org/HEARTORG/Conditions/HighBloodPressure/WhyBloodPressure Matters/Why-Blood-Pressure-Matters_UCM_002051_Article.jsp. Accessed January 28, 2011.

18. Centers for Disease Control and Prevention. High blood pressure facts. Available at: http://www.cdc.gov/bloodpressure/facts.htm. Accessed August 31, 2010.

19. Hyduk A, Croft JB, Ayla C, Zheng K, Zheng Z, Mensah GA. Pulmonary hypertension surveillance—United States, 1980–2002. Morbidity and Mortality Weekly Report 54(5). Atlanta, GA: Centers for Disease Control and Prevention; 2005. Available at: http://www.cdc.gov/mmwR/preview/mmwrhtml/ss5405a1.htm. Accessed August 31, 2010.

20. Lohri-Posey B. Middle-aged Appalachians living with diabetes mellitus: a family affair. *Fam Community Health.* 2006;29:214–220.

21. American Diabetes Association. Diabetes statistics. Available at: http://www.diabetes.org/diabetes-basics/diabetes-statistics/. Accessed August 31, 2010.

22. Wood LE. The economic impact of tobacco production in Appalachia. Washington, DC: Appalachian Regional Commission; 1998. Available at: http://www.arc.gov/research/researchreportdetails.asp?REPORT_ID=59.

23. American Heart Association. Cigarette smoking and cardiovascular diseases. Available at: http://www.americanheart.org/presenter.jhtml?identifier=4545. Accessed August 31, 2010.

24. Ohio Tobacco Prevention Foundation. Ohio tobacco statistics. Available at: http://www.standohio.org/resources/ohiotobaccostatistics.aspx. Accessed March 5, 2007.

25. Toborg MA, Meyer MG, Mande MJ. An assessment of tobacco prevention and control materials used in the Appalachian mountain region. Washington, DC: Toborg Associates; 1997. Available at: https://toborg.net/pdf/AssessTobacco_Appal .pdf. Accessed March 5, 2007.

26. Mayo Clinic. Exercise: 7 benefits of regular physical activity. Available at: http://www.mayoclinic.com/health/exercise/HQ01676. Accessed August 31, 2010.

27. Dorn J, Naughton J, Imamura D, Trevisan M. Results of a multicenter randomized clinical trial of exercise and long-term survival in myocardial infarction

patients: the National Exercise and Heart Disease Project (NEHDP). *Circulation.* 1999;100:1764–1769.

28. Parks SE, Housemann RA, Brownson RC. Differential correlates of physical activity in urban and rural adults of various socioeconomic backgrounds in the United States. *J Epidemiol Community Health.* 2003;57:29–35.

29. Keefe SE, Parsons P. Health and life-style indicators in a rural Appalachian county: implications for health-care practice. In: Keefe SE, ed. *Appalachian Cultural Competency: A Guide for Medical, Mental Health, and Social Service Professionals.* Knoxville, TN: University of Tennessee Press; 2005:183–195.

30. Abramson JL, Williams SA, Krumholz HM, Vaccarino V. Moderate alcohol consumption and risk of heart failure among older persons. *JAMA.* 2001;285:1971–1977.

31. Rimm EB, Williams P, Fosher K, Criqui M, Stampfer MJ. Moderate alcohol intake and lower risk of coronary heart disease: meta-analysis of effects on lipids and haemostatic factors. *BMJ.* 1999;319:1523–1528.

32. American Heart Association. Alcohol, wine and cardiovascular disease. Available at: http://www.americanheart.org/presenter.jhtml?identifier=4422. Accessed August 31, 2010.

33. Casto BC, Sharma S, Fisher JL, Knobloch TJ, Agrawal A, Weghorst CM. Oral cancer in Appalachia. *J Health Care Poor Underserved.* 2009;20:274–285.

34. Zhang Z, Infante A, Meit M, English N, Dunn M, Bowers KH. An analysis of mental health and substance abuse disparities and access to treatment services in the Appalachian region. Washington, DC: Appalachian Regional Commission; 2008. Available at: http://www.arc.gov/assets/research_reports/AnalysisofMentalHealthandSubstanceAbuseDisparities.pdf. Accessed February 17, 2010.

35. American Institute of Stress. What is stress? Available at: http://www.stress.org/topic-definition-stress.htm. Accessed January 28, 2011.

36. American Institute of Stress. Effects of stress. Available at: http://www.stress.org/topic-effects.htm. Accessed January 28, 2011.

37. National Heart, Lung, and Blood Institute. What is coronary artery disease? Available at: http://www.nhlbi.nih.gov/health/dci/Diseases/Cad/CAD_WhatIs.html. Accessed August 31, 2010.

38. Blumenthal JA, Sherwood A, Babyak MA, et al. Effects of exercise and stress management training on markers of cardiovascular risk in patients with ischemic heart disease: a randomized controlled trial. *JAMA.* 2005;293:1626–1634.

39. Adler NE, Ostrove JM. Socioeconomic status and health: what we know and what we don't. *Ann NY Acad Sci.* 1999;896:3–15.

40. Halverson JA, Barnett E, Casper M. Geographic disparities in heart disease and stroke mortality among black and white populations in the Appalachian region. *Ethn Dis.* 2002;12(S3):82–91.

41. Winkleby MA, Kraemer HC, Ahn DK, Varady AN. Ethnic and socioeconomic

differences in cardiovascular disease risk factors: findings for women from the third National Health and Nutrition Examination Survey, 1988–1994. *JAMA.* 1998;280:356–362.

42. Mary Babb Randolph Cancer Center/Office for Social Environmental and Health Research. Underlying socioeconomic factors influencing health disparities in the Appalachian region. Final Report Contract No. CO-15198. Morgantown, WV: Department of Community Medicine, Robert C. Byrd Health Sciences Center, West Virginia University; 2008.

43. Huttlinger K, Schaller-Ayers J, Lawson T. Health care in Appalachia: a population-based approach. *Public Health Nurs.* 2004;21:103–110.

44. Barnett E, Halverson JA, Elmes GA, Braham VE. Metropolitan and nonmetropolitan trends in coronary heart disease mortality within Appalachia, 1980–1997. *Ann Epidemiol.* 2000;10:370–379.

45. Abramson R, Haskell J. *Encyclopedia of Appalachia.* Knoxville, TN: University of Tennessee Press; 2006.

46. Stensland J, Mueller C, Sutton J. An analysis of the financial conditions of health care institutions in the Appalachian region and their economic impacts. Washington, DC: Appalachian Regional Commission; 2002. Available at: http://www.arc.gov/researchreports.asp?F_CATEGORY=13. Accessed March 5, 2007.

47. Bureau of Health Professions. Area resource file (ARF). Rockville, MD: U.S. Department of Health and Human Services, Health Resources and Services Administration, Bureau of Health Professions; 2008.

48. French MT, Zavala SK. The health benefits of moderate drinking revisited: alcohol use and self-reported health status. *Am J Health Promot.* 2007;21:484–491.

49. U.S. Department of Health and Human Services. *Healthy People 2010.* 2nd ed. Available at: http://www.healthypeople.gov/Publications/. Accessed August 31, 2010.

50. Neal WA, Demerath E, Gonzales E, et al. Coronary Artery Risk Detection in Appalachian Communities (CARDIAC): preliminary findings. *WV Med J.* 2001;97:102–105.

51. Be Active North Carolina. Appalachian partners with Be Active North Carolina to increase region's physical activity. Available at: http://www.beactivenc.org/mediacenter/news_asupartnership.cfm. Accessed March 23, 2007.

52. CareSpark. We are CareSpark. Available at: http://www.carespark.com. Accessed March 23, 2007.

53. Appalachian Regional Commission. Appalachian regional employment report—2009 Q3. Washington, DC: Appalachian Regional Commission; 2009. Available at: http://www.arc.gov/images/appregion/AppalachianRegion EmploymentReport2009Q3.pdf. February 10, 2010.

54. Hall MA, Wicks EK, Lawlor JS. HealthMarts, HIPCs (health insurance purchasing cooperatives), MEWAs (multiple employee welfare arrangements), and

AHPs (association health plans): a guide for the perplexed. *Health Aff (Millwood)*. 2001;20:142–153.

55. Mayo Clinic. Heart disease. Available at: http://www.mayoclinic.com/health/heart-disease/DS01120. Accessed August 31, 2010.

6

Diabetes and Its Management

Sharon A. Denham

According to the Centers for Disease Control and Prevention,[1] 25.8 million children and adults in the United States, or 8.3 percent of the nation's population, have been diagnosed with diabetes, a figure that has more than doubled since 1980. In addition, an estimated 7 million people are unaware that they have the disease, and as many as 79 million people may have prediabetes. It is important to note, however, that these estimates may understate diabetes' prevalence. For example, death certificates are likely to state the immediate cause of death and ignore diabetes, which may be a contributing factor. Diabetes is now the seventh leading cause of death in the United States[1] and imposes a substantial cost burden on society, on those with diabetes, and on their families. Rates of work loss due to diabetes-related complications are higher than for other disease groups.[2]

This chapter discusses diabetes and its risk factors, as well as the prevalence of diabetes in the Appalachian region and specifically in Appalachian Ohio. The management of diabetes is examined from the medical, self, and family perspectives, and models for diabetes interventions are presented. The chapter concludes with recommendations for future research and policies that address diabetes in Appalachia.

Diabetes

Diabetes mellitus, or diabetes, is a group of diseases characterized by uncontrolled blood glucose levels. This metabolic syndrome results when the body fails to produce or use insulin effectively. Insulin, a hormone manufactured by the pancreas, is essential for glucose uptake into body cells. Under current guidelines, the diagnosis of diabetes is dependent on an elevated glycosylated hemoglobin (HbA1c) level of 6.5 percent or higher. Levels from 5.7 to 6.4 percent point to a high risk of developing both diabetes and cardiovascular disease.[3] Diabetes is widely known to be a major contributor to amputations, vision loss, and kidney disease.

Types of Diabetes. The two major classifications of diabetes are type 1 and type 2. Type 1 diabetes is an autoimmune disease caused by the immune system attacking and destroying the insulin-producing beta cells in the pancreas, resulting in little or no insulin production in the body.[4] This form of diabetes accounts for 5 to 10 percent of all diabetes cases.[5] Symptoms are usually severe and occur rapidly. It is a lifelong condition that is treated with insulin. If not diagnosed and properly treated, a person with type 1 diabetes can lapse into a life-threatening diabetic coma.

The most common form of diabetes is type 2 diabetes, accounting for 90 to 95 percent of all diagnosed cases.[5] With type 2 diabetes, the pancreas is usually producing enough insulin, but for unknown reasons, the body cannot use the insulin effectively—a condition called insulin resistance. After several years, insulin production decreases. In contrast to type 1 diabetes, the symptoms of type 2 diabetes develop gradually. Type 2 diabetes can be prevented and is potentially reversible unless permanent beta cell failure has occurred.

Diabetes Risk Factors. Type 1 diabetes, referred to as juvenile-onset diabetes, can occur at any age but is usually diagnosed in people younger than 30 years. Type 2 diabetes is generally associated with people older than 45, although it is increasingly being diagnosed in children and adolescents. Because genetic makeup plays a large role in type 2 diabetes, a family history of the disease is a risk factor, but lifestyle and social determinants have become increasingly important concerns. Other major risk factors for type 2 diabetes include inadequate physical activity, poor diet, excess body weight (body mass index greater than 30), race or ethnicity (African Americans, Hispanic Americans, and Native Americans all have high rates of diabetes), high blood pressure, high-density lipoprotein (HDL) cholesterol levels less than 35 or triglyceride levels greater than 250, and, for women, a history of diabetes during pregnancy. Another concern is pre-diabetes, a condition in which individuals have elevated blood glucose or HbA1c levels that are not high enough to be classified as diabetes.[1] People with pre-diabetes have an increased risk of developing type 2 diabetes, heart disease, and stroke.

Diabetes Prevalence in Appalachia

Appalachian Region Overall. Diabetes is more prevalent in Appalachia than in other parts of the United States.[6] Combined data from the National Health and Nutrition Examination Survey (NHANES) and the Behavioral Risk Factor Surveillance System (BRFSS)[a] indicate that states with Appalachian counties have the highest diabetes prevalence, with Mississippi faring the worst in the nation.[7] Reports indicate that 81 percent of the Appalachian counties in West Virginia, Kentucky, and Tennessee, as well as 77 percent of the Appalachian counties in Alabama, Georgia, Mississippi, and South Carolina, have the highest diabetes rates in the country. The disease affects more than 20 percent of residents in the "Stroke Belt," a region that contains much of Southern Appalachia.[8] Regression analysis of BRFSS data from 2006–2007 found that those living in the distressed counties of Appalachia were at the greatest risk for diabetes.[9]

Over the last thirty years, evidence has been accumulating that depression is a serious comorbidity for those living with diabetes.[10] A study conducted among 201 rural Appalachian clinic attendees found that 31 percent reported both diabetes and depression.[11] Depression was associated with a younger age group, high unemployment, and multiple prescribed medications. A major concern is that among individuals with type 2 diabetes, those with depression have worse blood glucose levels, lower adherence to prescribed medical regimens, greater functional disabilities, more comorbidities, and increased mortality than those without depression.[2]

Appalachian Ohio. The Appalachian Rural Health Institute (ARHI) at Ohio University conducted random telephone surveys of adults in 2003, 2006, and 2008 to establish diabetes prevalence rates and comorbid conditions in Appalachian Ohio. The 2003 survey of four Ohio counties found that 8.3 percent of respondents reported a current diagnosis of type 2 diabetes, a rate that exceeded the 2002 BRFSS rates in the nation (6.2 percent) and in Ohio (7.5 percent).[12] The 2006 survey in seven additional Appalachian counties found an 11.3 percent prevalence rate, which exceeded the 2004 BRFSS national (7.2 percent) and Ohio (7.8 percent) rates.[13] The 2008 survey in nine different Appalachian Ohio counties found the diabetes rate to be 12.5 percent, exceeding both the Ohio (9.5 percent) and the national (8.6 percent) rates in the 2007 BRFSS.[14] In addition, a separate study of eleven rural Appalachian Ohio counties found a higher self-reported prevalence of diabetes (12.5 percent) compared with the 2004 BRFSS rates for Ohio (7.8 percent) and the nation (7.2 percent).[15] These surveys also found that those who reported having diabetes (23 percent) were more likely to report comorbid depression than were those without diabetes; that cost prevented 28 percent of those diagnosed with diabetes from taking oral medications, 29.5 percent from checking glucose levels, and 14.5 percent from attending diabetes education programs; and that prevalence rates were significantly associated with lower income levels and decreased access to medications and glucose monitoring supplies. A recent study involving 3,841 adults in nine Appalachian Ohio counties found that 49.2 percent of those with a diabetes diagnosis were younger than 40 years,[14] a rate substantially higher than the 19 percent rate for this age group reported in the 2008 National Health Interview Survey.[16]

Medical Management of Diabetes

Medical management is defined as an interaction between a person with a disease and health care professionals. In the case of diabetes, these professionals may include physicians, nurses, medical specialists, pharmacists, ophthalmologists, podiatrists, psychologists, dentists, nurse practitioners, and diabetes educators. The medical management of diabetes focuses on activities that keep blood glucose levels within normal ranges, the prevention and treatment of complications, and education that assists with daily self-management. The quality of medical management can vary widely based on access to health care providers, provider knowledge about diabetes, health insurance or the ability to pay for care, and the ability to access educational information.

To examine the medical management of diabetes in Appalachia, an environmental scan[b] was completed with health care providers from federally qualified health centers, county health departments, and certified diabetes educators working in 182 agencies in the Appalachian region.[17, 18] Survey data were linked with county socioeconomic status based on the Appalachian Regional Commission's five categories of economic health: distressed, at-risk, transitional, competitive, and attainment. Almost half the surveys came from participants in counties identified as distressed or at-risk. Findings indicated that facilities located in distressed counties were significantly less likely to employ certified diabetes educators. In addition, the environmental scan pointed out the need for earlier diagnosis, better continuity of care, timelier referral to specialists, improved diabetes education, and improved coordination among hospitals, community providers, and home care settings. Health professionals' lack of knowledge about standards of care for diabetes was often cited as a problem. For example, one participant said physicians need to "stop telling patients they are 'borderline' and give them meal and exercise plans to prevent getting diabetes." Another participant said, "Oftentimes, patients are newly diagnosed with type 2 diabetes, given a prescription for medications or insulin, and sent home with little or no education. Many patients have the misconception that if they 'stay away from sweets' they are managing their disease."

Clear communication between health care providers and persons with diabetes and their families is important to achieve optimal diabetes outcomes. A person's knowledge, needs, and competencies must be clearly understood by health care providers, and appropriate information must be provided to the patient and family members. Some Appalachians are at high risk for communication impairment and low literacy levels.[19] Lower levels of literacy have been linked with poorer health, and low levels of health literacy—the ability to read, understand, and act on health information—are associated with poor health outcomes, including lack of screening and early detection.[20] Consequently, low health literacy in persons with diabetes may cause them to be labeled noncompliant, experience repeated hospital admissions, and have multiple complications due to poor disease control.[21]

It is important that health care providers in the region not judge their patients' intellectual capacity based on dialect or speech patterns. Clear communication should be devoid of stereotypes associated with being Appalachian. Health education materials designed for Appalachian populations should be written at an appropriate reading level and include suitable language, photos, and information.[22]

Diabetes Self-Management

Most diabetes management occurs outside the purview of medical professionals and entails self-management and family-supported management, as well as alterations in daily life routines.[23] Self-management implies the integration of multiple self-care activities, such as adherence to a medical regimen, diet management, and physical activity, into daily life. Although pharmacotherapy is important, lifestyle modifications are critical in preventing and managing type 2 diabetes.[24]

Education is essential to the self-management of diabetes because it plays a central role in improving glycemic control, reducing the risks of long-term complications, and enhancing the quality of life.[25] However, lack of personal motivation, a limited number of health professionals, difficulty obtaining physician referrals, lack of adequate health insurance, and transportation problems may prevent many patients from obtaining diabetes education[26] as well as the supplies and care they need for good self-management of the disease.

There are many concerns about the availability and adequacy of diabetes education in the Appalachian region.[17, 18] Earlier referral to formal classes, better and more comprehensive community prevention efforts, healthy lifestyle management, increased inpatient health education, ongoing self-management classes for those already experiencing complications, sufficient space for education, and adequate teaching resources are viewed as essential but may be problematic in Appalachia. Although reimbursement for diabetes education and prevention programs varies among states and health insurance plans, these factors greatly impact education availability and delivery.

Diabetes Management from a Family Perspective

A significant portion of diabetes management takes place in the home setting,[27] with family members playing a vital role.[28] Social support has long been identified as a critical factor associated with diabetes management[27]; along with the family environment, it can either facilitate or hinder diabetes self-care.[29] Family support has been associated with treatment adherence, illness adaptation, and blood sugar control.[30–32] Studies of patients with type 1 diabetes have shown that family-focused interventions can be cost-effective, improve HbA1c results, and have a positive effect on quality of life.[33] Thus, family and household member support can reinforce individual behaviors with regard to nutrition and dietary routines, activity patterns, and adherence to prescribed medical regimens.[34, 35] However, alterations in family routines can affect health outcomes and alter behaviors linked to diabetes care either negatively or positively.[36, 37] For example, studies of self-management support by married couples with either type 1 or type 2 diabetes indicated that some partners positively supported their spouses' nutritional health through food procurement, meal preparation, and shared meal plans[38]; others gave negative feedback through critical comments and were unable to effectively communicate concern and support.

Family has long been recognized as an important component in the lives of Appalachians. Studies of Appalachian families have found that gender, traditions, family routines, and intergenerational links have the potential to influence diabetes self-management behaviors.[34, 39–41] Findings from three qualitative research studies indicated that family health routines among those living in Appalachia were used to support health processes related to individual and family development; avoid illness, disease, and injury; cooperate to attain, sustain, and regain health; communicate with health experts; obtain resources for health needs; distribute family health resources; and structure behaviors related to health.[42–44] In these studies, family members were aware of one another's health behaviors and could consistently and reliably describe them.

Based on this research, the Family Health Model was developed to address health processes,[45] a framework especially pertinent to Appalachian families. Family health is a collective experience influenced by individual and family factors that are supported and challenged by the beliefs, values, goals, and resources of the larger society. This model uses an ecological framework to better understand the interrelations among families, individual health, and health as a whole. Three domains (contextual, functional, and structural) are used to articulate the processes pertinent to family health. Family health is influenced to a greater extent by household and member variables, member interactions, and routine behaviors than by occasional medical encounters. Research with Appalachian families suggests that mothers and other family members play more important roles in health than do physicians, nurses, or other health professionals.

Two subsequent qualitative studies used the Family Health Model as a conceptual framework to learn how persons with type 2 diabetes and their family members self-manage prescribed medical care.[34, 39] The first study, which focused on thirteen Appalachian Ohio families, found that family members provided some assistance with diabetes self-management;

gender differences seemed to influence some types of support; food preferences, family traditions, and intergenerational dietary patterns influenced the ways behavioral changes occurred; and dietary routines were of special concern.[34] These findings were supported by another study that identified the importance of including family members of those with type 2 diabetes in discussions and education about diabetes management.[46]

The second study, involving a different group of fourteen Appalachian Ohio and West Virginia families, found that families often have concerns about the daily management of diabetes.[39] Although many of the study participants with diabetes had been diagnosed at least ten years earlier, more than half had never received disease management education; most family members had no formal diabetes education, and the diabetes education provided was not regularly updated. Even those who had obtained diabetes education at the time of the initial diagnosis acknowledged that they had a poor understanding of and limited knowledge about what was required for proper self-management. Although many were clear about medication use, other practices related to daily management and complication prevention were less clear. Stories told by individuals and family members indicated that inconsistent care was common; these stories revealed health legacies that included misinformation, out-of-date medical information, uncertainties about prevention, and a sense that efforts to make changes would be futile. Although the disease was viewed as a serious one that needed special daily attention, individuals with diabetes, as well as their family members, often lacked information about how best to manage the disease. A mixture of correct and incorrect medical knowledge about diabetes existed within single families, often resulting in conflict, inadequate family support, blame and shame for errant behaviors, and uncertainty about where to obtain information for problem solving and decision making. For some families, the lack of health insurance or limited access to health care providers was a deterrent to seeking medical care; limited economic resources, misinformation, and an unwillingness to ask questions or seek assistance from others were often observed. Study participants often believed that little could be done to alter the outcome once the diagnosis had been made. This study suggested that a wall of silence and shame linked to diabetes may keep the larger community from openly addressing disease concerns through social networks or groups such as church congregations.

Models for Diabetes Intervention in Appalachia

Over several years, fifty-two separate focus groups were conducted in the Appalachian portions of ten states to discern themes relevant to health education. They concluded that "health education in the region that respects the key role of the family in the lives of its members shows promise as an effective means to intervene against behaviors that dispose individuals to increased risk for disease."[22] Furthermore, specific styles of health education were identified as being important to Appalachians, particularly efforts involving one-on-one contact, polite messages, and reliance on facts. Families use routines to arrange their ordinary day-to-day lives and to cope with illness.[47] A diabetes diagnosis impacts previously constructed health routines; thus, old behaviors often need to be deconstructed and new ones created to meet unique family needs.[39]

A small 2006 pilot study investigated the feasibility of including family members in diabetes education classes for rural Appalachians.[48] Family members who participated in the study reported higher overall scores in diabetes-related distress than the persons who actually had type 2 diabetes, suggesting that diabetes has a greater relative impact on family members. However, family distress scores were lower and diabetes knowledge was improved after education, suggesting the utility of a family intervention approach. A more recently published study had two important findings: (1) family members believed that diabetes is controlled mostly by treatment and is less influenced by individual behaviors, and (2) family members needed more emotional and informational support from health care providers.[46]

Many Appalachians appreciate narrative formats such as storytelling, indicating that this method can aid their understanding of diabetes and diabetes management. DeBord[49] utilized a specific five-step method of storytelling to create a personal narrative for participants in a variety of workshops involving Appalachians. The involvement of multiple group members is an informal way to increase the visibility and meaning of diabetes among people from a common geographic area. This method results in the cocreation of a single narrative with the potential to raise awareness, correct outdated information, share the latest management and prevention techniques, increase understanding about disease self-management, and develop a supportive community. A diabetes educator or a knowledgeable health professional acts as a resource for distinguishing between fact and fiction, correcting myths or inaccuracies, sharing information about other resources, answering specific disease- or management-related questions, and helping group members realize the social capital they offer one another.

Community-minded, locally attuned approaches are needed to address diabetes in Appalachia. Traditional methods have not been effective in slowing or reversing the disparate prevalence of diabetes in the region. Blaming individuals who are caught in social environments where factors linked with diabetes are complex and often outside their control has not solved the problem. It is important to address diabetes prevention and self-management and the promotion of healthy lifestyles where people work, play, pray, and stay. Awareness of personal routines tied to family traditions; of the expectations of extended kin networks; of stories that relate local beliefs, values, and perceived needs; of available resources; and of clear communication styles is just as important as remediating shortages of health professionals and improving the availability of health insurance. The following are four examples of community-based intervention efforts.

Appalachian Diabetes Control and Translation Project. This joint project is supported by the Centers for Disease Control and Prevention, the Appalachian Regional Commission, and Marshall University's Robert C. Byrd Center for Rural Health.[50] Since 2001 this consortium has mobilized sixty-seven coalitions across Appalachia. Community and local resources, leadership, education, and support are used to emphasize lifestyle changes.

Diabetes: A Family Matter. This translational program and toolkit package,[c] based on the Family Health Model,[45] is intended to increase Appalachian residents' awareness of healthy lifestyles, diabetes prevention, and self-management.[51] Based on best practices and research findings, the toolkit employs an "edutainment" approach to diabetes education, including ideas about family fun, entertainment, rural perspectives, real-life experiences, storytelling, and health literacy. The program focuses on citizen action, education, support, and the mobilization of family and friends and neighborhood and community resources to make the problem of diabetes visible. This kind of citizen action is based on the idea that residents need to be informed about local problems and assume responsibility for their personal and collective well-being. In addition, the program encourages participation by a local leader, preferably a diabetes educator or someone with knowledge and expertise about diabetes, and the use of community coalitions and SUGAR (Support to Unite Generations in the Appalachian Region) volunteers.

A two-year evaluation study is currently under way in one West Virginia, three Kentucky, and eleven Appalachian Ohio counties to disseminate the program and toolkit materials and evaluate the outcomes of community team actions. A train-the-trainer model is used to prepare and support county teams of four or five community representatives, who in turn recruit and train six to ten volunteers in each county. Project participants spread the word about healthy lifestyles, diabetes prevention, and diabetes self-management. The team members work individually and collectively to make diabetes more visible in the community by sharing knowledge with family members, friends, and local groups. Teams cooperate with others to hold special events to inform the community about diabetes. Local empowerment through information, skills, resources, and support is an important way to increase knowledge about diabetes risks and suggest how people can help themselves.

The Asheville Model. This model focuses on the idea that diabetes is best treated through self-management activities, lifestyle routines, and pharmaceutical therapy. Initiated by the city of Asheville, North Carolina, in 1996 and replicated in Polk County, Florida, this employer-based program provides education and personal oversight for employees with chronic health problems, including diabetes.[52] A structured curriculum is used, and employees are offered the opportunity to participate in several face-to-face discussions with pharmacists. At the end of one year, participants had improved HbA1c levels, reduced systolic and diastolic blood pressure, and decreased hospitalizations and emergency room visits. This type of intervention, using either nurse practitioners or pharmacists, could be used to satisfy the ongoing need for diabetes education in Appalachia, monitor lifestyle changes, clarify misinformation, and intervene earlier to prevent comorbidities.

Strengthening Communities to Prevent Diabetes in Rural Appalachia. With funding from the Centers for Disease Control, this five-year project was started in September 2010 to develop diabetes coalitions, mobilize partnerships, develop strategic plans, and use interventions with the broadest sustainable impact to evaluate behavioral changes, policies, and environmental improvements to promote healthy lifestyles and reduce diabetes risks. Teams from Ohio University, Marshall University, and the Center for Appalachian Philanthropy will collaborate to reduce morbidity and premature mortality and eliminate health disparities associated with diabetes in rural Appalachian communities. The project will assist eleven county partners from Kentucky, Mississippi, Ohio, Virginia, and West Virginia to reduce the disproportionate burden of diabetes in the vulnerable populations of rural Appalachia. Working with community volunteers and supporters, Strengthening Communities will draw on existing coalitions to form a collaborative network that mobilizes and empowers local citizen action in the eleven counties.

Further Research

Designing and implementing cost-effective interventions to address the problems of diabetes in Appalachia will require additional research in several areas. First, more research is needed to identify specific variables linked to diabetes risk, prevalence, and self-management in the various geographic areas of Appalachia. Although awareness of disparities between Appalachian and non-Appalachian regions is growing, more needs to be known about the sociocultural and environmental factors that result in a higher incidence of diabetes in some Appalachian counties. State prevalence data and underlying risk factors need to be aggregated and differentiated by the Appalachian Regional Commission's economic designations. Longitudinal research designs that compare cohorts from different geographic regions (including environmental variables) and that consider interactions of multiple household members would be useful in identifying how literacy, health literacy, family history, traditions, and beliefs correlate with diabetes prevalence and comorbidities. Comparison of the risks associated with rural and urban places would be another useful contribution to the literature. In addition, more needs to be known about diabetes' link to obesity and a sedentary lifestyle in both younger and older residents of the region and throughout the life span.

Second, more information is needed about the way families support or hinder type 2 diabetes self-management, and intervention studies involving families must be conducted. Although the literature identifies the importance of family support for those with type 1 diabetes, little research has been conducted on how family processes influence type 2 diabetes self-management[27] and how family members support self-care regimens.[33] The important questions to be answered are: What mechanisms do Appalachian families use to support a member with type 2 diabetes? What family characteristics are the most important indicators of good diabetes self-management? What changes in the social environment need to occur?

Third, education is needed to empower individuals to successfully self-manage diabetes outside the purview of health care providers and to address the changing care needs and risks occurring over a lifetime. It is important to know the most efficacious and cost-effective ways to structure and deliver diabetes education in Appalachia. Studies that consider various types of interventions with individuals, groups, and families are needed, in addition to longitudinal studies that compare interventions utilizing different formats with more conventional formats currently in use. Because cost and availability are of concern to many in Appalachia and other parts of the nation, investigations are needed to examine the financial resources required to provide diabetes education versus the potential costs if it is not provided.

Another area of inquiry involves the lack of health professionals, specialists, and expert services in some parts of Appalachia. Studies that test the effectiveness of using nurse practitioners to deliver diabetes care and self-management education to remote areas of Appalachia would be useful in determining long-term feasibility. Finally, the training and use of local health coaches to educate and support residents could be a good way to increase the visibility of diabetes and disseminate information about diabetes risks, healthy lifestyles, and diabetes self-management.

Policy Recommendations

Policies to address and better understand diabetes in Appalachia must begin with support for electronic data-collection systems in which complex risk factor information is linked with diabetes diagnosis, medical treatment, education provided, care management, and disease outcomes. Currently, most information about diabetes comes from state BRFSS telephone surveys; this is a useful survey mechanism, but it is based on self-reports. In addition, this method of data collection fails to capture the risks associated with an increasing number of children and youths being diagnosed with type 2 diabetes, as well as information about those who may have the disease but have not been diagnosed. It is time to institute replicable statewide systems to track medical care, medical costs, risk variables, economic costs, and health outcomes at the point of care over time. Implementing such systems will be costly initially, but they are needed to obtain a true picture of diabetes in Appalachia.

The use of technologies to deliver public health messages must be re-envisioned. Webcasts, social networks, DVDs, the Internet, and cell phones should all be used to increase local knowledge, community health training, and leadership development with regard to diabetes. The challenge is to use these technologies in a cost-effective manner in areas of Appalachia where technology access might be limited. Assuring that the region is not disadvantaged by a "digital divide" that limits information access should be at the forefront of policy considerations.

Policies are needed that approach diabetes prevention from a family-focused perspective. Effective interventions to reduce the prevalence of diabetes or to manage the disease come down to getting individuals and families to alter their health routines to favor well-being, prevent disease risks, and enhance quality of life. Households are where self-management occurs. Thus, programs that address nutrition, portion sizes, food preparation, healthy lifestyles, and physical activity for the entire family are needed.

Communities in Appalachia must assume responsibility for the health of their residents. Waiting for the federal and state governments to act or expecting health professionals and services to relocate to the region has proved ineffective. It is time for policies that mobilize schools, businesses, coalitions, faith-based ministries, social groups, workplaces, community-based organizations, and local leadership to act as avenues of health promotion and risk reduction. Links among chronic care programs and the faster diffusion of effective interventions are needed. City and county government policies must drive change at the local level to promote healthy communities; these initiatives might include creating community gardens, developing local food markets, assuring that food pantries carry items with high nutritional value, educating food stamp recipients about good nutrition, addressing environmental concerns, encouraging physical activity, and creating school and workplace policies to address families.

Notes

a. The BRFSS is an annual state-based system of health surveys used to assess key behavioral risk factors and chronic conditions in noninstitutionalized U.S. adults aged 18 years and older. The BRFSS response rate varies across states and counties; this may affect state comparisons if the determinants of nonresponse are associated with diabetes prevalence. The BRFSS data are based on self-reports and do not provide estimates of undiagnosed diabetes.

b. An environmental scan is a survey method that uses a variety of techniques to examine the scope of a problem from many different perspectives. In this case, professionals and clinicians employed in health departments and clinics gathered diabetes educational materials, and a qualitative study was conducted with fourteen families.

c. The free downloadable program and toolkit materials are available at www .diabetesfamily.net. The Diabetes: A Family Matter website is intended to be a one-stop portal for those with diabetes living in the Appalachian region. It provides educational information, resources, and social networking capacities for persons with diabetes, family members, health care providers, and others.

References

1. Centers for Disease Control and Prevention. National diabetes fact sheet. Available at: http://www.cdc.gov/diabetes/pubs/pdf/ndfs_2011.pdf. Accessed February 24, 2011.

2. Egede LE, Zheng D, Simpson K. Comorbid depression is associated with increased health care use and expenditures in individuals with diabetes. *Diabetes Care.* 2002;25:464–470.

3. American Diabetes Association. Summary of revisions for the 2010 clinical practice recommendations. *Diabetes Care.* 2010;13(Supplement I):S3.

4. National Institute for Digestive and Kidney Diseases. National diabetes information clearinghouse. Available at: http://diabetes.niddk.nih.gov. Accessed November 2, 2006.

5. Centers for Disease Control and Prevention. Number of people with diabetes increases to 24 million. Available at: http://www.cdc.gov/media/pressrel/2008/r080624.htm. Accessed October 25, 2008.

6. Centers for Disease Control and Prevention. Number (in millions) of civilian/non-institutionalized persons with diagnosed diabetes, United States, 1980–2006. Available at: www.cdc.gov/diabetes/statistics/prev/national/figpersons.htm. Accessed March 11, 2010.

7. Danaei G, Friedman AB, Oza S, Murray CJ, Ezzati M. Diabetes prevalence and diagnosis in U.S. states: analysis of health surveys. *Popul Health Metr.* 2009;7:16.

8. Voeks JH, McClure LA, Go RC, et al. Regional differences in diabetes as a possible contributor to the geographic disparity in stroke mortality: the reasons for geographic and racial differences in stroke study. *Stroke.* 2008;39: 1675–1680.

9. Barker L, Crespo R, Gerzoff RB, Denham S, Shrewsberry M, Cornelius-Averhart D. Residence in a distressed county in Appalachia as a risk factor for diabetes, Behavioral Risk Factor Surveillance System, 2006–2007. *Prev Chronic Dis.* 2010;7:A104.

10. Eaton WW. Epidemiologic evidence on the comorbidity of depression and diabetes. *J Psychosom Res.* 2002;53:903–906.

11. de Groot M, Doyle T, Hockman E, et al. Depression among type 2 diabetes rural Appalachian clinic attendees. *Diabetes Care.* 2007;30:1602–1604.

12. Appalachian Rural Health Institute (ARHI). Prevalence of diabetes. Athens, OH: Voinovich School of Leadership and Public Affairs at Ohio University; June 2004. Available at: http://www.ohio.edu/voinovichschool/news_info/publications/docs/upload/Diabetes-Factors-Final.pdf. Accessed August 28, 2011.

13. Appalachian Rural Health Institute (ARHI). Diabetes. Athens, OH: Voinovich School of Leadership and Public Affairs at Ohio University; June 2006. Available at: http://www.ohio.edu/voinovichschool/news_info/publications/docs/upload/Diabetes-06-Final.pdf. Accessed August 28, 2011.

14. Appalachian Rural Health Institute (ARHI). Health needs assessment survey III, research report. Athens, OH: Voinovich School of Leadership and Public Affairs at Ohio University; December 2009. Available at: http://www.ohio.edu/voinovichschool/news_info/publications/docs/upload/Diabetes_TO-PRINT.pdf. Accessed August 28, 2011.

15. Schwartz F, Ruhil AV, Denham S, Shubrook J, Simpson C, Boyd SL. High self-reported prevalence of diabetes mellitus, heart disease, and stroke in 11 counties of rural Appalachian Ohio. *J Rural Health.* 2009;25:226–230.

16. Centers for Disease Control and Prevention. Distribution of age at diagnosis of diabetes among adult incident cases aged 18–79 years, United States, 2008. Available at: http://www.cdc.gov/diabetes/statistics/age/fig1.htm. Accessed March 11, 2010.

17. Denham SA, Wood LE, Remsberg K. Diabetes care: provider disparities in the U.S. Appalachian region. *Rural Remote Health.* 2010;10:1320.

18. Denham SA, Remsburg K, Wood L. Diabetes education in the Appalachian region: providers' views. *Rural Remote Health.* 2010;10:1321.

19. Roark A, Wallace G. Appalachian culture: a thumbnail sketch. Memphis, TN: University of Tennessee–Knoxville, Department of Audiology and Speech Pathology; 1996.

20. Rudd RE, Moeykens BA, Colton TC. Health and literacy: a review of medical and public health literature. In: Comings J, Garner B, Smith C, eds. *Annual Review of Adult Learning and Literacy.* Vol. 1. San Francisco, CA: Jossey-Bass; 2000:158–199.

21. Kleinbeck C. Reaching positive diabetes outcomes for patients with low literacy. *Home Healthcare Nurse.* 2005;23:16–22.

22. Denham SA, Meyer MG, Toborg MA, Mande MJ. Providing health education to Appalachia populations. *Holist Nurs Pract.* 2004;18:293–301.

23. Nagelkerk J, Reick K, Meengs L. Perceived barriers and effective strategies to diabetes self-management. *J Adv Nurs.* 2006;54:151–158.

24. Knowler WC, Barrett-Connor E, Fowler SE, et al. Reduction in the incidence of type 2 diabetes with lifestyle intervention or metformin. *N Engl J Med.* 2002;346:393–403.

25. Visser A, Snoek F. Perspectives on education and counseling for diabetes patients. *Patient Educ Couns.* 2004;53:251–255.

26. Funnell MM, Anderson RM, Arnold MS, et al. Empowerment: an idea whose time has come in diabetes education. *Diabetes Educ.* 1991;17:37–41.

27. Fisher L, Chesla CA, Bartz RJ, et al. The family and type 2 diabetes: a framework for intervention. *Diabetes Educ.* 1998;24:599–607.

28. Rolland JS. *Families, Illness, and Disabilities: An Integrative Treatment Model.* New York, NY: Basic Books; 1994.

29. Epple C, Wright AL, Joish VN, Bauer M. The role of active family nutritional support in Navajos' type 2 diabetes metabolic control. *Diabetes Care.* 2003;26:2829–2834.

30. Cardenas L, Vallbona C, Baker S, Yusim S. Adult onset diabetes mellitus: glycemic control and family function. *Am J Med Sci.* 1987;293:28–33.

31. Garay-Sevilla ME, Nava LE, Malacara JM, et al. Adherence to treatment and social support in patients with non-insulin dependent diabetes mellitus. *J Diabetes Complications.* 1995;9:81–86.

32. Primomo J, Yates BC, Woods NF. Social support for women during chronic illness: the relationship among sources and types to adjustment. *Res Nurs Health.* 1990;13:153–161.

33. Anderson LM, Shinn C, Charles, JS, et al. Community interventions to promote healthy social environments: early childhood development and family housing. A report on recommendations of the Task Force on Community Preventive Services. *MMWR Recomm Rep.* 2002;51:1–8.

34. Denham SA, Manoogian M, Schuster L. Managing family support and dietary routines: type 2 diabetes in rural Appalachian families. *Families, Systems and Health.* 2007;25(1):36–52.

35. Schuster L. Family support in dietary routines in Appalachians with type 2 diabetes [master's thesis]. Athens, OH: Ohio University; 2005.

36. Chesla CA, Fisher L, Skaff MM, Mullan JT, Gilliss CL, Kanter R. Family predictors of disease management over one year in Latino and European American patients with type 2 diabetes. *Fam Process.* 2003;42:375–390.

37. Keltner B, Keltner NL, Farren E. Family routines and conduct disorders in adolescent girls. *West J Nurs Res.* 1990;12:161–170; discussion 170–174.

38. Trief PM, Sandberg J, Greenberg RP, et al. Describing support: a qualitative study of couples living with diabetes. *Families, Systems and Health.* 2003;21:57–67.

39. Manoogian MM, Harter LM, Denham SA. The storied nature of health legacies in the familial experience of type 2 diabetes. *Journal of Family Communication.* 2010;10:1–17.

40. Denham SA. Family health in a rural Appalachian Ohio county. *Journal of Appalachian Studies.* 1996;2(2):299–310.

41. Denham SA. An ethnographic study of family health in Appalachian microsystems [PhD dissertation]. Birmingham, AL: University of Alabama at Birmingham; 1997.

42. Denham SA. The definition and practice of family health. *J Fam Nurs.* 1999;5(2):133–159.

43. Denham SA. Family health: during and after death of a family member. *J Fam Nurs.* 1999;5(2):160–183.

44. Denham SA. Family health in an economically disadvantaged population. *J Fam Nurs.* 1999;5(2):184–213.

45. Denham SA. *Family Health: A Framework for Nursing.* Philadelphia, PA: F. A. Davis; 2003.

46. White P, Smith SM, Hevey D, O'Dowd T. Understanding type 2 diabetes: including the family member's perspective. *Diabetes Educ.* 2009;35:810–817.

47. Fiese BH, Wamboldt FS. Family routines, rituals, and asthma management: a proposal for family-based strategies to increase treatment adherence. *Families, Systems and Health.* 2000;18(4):405–418.

48. deGroot M, Denham SA. Pilot and feasibility of "The Caring for Diabetes" family diabetes intervention. Funded by the Appalachian Rural Health Institute Diabetes Research Initiative; 2006.

49. DeBord A. Telling your own story: a story illumination project. *Journal of Appalachian Studies.* 2003;9(2):363–376.

50. Centers for Disease Control and Prevention. Appalachian diabetes control and translation project. Available at: http://www.cdc.gov/diabetes/projects/appalachian .htm. Accessed May 25, 2011.

51. Denham SA, Rathbun A. ARHI community health assessment: diabetes findings. Athens, OH: Appalachian Regional Health Institute, Ohio University; 2005.

52. Iyer R, Coderre P, McKelvey T, et al. An employer-based, pharmacist intervention model for patients with type 2 diabetes. *Am J Health Syst Pharm.* 2010;67:312–316.

7

Obesity and Food Insecurity

Jennifer Chubinski and Mark A. Carrozza

Obesity has increased dramatically in the United States since 1980.[1] It is now the second leading cause of preventable death, contributing to more than 100,000 deaths annually.[2] The health effects of obesity are well documented, including increased rates of cancer, diabetes, and heart disease. These conditions lead to greater health care spending, disability, and death.[3–7] Because obesity is not distributed randomly across the population, certain groups are more likely than others to be obese.[8] Minorities, women, the poor, and the less educated generally have a higher risk of being obese.[8, 9] In addition, rural Americans tend to have higher levels of obesity than those living in urban areas.[10, 11]

This chapter examines obesity in the Appalachian region by compiling data from various sources on the topic, and it presents recommendations for future research and policy directions. The scarcity of data on obesity in Appalachia is striking, particularly for children. Thus, a variety of data are used to document findings, drawing on a broad spectrum of national, state, and local sources.[a] In addition, this chapter examines the linkages between food scarcity and obesity in Appalachian rural and urban areas. Although it may seem counterintuitive, it has been posited that food scarcity can lead to increased rates of obesity[11–13] through several mechanisms, including binge eating when food is available, poor nutritional habits, and barriers to food purchase, such as distance to the closest supermarket and limited food choice in local grocery stores. This chapter distinguishes between Appalachian migrants—that is, those who reside outside the region but were born in or have a parent who was born in one of the 420 Appalachian counties—and Appalachians who currently reside in an Appalachian county.[b] Locating data on obesity or any health status indicator in which Appalachian status is known is quite difficult. Most of the comparisons in this chapter are between individuals living in Appalachian counties and those living in non-Appalachian counties rather than between Appalachians and non-Appalachians. Although this is not ideal, it shows the regional differences in obesity and clearly indicates a serious need for better data on Appalachians.

Obesity among Appalachian Adults

The standard measurement of obesity is the body mass index (BMI). For adults, BMI is an individual's weight in kilograms divided by the square of their height in meters (kg/m^2). A BMI of 25 or greater is considered overweight, and a BMI of 30 or greater is considered obese. BMIs for children (aged 2 to 17 years) are calculated and then plotted on growth charts by age and sex to obtain a percentile ranking. This percentile ranking classifies the child as underweight, healthy weight, overweight, or obese. BMI is a controversial measure of obesity because it does not account for differences in sex and age (except for children), race, or ethnicity, or for variances in bone density, muscle mass, or body fat. Although there is much academic debate about whether BMI is an accurate measure, it is the current standard for obesity studies.[c]

The Appalachian Region as a Whole. The Centers for Disease Control and Prevention (CDC) identifies Appalachia, along with parts of some southern states and tribal lands, as having the highest rates of obesity and diabetes in the nation.[14] In 2008 Alabama, Mississippi, and West Virginia had the highest levels of adult obesity among the thirteen Appalachian states, with rates exceeding 30 percent (figure 7.1). Although New York, Virginia, and Maryland had the lowest levels of obesity, with rates around 25 percent, this still represents a major concern. In the nation as a whole, seven of the ten states with the highest adult obesity levels were Appalachian states. Within the Appalachian region, Appalachian counties have a slightly higher rate of obesity than non-Appalachian counties (table 7.1).

Obesity status in Appalachia varies by subregion and by county economic status. According to the economic status classification developed by the Appalachian Regional Commission, distressed and at-risk counties have obesity rates considerably higher than those in transitional,

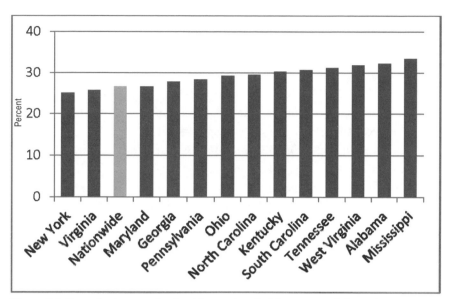

Figure 7.1. State obesity rates for the thirteen Appalachian states and the nation, 2008.

Table 7.1. Average Obesity Rates by Appalachian County Status, Economic Status, and Subregion

	% Obese
Thirteen-state region	27.6
Non-Appalachian counties	27.2
Appalachian counties	28.8
Appalachian county economic status	
Distressed	32.7
At-risk	30.7
Transitional	28.8
Competitive	27.0
Attainment	26.5
Appalachian subregion	
Northern	28.5
Central	31.2
Southern	28.6

Source: Centers for Disease Control and Prevention. Behavioral Risk Factor Surveillance System data, 2007.

competitive, and attainment counties (table 7.1). As such, Central Appalachia, with a higher number of distressed and at-risk counties, has the highest obesity rate.

Rural-Urban Variations. Both urban and rural regions of Appalachia are experiencing sizable increases in the percentage of adults and children who are overweight and obese, but rural populations seem to be at higher risk. A recent study by the Ohio Department of Health identified the rural counties of Appalachian Ohio as being at risk for obesity.[15] The report expressed particular concern about the changing perception of what is normal: "because the prevalence of obesity is very high in Ohio's rural populations, and in particular Ohio's Appalachian populations, a new norm may have emerged for what is considered a normal body weight" (p. 29).[15] In addition, the National Association of Counties found rural populations to be at higher risk of obesity because of their limited access to health care, the presence of food insecurity and food deserts (defined later in this chapter), and the existence of few opportunities for physical activity, among other issues.[11]

Appalachian Ohio. Of Ohio's eighty-eight counties, thirty-two in the southern and eastern portions of the state are classified as Appalachian. According to the 2008 Ohio Family Health Survey,[16] 31 percent of the adult residents of these Appalachian counties had BMIs greater than 30, based on self-reported height and weight. This compares to 27 percent in metropolitan counties, 29 percent in rural counties, 29 percent in suburban counties, and 28 percent statewide. Five of the ten most obese counties in Ohio were Appalachian counties, with Monroe County ranking highest at 42 percent. There was a similar phenomenon among children (discussed later).

Cincinnati Region. Data from the 2005 Greater Cincinnati Community Health Status Survey[17] show that approximately 68 percent of first- and second-generation white Appalachians were considered obese, based on self-reported height and weight—almost 11 percentage points higher than the rate for white non-Appalachians (table 7.2). The percentage of white Appalachians with severe or very severe obesity was almost double that of white non-Appalachians.

These data, collected from various sources and at different times using different instruments, all point to a higher obesity rate in low-income

Table 7.2. Adult Obesity Status in Greater Cincinnati				
	Severely Obese (%)	Very Severely Obese (%)	Total Obese (%)	No. of Respondents
White Appalachians	6.3	5.0	67.7	464
White non-Appalachians	3.8	2.8	57.1	1,234
Source: Greater Cincinnati Community Health Status Survey, 2005.				

Appalachian counties and among migrants from Appalachia. Nonetheless, there are insufficient data to infer a direct link between Appalachian heritage and obesity.

Obesity among Appalachian Children

Studying adult obesity is important, but understanding childhood obesity is critical because overweight children are at a high risk of developing major health problems as adults.[18] According to the U.S. surgeon general, overweight adolescents have a 70 percent chance of becoming overweight or obese adults.[19]

Similar to adults, overweight and obesity rates for children have increased dramatically. Over the last thirty years, obesity has risen for all childhood age groups.[20, 21] Like adults, children are eating outside the home more frequently; have greater access to calorie-dense, nutrition-poor foods; and have fewer opportunities for physical activity. Rural children, in particular, have a higher risk of obesity because they have lower levels of physical activity. Children in Appalachia often eat a traditional high-fat, high-calorie diet.[11] Schools are also being built farther away from city centers, which, along with other factors, has significantly reduced the number of children who walk or ride bicycles to school.[21]

The data available to study childhood obesity are scarce. The Behavioral Risk Factor Surveillance System (BRFSS), used extensively to evaluate the public health system, currently provides limited information on children and youths, leaving researchers with an incomplete picture of what childhood obesity really looks like.[d] The difficulty is compounded when seeking data on children of Appalachian decent.

Appalachian Ohio. Based on the 2008 Ohio Family Health Survey,[16] adolescents (aged 12 to 17 years) in Ohio's Appalachian counties have an obesity rate of 22 percent, compared with 18 percent in metropolitan counties, 19 percent in rural counties, 16 percent in suburban counties, and 18 percent in the state as a whole. Similar to the results for adults, the Appalachian counties lead the state in adolescent obesity rates. Six of the ten most obese counties in Ohio for adolescents are Appalachian, with Meigs County number one at 53 percent.

Cincinnati Region. When the 2005 Greater Cincinnati Child Well-Being Survey[22] asked adult respondents whether their children were over-weight, underweight, or about the right weight, 14.6 percent of parents of first- and second-generation white Appalachians reported that their children were overweight, compared with 7.4 percent of white non-Appalachians.

Researchers at Cincinnati Children's Hospital Medical Center con-ducted a study in 2006 using a matched parent-child sample from pedia-tricians' offices to examine the accuracy of parental perceptions of their children's weight.[23] Based on 41 Appalachian (that is, either the child, a parent, or both were born in an Appalachian county) and more than 350 non-Appalachian participants, the researchers found that most par-ents were fairly accurate at determining their children's actual weight and obesity status. The Appalachian children had slightly but not significantly higher estimated and actual BMIs than non-Appalachian children.

Thus, based on the available data, it is not possible to state confident-ly whether Appalachian children, regardless of location, have increased obesity rates. However, Appalachian-born adults in Kentucky expressed greater concern about childhood obesity than did non-Appalachians when asked, "Would you say childhood obesity in Kentucky is a serious prob-lem, a problem but not serious, or not a problem?"[24] Sixty-five percent of Kentucky adults who were first- or second-generation Appalachians con-sidered childhood obesity a serious problem, compared with 51 percent of non-Appalachian respondents.

Food Security and Obesity

In 2008, 15 percent of U.S. households were food insecure.[25] The U.S. Department of Agriculture defines food insecurity as "households that were uncertain of having, or unable to acquire, enough food to meet the needs of all their members because they had insufficient money or other resources for food."[25] Holben and Pheley[12] found that BMI was greater for individuals from food-insecure households in the six rural Ohio Appalachian counties they studied.

Data from a Current Population Survey conducted in December 2006 showed that respondents from nonmetropolitan areas had higher levels of low or very low food security in the last thirty days and twelve months than those from metropolitan areas (table 7.3).[26] Adults in metropolitan areas of Appalachia had higher rates of low or very low food security than adults in metropolitan areas outside of Appalachia at both thirty days and twelve months. Children living in Appalachian metropolitan areas had lower rates of low or very low food security than non-Appalachian children. In all cases, respondents in nonmetropolitan areas reported higher rates of low or very low food security. The rates among adults living in Appalachian metropolitan areas resembled those in nonmetropolitan areas, while children in Appalachian metropolitan areas were less likely to have low and very low food security than their counterparts in non-Appalachian metropolitan areas. This difference may be due to the food safety net system in place in many Appalachian metropolitan areas, which includes school-based food programs for children. In many communities, children eat two or three meals a day at school and are often provided with food to take home for the weekend.

Access to Food. Access to food is a critical factor in food security. Research has shown that poor food choices are more prevalent in low-income areas,[11] where the phenomenon of food deserts is often to blame. Food

Table 7.3. Respondents with Low or Very Low Food Security

	Last 30 Days			Last 12 Months		
	Non-metropolitan	Non-Appalachian Metropolitan	Appalachian Metropolitan	Non-metropolitan	Non-Appalachian Metropolitan	Appalachian Metropolitan
Children (%)	5.5	4.4	3.3	10.1	7.9	5.6
Adults (%)	6.1	4.6	6.0	12.0	9.1	10.9
Total (%)	6.6	5.1	6.3	13.3	10.1	11.9

Source: Current Population Survey (Food Security Supplement File), December 2006.

Table 7.4. Prevalence of Supermarkets, Grocery Stores, and Convenience Stores per 10,000 by Appalachian County Economic Status

Economic Status	Supermarkets	Grocery Stores	Convenience Stores
Distressed	3.3	4.2	0.9
At-risk	2.7	3.6	0.9
Transitional	2.1	3.0	0.8
Competitive	1.7	2.7	0.9
Attainment	1.7	2.1	0.5
Remainder of U.S.	2.2	3.2	1.0

Source: County Business Patterns, 2006.

deserts are areas where a significant portion of the population spends its food budget in locations that do not have fresh fruits and vegetables.[15] Studies have shown that living close to supermarkets can be linked to lower obesity rates, while living close to small convenience stores can be linked to higher obesity rates.[27] Similarly, living close to fast-food restaurants can increase the risk of obesity.[6, 15, 28] Being able to shop at grocery stores with a good selection of fresh produce, and being able to afford that produce, decreases the likelihood of an individual being overweight or obese.

Table 7.4 shows the number of supermarkets, grocery stores, and convenience stores per 10,000 population by Appalachian county economic status. As economic conditions improve (moving from distressed to attainment), the supermarkets and grocery stores per 10,000 population decrease, while the number of convenience stores remains relatively flat. There are more grocery stores per capita than supermarkets in all regions of Appalachia. Grocery stores can vary significantly in size and range of goods sold, while supermarkets typically sell a wide variety of food items and general merchandise. On the whole, individuals living in areas with higher poverty cannot travel as far to do their grocery shopping; thus there are more, probably smaller, grocery stores in these counties than in counties with less poverty.

The economically distressed and at-risk regions of Appalachia have higher densities of grocery stores and supermarkets than other Appalachian counties and the remainder of the United States. Although there is some difference in the number of grocery stores and supermarkets per person, the rate of convenience stores is similar across the board in Appalachian counties. A visual review of a map of fast-food restaurants, full-service restaurants, and drinking establishments per capita (not shown) reveals no clear spatial difference between Appalachian and non-Appalachian counties.

Based on the aforementioned research, high per capita rates of super-markets and grocery stores should be linked to lower rates of obesity. In Appalachia, however, the data suggest the opposite: in poor regions, obe-sity rates are higher, despite the presence of more supermarkets and gro-cery stores per capita. In the absence of information on the quality of food available at all the retail food establishments, there is no way of knowing whether residents have access to nutrition-dense, healthy, fresh food. In ad-dition, there are currently no data on Appalachian and non-Appalachian food purchase patterns. These and other factors might help explain the conflict between Appalachian obesity rates and food store patterns and previous research.

Food Security for Children in Greater Cincinnati. The 2005 Greater Cincinnati Child Well-Being Survey,[22] conducted in the twenty-two coun-ties surrounding the city, asked four questions about food security for chil-dren. The results showed that first- and second-generation Appalachian children had higher rates of food insecurity than non-Appalachians on all four questions; however, the differences on three of the four questions were not statistically significant. The only question with statistically significant results is shown in table 7.5, which suggests that Appalachians more often than non-Appalachians lacked the money to purchase sufficient food.

Table 7.5. Responses to: "The Food that I Bought Just Didn't Last, and I Didn't Have Money to Get More"

	Often True (%)	Sometimes True (%)	Never True (%)	No. of Respondents
Appalachians*	9	9	82	194
Non-Appalachians	5	13	83	1,345

Source: Greater Cincinnati Child Well-Being Survey, 2005.
* Difference is significant with a Pearson chi-square of 0.033.

Findings

The CDC has identified Appalachia as one of the nation's most obese regions. It is not clear from the data whether individuals of Appalachian descent who have migrated from the region are more or less obese than their non-Appalachian counterparts; however, there may be increased rates of obesity and a poorer diet among the population living in the Appalachian region. The data also imply that parts of Appalachia have higher rates of food insecurity than the rest of the country: rural and economically challenged areas seem to be at higher risk. The data also suggest that Appalachians in the Cincinnati area have higher levels of food insecurity. These conclusions are quite tenuous, however, because establishing links between obesity and food scarcity for the whole region is difficult, given that the available data are based on small sample sizes and incomplete coverage of the Appalachian population.

Model Programs

A number of community-based programs can be used as best-practice models for addressing the issues surrounding obesity. The following case studies describe two such strategies, one in Appalachia and one outside the region.

The Appalachian Sustainable Agriculture Project (ASAP).[29] ASAP is designed to increase access to fresh food and support local agriculture and food production in Appalachia. Linking food producers with consumers at both the individual and the institutional levels, ASAP includes 76 tailgate markets, 82 restaurants and bakeries, 23 grocers, and 14 bed-and-breakfasts where one can buy locally produced food. ASAP describes this as neighbors selling to neighbors, and it is a sustainable model because purchasing dollars remain in the community. ASAP also tries to connect food suppliers with institutions looking to buy local food, linking 2 schools, 4 hospitals, 7 distributors, and 19 other food-related organizations with 246 food suppliers. ASAP's system of connecting buyers with sellers has the potential to make high-quality fresh, locally grown foods more available (and possibly more affordable) to urban and rural Appalachian populations. These efforts are based on the assumption that the availability of better food helps fight obesity.

Shape Up Somerville.[30–34] The Shape Up Somerville project was a community intervention designed to fight childhood obesity in Somerville, Massachusetts. It is one of the best-documented cases of a community-wide intervention to fight childhood obesity. Somerville is a densely populated, culturally and socioeconomically diverse community of mostly young families, blue-collar workers, and immigrants. The project targeted first- to third-grade students, 46 percent of whom were at risk for being overweight or obese, and included the following key elements:

- Improved food service: elimination of unhealthy snacks and increased availability of fresh fruits and vegetables, along with educational programs on new fruits and vegetables
- Curriculum changes: teacher-created curriculum to educate students on the benefits of eating better and to provide increased opportunities for physical activity
- Health report cards: records of the children's health, including BMI scores, sent home by the school
- Change in school culture: a ban on before-lunch fund-raisers involving the sale of baked goods, candy, and other sugary snacks
- After-school changes: a modified after-school curriculum that included more cooking classes and games involving physical activity
- Parent and community outreach: a newsletter, coupons, and sponsored community events that focused on eating better and increasing physical activity
- Shape Up–approved restaurants: collaborative effort involving the city, program researchers, and twenty-one local restaurants to offer lower-calorie items, smaller portions, and fruits and vegetables as side dishes
- Safe routes to school: hiring a pedestrian-bike coordinator and creating safe routes so more children could walk or bike to school
- School nurses: training more than fifty local clinicians and school nurses on how to assess and deal with overweight children

Outcomes of the program included greater fruit and vegetable consumption at lunch and reductions in the children's weight.

Further Research

This chapter is only an initial look at the link between obesity and food security in Appalachia. There is a tremendous need for additional research in the following areas.

Better Data. There is an urgent need for more and better data. Appalachians are a large enough group that they should be identified in national data sets. None of the national, federally funded data used to examine obesity and food scarcity issues include an indicator of Appalachian descent that can identify Appalachians within or outside the region. Most data do, however, include a county identifier, which could be used to establish a regional indicator, under the assumption that all persons within the county are Appalachian. Although small-area projects such as the Greater Cincinnati Community Health Status Survey,[17] the Greater Cincinnati Child Well-Being Survey,[22] and the Kentucky Health Issues Poll[24] include indicators of Appalachian descent, these projects are limited in scope due to cost constraints; this makes it difficult to collect sufficient data, and the resulting estimates of obesity and obesity-related illness are tenuous at best. Also, non–federally funded data-collection efforts that provide comprehensive coverage of the thirteen-state Appalachian region are nonexistent. Projects such as the Ohio Family Health Survey,[16] the Greater Cincinnati Community Health Status Survey,[17] and the Kentucky Health Issues Poll[24] permit a patchwork analysis of the region, but separately, they are inadequate for such a large area with such a diverse population. Without reliable, national data sets that identify Appalachians, it is nearly impossible to determine conclusively whether obesity is higher among Appalachians than non-Appalachians.

Food Choice versus Food Scarcity. Some local and regional researchers have suggested that Appalachian lifestyles include a diet rich in fried and fatty foods. Thus, even with a full-service grocery store full of affordable fruits and vegetables, obesity rates may not decrease. It is important to study to what extent obesity derives from a lack of choice and to what extent it is based on a certain type of diet.

Rural versus Urban. There are insufficient data to compare urban and rural Appalachians. The development of benchmarks on obesity and food availability for urban versus rural populations would help define and refine public health programming.

Policy Recommendations

Several national organizations are working to identify and implement policy solutions to food access and obesity issues in America. These policies would improve not only access to healthy food but also the health of many communities. Some of these policy solutions could be implemented in Appalachian communities even during difficult financial times.

Many leading experts suggest that changes to federal food policy are required to ensure that families have access to nutritious food. These include monitoring implementation of the 2007 changes to the Women, Infants, and Children (WIC) program and changes to the funding of the Supplemental Nutrition Assistance Program (SNAP; formerly food stamps). Recent changes to WIC are expected to increase the demand for fresh food,[35] but policy makers should ensure that WIC-authorized stores are following the guidelines to guarantee a reasonable supply of healthy choices. Experts also suggest that federal policy should encourage farmers' markets to accept SNAP and WIC by authorizing funding and support for the adoption of these practices.

Although federal policy is important, community-level action is critical for real change. Experts across the board suggest a variety of local strategies for improving health status and food security. These strategies include public-private partnerships to open and sustain full-service grocery stores in communities without access to healthful foods. However, this is a major project with a long timeline. Smaller entrepreneurial ventures are often easier to get up and running quickly. Thus, many successful neighborhood campaigns focus on small-scale innovations such as mobile vendors, farmers' markets, vending machines, farm stands, and community gardens. These operations often produce additional local benefits, such as supporting local farmers or providing flexible employment to area residents. Along with adding food options to the local market, many national experts suggest limiting the number of fast-food restaurants in communities where they are already abundant. This has been done by implementing zoning regulations to achieve a balance between fast-food restaurants and convenience stores and those establishments that offer fresh fruit and vegetables. Zoning and land-use controls can also be utilized to promote potential sites for community gardens and farmers' markets.

Dealing with childhood obesity is critical because obese children face a lifetime of adverse health effects if their weight is not controlled. Children spend most of their day at school, so most food policy experts suggest changes to school policies. These changes fall into two categories: (1) providing only healthy foods in schools by improving the quality of meals served at breakfast and lunch and removing unhealthy foods from vending machines, and (2) requiring all schools (K–12) to set aside time each day for all children to be physically active.

Acknowledgment

The authors would like to thank Diana Trapp, Program Assistant at The Health Foundation of Greater Cincinnati, for her help on this project.

Notes

a. This chapter draws on multiple data sources to describe the causes and consequences of obesity in Appalachia and examines national surveys of both people and businesses, national administrative databases of governmental support, and state and regional surveys of individual health status. Specifically, the following sources were used: (1) The Current Population Survey (CPS)[26] is a monthly survey of approximately 60,000 households in the United States that includes detailed data on food insufficiency and food insecurity. Because the CPS does not identify respondents by Appalachian birth and does not clearly identify Appalachian counties, the Appalachian population was approximated by selecting survey respondents from any state with Appalachian counties. Respondents from the Office of Management and Budget's defined metropolitan statistical areas that are predominantly (at least 50 percent) in Appalachia were assumed to be Appalachian. (2) County Business Patterns (CBP) is an annual accounting of economic activity by industry for all counties in the United States. The 2006 CBP data[36] were used to measure the availability of food through estimates of the number of supermarkets or grocery stores, convenience stores, fast-food restaurants, and full-service restaurants in the thirteen Appalachian states. (3) The U.S. Department of Agriculture's Economic Research Service[37] publishes nationwide data on food stamp participation, cash benefits, and poverty for all counties. (4) The Behavioral Risk Factor Surveillance System (BRFSS),[38] conducted annually by the Centers for Disease Control and Prevention (CDC), is a nationwide survey of 350,000 adults regarding health risk behaviors, preventive health practices, and access to health care for chronic disease and injury. In November 2009 the CDC employed Bayesian multilevel models to produce reliable county-level measures of diabetes and obesity for all counties in the United States. This measure is the primary indicator of obesity used in this chapter, unless otherwise noted. (5) In late 2008 the Ohio Department of Jobs and Family Services conducted the Ohio Family Health Survey (comprising more than 50,000 adult telephone responses and more than 13,000 child proxy responses).[16] First- and second-generation Appalachian status was based on county of birth for the respondent and his or her parents. (6) The Kentucky Health Issues Poll (this chapter uses data from the 2009 poll)[24] is conducted annually by The Foundation for a Healthy Kentucky and The Health Foundation of Greater Cincinnati. It addresses issues that affect the health and health care of Kentucky residents. (7) The Greater Cincinnati Community Health Status Survey is conducted every five years (this chapter uses data from the 2005 survey)[17] and provides a snapshot of how Appalachians in the area differ from non-Appalachians. (8) The 2005 Greater Cincinnati Child Well-Being Survey[22] was conducted in the twenty-two counties surrounding Cincinnati through adult proxy interviews.

b. This chapter uses county of birth to determine Appalachian status. When that information was not available, residence in an Appalachian county was used as a substitute.

c. Many of the BMI data presented in this chapter are based on self-reported height and weight. There is some evidence that people overreport height and underreport weight, meaning that the figures in this chapter could underestimate actual obesity rates.[39, 40] Only a limited number of studies have actually measured the participants' height and weight to get accurate BMI numbers. The findings of one such study are discussed in the children's section of this chapter.

d. The limited data on children and youths could not be aggregated or separated by county or Appalachian status. Data were available for Kentucky and Mississippi high school students, Ohio youths, New York children younger than 5 years by county, and North Carolina children aged 2–18 years who were receiving services in the public health–sponsored WIC clinic. The CDC also has some statewide aggregate data for West Virginia, South Carolina, North Carolina, New York, Georgia, and Tennessee.

References

1. National Center for Health Statistics. Health, United States, 2007 with chartbook on trends in the health of Americans. Hyattsville, MD: National Center for Health Statistics; 2007.

2. Williams CH. The built environment and physical activity: what is the relationship? Princeton, NJ: The Robert Wood Johnson Foundation; 2007.

3. Finkelstein EA, Fiebelkorn IC, Wang G. State-level estimates of annual medical expenditures attributable to obesity. *Obes Res.* 2004;12:18–24.

4. Finkelstein EA, Fiebelkorn IC, Wang G. National medical spending attributable to overweight and obesity: how much, and who's paying? *Health Aff (Millwood).* 2003;Suppl Web Exclusives (W3): 219–226.

5. Wolf AM, Colditz GA. Current estimates of the economic cost of obesity in the United States. *Obes Res.* 1998;6:97–106.

6. National Center for Health Statistics. Health, United States, 2008 with chartbook. Hyattsville, MD: National Center for Health Statistics; 2009.

7. U.S. Department of Health and Human Services. The surgeon general's call to action to prevent and decrease overweight and obesity. Rockville, MD: U.S. Department of Health and Human Services, Public Health Service, Office of the Surgeon General; 2001.

8. Lopez RP. Neighborhood risk factors for obesity. *Obesity (Silver Spring).* 2007;15:2111–2119.

9. Cuttler L, Singer M, Simpson L, Gallan A, Nevar A, Silvers JB. Obesity in children and families across Ohio: results from the 2008 Ohio Family Health Survey. Cincinnati, OH: Child Policy Research Center. Available at: http://www.cincinnatichildrens.org/assets/0/78/1067/1395/1833/1835/9810/9d85d8b3–3373–40f6–9c5b-64d549bfc85b.pdf. Accessed May 12, 2010.

10. Appalachian Ohio Healthy Living Task Force. Report to the governor on addressing obesity in Appalachian Ohio. Nelsonville, OH: Osteopathic Heritage Foundation of Nelsonville; 2006. Available at: http://www.osteopathicheritage.org/UserUploads/HLTF_Executive_Summary.pdf. Accessed April 2, 2009.

11. Dillon C, Rowland C. Rural obesity—strategies to support rural counties in building capacity. Washington, DC: National Association of Counties; 2008.

12. Holben DH, Pheley AM. Diabetes risk and obesity in food-insecure households in rural Appalachian Ohio. *Prev Chronic Dis.* 2006;3:A82.

13. Babey SH, Diamant AL, Hastert TA, et al. Designed for disease: the link between local food environments and obesity and diabetes. Davis, CA: California Center for Public Health Advocacy, PolicyLink, and the UCLA Center for Health Policy Research; 2008.

14. Centers for Disease Control and Prevention. Press release: highest rates of obesity, diabetes in the South, Appalachia, and some tribal lands. Available at: http://www.cdc.gov/media/pressrel/2009/r091119c.htm. Accessed February 28, 2010.

15. Ohio Department of Health. The Ohio obesity prevention plan. Columbus, OH: Ohio Department of Health; 2009. Available at: http://healthyohioprogram.org/ASSETS/0B9A7DFFF7E64202AE5A704AEB9A9EC0/ohobespln.pdf. Accessed April 2, 2009.

16. The Ohio State University. 2008 Ohio Family Health Survey. Available at: http://grc.osu.edu/ofhs/. Accessed February 9, 2009.

17. The Health Foundation of Greater Cincinnati. 2005 Greater Cincinnati Community Health Status Survey. Available at: http://www.healthfoundation.org/data_publications/gcchss/2005.html. Accessed February 9, 2009.

18. Schuchter J, Besl J, Simpson L. Child health in northern Kentucky. Cincinnati, OH: Child Policy Research Center; 2010. Available at: http://www

.cincinnatichildrens.org/assets/0/78/1067/1395/1833/1835/1849/1853/1190f79b-fecb-40e1–988c-04939bb11db2.pdf. Accessed May 12, 2010.

19. Office of the Surgeon General, U.S. Department of Health and Human Services. The surgeon general's call to action to prevent and decrease overweight and obesity. Available at: http://www.surgeongeneral.gov/topics/obesity/calltoaction/fact_adolescents.htm. Accessed May 12, 2010.

20. Institute of Medicine (U.S.). Committee on Prevention of Obesity in Children and Youth, Koplan J, Liverman CT, Kraak VI, eds. *Preventing Childhood Obesity: Health in the Balance.* Washington, DC: National Academies Press; 2005.

21. Centers for Disease Control and Prevention. KidsWalk-to-School: Resource Materials|DNPAO|CDC. Available at: http://www.cdc.gov/nccdphp/dnpa/kidswalk/then_and_now.htm. Accessed April 2, 2009.

22. The Health Foundation of Greater Cincinnati and The Child Policy Research Center at Cincinnati Children's Hospital Medical Center. 2005 Greater Cincinnati Child Well-Being Survey. Available at: http://www.cincinnatichildrens.org/assets/0/78/1067/1395/1833/1835/9811/9813/9818/9aadc334–053d-4d27-a169–8280b9c8e55b.pdf. Accessed February 9, 2009.

23. Ritchey M, Bolling C, Hornung R, Buchholz R, Donovan E. Caregivers' accuracy in reporting their child's height and weight, and their perceptions about their child's weight status. Cincinnati, OH: The Health Foundation of Greater Cincinnati; 2008.

24. The Foundation for a Healthy Kentucky and The Health Foundation of Greater Cincinnati. 2009 Kentucky Health Issues Poll. Available at: http://www.healthfoundation.org/data_publications/khip.html. Accessed February 9, 2009.

25. Nord M, Andrews M, Carlson S. Household food security in the United States, 2008. Washington, DC: U.S. Department of Agriculture, Economic Research Service; 2009:ERR-83.

26. Bureau of Labor Statistics, U.S. Department of Labor. Current Population Survey (CPS), 2006. Available at: http://www.bls.gov/cps/home.htm. Accessed February 9, 2009.

27. Morland K, Diez Roux AV, Wing S. Supermarkets, other food stores, and obesity: the atherosclerosis risk in communities study. *Am J Prev Med.* 2006; 30:333–339.

28. Davis B, Carpenter C. Proximity of fast-food restaurants to schools and adolescent obesity. *Am J Public Health.* 2009;99:505–510.

29. The Appalachian Sustainable Agriculture Project. Available at: http://www.buyappalachian.org/. Accessed September 2, 2010.

30. Economos CD, Irish-Hauser S. Community interventions: a brief overview and their application to the obesity epidemic. *J Law Med Ethics.* 2007;35:131–137.

31. Cluggish S, Kinder G. Shape Up Somerville: a district tackles childhood obesity. *School Administrator.* 2008;65(1):12–16.

32. Shape Up Somerville—Friedman School of Nutrition Science and Policy—Tufts University. Available at: http://nutrition.tufts.edu/1174562918285/Nutrition-Page-n12w_1179115086248.html. Accessed September 2, 2010.

33. New England Cable News. Call to revolution crisis and opportunity in Boston: Shape Up Somerville. Available at: http://www.youtube.com/watch?v=71V12zS7nQU. Accessed February 23, 2009.

34. *The Today Show,* NBC News. Shape Up Somerville. Available at: http://video.msn.com/video.aspx?mkt=en-us&vid=fef93a9e-3a61–4dea-8e6c-4b2951dd41f3. Accessed February 23, 2009.

35. Public Health Law and Policy. Changes in the WIC food packages, a toolkit for partnering with neighborhood stores. Oakland, CA: California WIC Association; 2009. Available at: http://www.calwic.org/docs/nfood/2009/vendor_toolkit.pdf. Accessed September 24, 2009.

36. U.S. Bureau of Census. County Business Patterns, 2006. Available at: http://www.census.gov/econ/cbp/index.html. Accessed February 9, 2009.

37. Economic Research Service, U.S. Department of Agriculture. ERS/USDA data—Supplemental Nutrition Assistance Program (SNAP) data system. Available at: http://www.ers.usda.gov/Data/SNAP/index.htm. Accessed February 9, 2009.

38. Centers for Disease Control and Prevention. Estimated county-level prevalence of diabetes and obesity—United States, 2007. *MMWR Morb Mortal Wkly Rep.* 2009;58(45):1259–1263.

39. Yun S, Zhu BP, Black W, Brownson RC. A comparison of national estimates of obesity prevalence from the Behavioral Risk Factor Surveillance System and the National Health and Nutrition Examination Survey. *Int J Obes (Lond).* 2006;30:164–170.

40. Flegal KM, Carroll MD, Ogden CL, Johnson CL. Prevalence and trends in obesity among U.S. adults, 1999–2000. *JAMA.* 2002;288:1723–1727.

8

Cancer-Related Disparities

*James L. Fisher, John M. McLaughlin, Mira L. Katz,
Mary Ellen Wewers, Mark B. Dignan,
and Electra D. Paskett*

This chapter describes disparities in cancer incidence, prevalence, and mortality in Appalachia, as well as differences in contributing factors such as cancer screening behaviors (e.g., mammography) and cancer-related behaviors (e.g., tobacco use). It focuses on the four leading anatomic sites of cancer (lung/bronchus, colon/rectum, female breast, and prostate) and the two cancers (cancer of the cervix and cancer of the oral cavity/pharynx) for which screening tests are available and for which data sources exist on potential disparities in Appalachia. Information on these disparities is drawn from published literature as well as from rates and proportions determined from six state-based central cancer registries, each containing an Appalachian area and each participating in the Appalachian Community Cancer Network (ACCN). The ACCN, discussed in more detail later, is a National Institutes of Health–funded project addressing cancer health[a] disparities in seven states containing Appalachian counties. The data presented on cancer incidence and mortality rates come from cancer registries maintained by state departments of health, and the data concerning cancer-related behaviors are taken from state-based Behavioral Risk Factor Surveillance System (BRFSS) surveys. The chapter concludes with recommendations for future research and policy directions.

Disparities in Cancer Incidence and Mortality

Previous reports of cancer-related disparities in Appalachia focused primarily on cancer incidence and mortality rates.[1–13] In the first study of cancer incidence rates in a large portion of the Appalachian population, Wingo and associates[14] reported the following: (1) rates were higher in Appalachia than in the rest of the United States; (2) rates for lung, colon/rectum, and other tobacco-related cancers were particularly high; (3) Central Appalachia had the highest rates for cancers of the cervix and lung/bronchus; (4) Northern Appalachia had the highest rates for cancers of the female breast and prostate, in addition to less common anatomic sites and types of cancer; and (5) Southern Appalachia had the lowest overall cancer incidence rates. The relatively consistent findings of the majority of studies assessing cancer-related disparities in Appalachia are corroborated by more recent analyses of the average annual, age-adjusted cancer incidence (table 8.1) and mortality rates (table 8.2) for six of the seven states participating in the ACCN. Table 8.1 shows that incidence rates for cancers of the cervix, colon/rectum, lung/bronchus, and oral cavity/pharynx were greater in the majority of the states' Appalachian areas versus non-Appalachian areas, and incidence rates for cancers of the female breast and prostate were generally lower in the Appalachian areas. Table 8.2 shows similar findings for mortality rates in these states. Wingo and associates[14] identified substantial variation in cancer incidence rates throughout Appalachia, supporting the notion that cancer incidence is not a homogeneous phenomenon in the region.

Although cancer incidence and mortality disparities among residents of Appalachia have consistently been confirmed, there has been limited research on the possible reasons for these disparities. There is some evidence that socioeconomic differences and differences in population density may partially explain these disparities—that is, people with lower incomes, with less education, and residing in more rural areas have higher cancer incidence and mortality rates.[11, 15] In examining cancer incidence rates among Appalachian and non-Appalachian Ohio residents, Fisher and colleagues[15] reported that lower household income and lower educational attainment contributed to disparities in the incidence of cervical and lung/bronchus cancers and might play a role in colon/rectum cancer but did not contribute to the slight disparity in oral cavity/pharynx cancer incidence. In addition, lower population density partially explained the disparity in the incidence of melanoma of the skin and might have been an important factor in cervical and colon/rectum cancer disparities.[15] Because so many

Table 8.1. Average Annual (2002–2006) Age-Adjusted Incidence of Selected Invasive Cancers per 100,000 Persons in Appalachian (App) versus Non-Appalachian (Non-App) Parts of Six States Participating in the Appalachian Community Cancer Network

Cancer Type	Kentucky		Ohio		New York		Pennsylvania		Virginia		West Virginia[*]	
	App	Non-App	App	Non-App	App	Non-App	App	Non-App	App	Non-App	App	Non-App[†]
Cervix[‡]	11.1	8.8	8.7	7.8	8.2	8.7	7.7	8.0	7.7	6.8	10.2	n/a
Colon/rectum	59.8	56.7	57.1	51.0	53.8	52.0	56.9	54.7	47.1	48.0	61.4	n/a
Female breast[‡]	112.2	122.8	115.5	121.9	126.5	123.9	119.2	126.5	113.7	122.3	115.4	n/a
Lung/bronchus	108.8	97.1	80.3	73.3	76.5	63.7	69.7	69.4	77.9	67.5	89.1	n/a
Oral cavity/pharynx	11.8	11.8	10.4	9.3	11.4	9.7	10.5	9.8	9.1	10.0	n/a	n/a
Prostate[‡]	134.2	146.0	138.4	143.6	181.7	164.8	148.5	164.2	116.8	160.4	139.5	n/a

[*] West Virginia rates are from 2001–2004.
[†] Not applicable (n/a) because all counties in West Virginia are Appalachian.
[‡] Incidence rates of cancers of the cervix, female breast, and prostate are sex specific.

Table 8.2. Average Annual (2002–2006), Age-Adjusted Mortality Rates for Selected Invasive Cancers per 100,000 Persons in Appalachian (App) versus Non-Appalachian (Non-App) Parts of Six States Participating in the Appalachian Community Cancer Network

Cancer Type	Kentucky		Ohio		New York		Pennsylvania		Virginia		West Virginia[*]	
	App	Non-App	App	Non-App	App	Non-App	App	Non-App	App	Non-App	App	Non-App[†]
Cervix[‡]	3.1	2.7	2.9	2.4	2.5	2.6	2.2	2.4	2.1	2.1	3.5	n/a
Colon/rectum	22.2	21.9	21.3	19.7	19.0	18.2	20.1	20.0	16.6	18.2	21.8	n/a
Female breast[‡]	26.4	25.2	26.6	27.1	23.4	24.6	25.9	26.6	25.7	25.9	25.6	n/a
Lung/bronchus	88.2	75.1	64.2	59.3	54.3	45.7	53.4	53.2	63.6	54.7	69.8	n/a
Oral cavity/pharynx	2.8	2.9	2.5	2.6	2.4	2.3	2.3	2.3	2.3	2.3	2.6	n/a
Prostate[‡]	26.6	26.6	25.1	27.4	25.2	24.3	25.8	29.1	23.6	29.0	26.6	n/a

[*] West Virginia rates are from 2001–2004.
[†] Not applicable (n/a) because all counties in West Virginia are Appalachian.
[‡] Mortality rates for cancers of the cervix, female breast, and prostate are sex specific.

complex and interacting factors may be involved in an individual being diagnosed with cancer, it is difficult to sort them out. A variety of geographic, demographic, social, behavioral, and psychological characteristics of individuals residing in Appalachia probably interact to produce higher incidence and mortality rates for many cancers.

Disparities in Cancer Diagnosis

It is well documented that a cancer diagnosis at an earlier stage increases the likelihood of survival. As shown in table 8.3, a comparison of Appalachian and non-Appalachian areas indicates slightly greater proportions of late-stage diagnoses of cancers of the cervix and prostate in Appalachian Pennsylvania, while late-stage diagnoses of colon/rectum cancer were higher in Appalachian Kentucky. For female breast cancer, there was a greater proportion of late-stage diagnoses in Appalachian Kentucky and a slightly greater proportion in the Appalachian counties of Virginia. With the exception of a greater proportion of late-stage diagnoses among females with oral cavity/pharynx cancer in Appalachia Ohio, the remaining disparities were slight. For the majority of cancers examined, the proportions of late-stage diagnoses were lower in Appalachian counties, but the proportions of patients diagnosed with cancer at an unknown stage were greater in the Appalachian counties in Ohio and Pennsylvania (not shown in table 8.3). It is likely that in many cases, lower proportions of late-stage diagnoses in Appalachian counties were the result of a higher proportion of diagnoses at an unknown stage.

Overall, research reporting disparities in cancer stage at diagnosis is limited. It is likely that such disparities are associated with race and urban or rural status (or population density) in addition to Appalachian residence. Lengerich and coauthors[8] reported that the rates of unstaged cancer for every examined anatomic site or cancer type were elevated in rural Appalachia, suggesting a lack of access to cancer health care in these areas. It is possible that previous research, as well as the results shown in table 8.3, failed to reveal important disparities because unstaged cancers are commonly removed from the denominators before calculating proportions; that is, it is possible that many unstaged cancers in Appalachia have not been properly accounted for when interpreting the proportion of late-stage diagnoses.

Table 8.3. Portions of Late-Stage* Diagnoses of Selected Cancers in Appalachian (App) versus Non-Appalachian (Non-App) Parts of Five States Participating in the Appalachian Community Cancer Network, 2002–2006

Cancer Type	Kentucky		Ohio		New York		Pennsylvania		Virginia	
	App	Non-App	App	Non-App	App	Non-App	App	Non-App	App	Non-App
Cervix	46.3	47.4	38.0	40.8	34.0	43.6	48.7	47.0	42.4	45.2
Colon/rectum	Male: 48.5	Male: 46.5	Male: 46.5	Male: 47.6	Male: 50.0	Male: 51.1	Male: 53.2	Male: 54.6	Male: 54.9	Male: 55.8
	Female: 49.7	Female: 47.1	Female: 46.7	Female: 48.1	Female: 51.4	Female: 52.7	Female: 54.1	Female: 55.6	Female: 55.2	Female: 55.5
Female breast	32.1	28.6	27.0	27.9	30.7	34.6	35.0	35.5	36.2	35.1
Lung/bronchus	Male: 73.1	Male: 75.1	Male: 65.9	Male: 67.7	Male: 66.9	Male: 68.2	Male: 75.6	Male: 75.4	Male: 66.0	Male: 74.3
	Female: 72.7	Female: 71.8	Female: 61.7	Female: 64.1	Female: 64.6	Female: 65.1	Female: 71.9	Female: 72.2	Female: 61.7	Female: 69.4
Oral cavity/ pharynx	Male: 52.9	Male: 55.1	Male: 57.9	Male: 60.2	Male: 58.1	Male: 60.8	Male: 64.7	Male: 66.5	Male: 60.0	Male: 65.8
	Female: 39.7	Female: 43.3	Female: 51.9	Female: 47.9	Female: 49.1	Female: 48.3	Female: 51.6	Female: 53.6	Female: 45.9	Female: 48.4
Prostate†	12.0	13.1	2.7	3.4	3.5	3.8	4.1	3.6	9.6	11.4

* Regional and distant stages combined.
† Late-stage prostate cancer is defined as only distant stage.

Disparities in Cancer Screening

Table 8.4 shows the prevalence of selected cancer screening tests in Appalachian versus non-Appalachian areas of five of the ACCN-participating states. The prevalence of mammography, digital rectal examination, and Pap smear was lower in each of the Appalachian areas, while the prevalence of colonoscopy or sigmoidoscopy and prostate-specific antigen testing was lower in three and two of the Appalachian areas, respectively.

It is generally well established that the prevalence of cancer screening within recommended guidelines is significantly lower among Appalachian than non-Appalachian adults.[5, 16–23] Barriers to cancer screening have been identified at the patient, provider, and system levels for each screening test. Many of the barriers identified for residents of Appalachia are similar to those identified in studies conducted throughout the United States. These include unawareness of screening guidelines, lack of provider recommendations, and absence of symptoms, as well as lack of health insurance and child care.[23] In addition, many rural Appalachians are low income or unemployed, live in remote locations, lack transportation, or have less access to medical care—each of which may play a role in a lower prevalence of cancer screening.[19, 22, 24–26] Patient-level barriers to breast, cervical, and colorectal cancer screening tests have been documented among individuals participating in studies conducted at clinics and churches, as well as from BRFSS data. Barriers to cancer screening reported in these studies included lower level of educational attainment, lower household income, lack of provider recommendations, lack of health insurance, and lack of a regular source of medical care.[19, 22, 25] Interviews of eighteen key informants (women who were longtime residents of Appalachia, had detailed knowledge about local cancer beliefs and prevention efforts, and represented a county-level American Cancer Society office) in Appalachian Ohio revealed that barriers to cervical cancer screening included cost, lack of insurance, transportation problems, fear, embarrassment, and privacy issues.[27] Rural Appalachians may initially be wary of unfamiliar health care providers and health care systems, putting up additional barriers to improved cancer screening rates.[24, 25]

To address the low prevalence of cancer screening among Appalachians, creative and effective strategies should be developed, implemented,

Table 8.4. Prevalence of Selected Cancer Screening Tests in Appalachian (App) versus Non-Appalachian (Non-App) Parts of Five States Participating in the Appalachian Community Cancer Network, Based on Data from the Behavioral Risk Factor Surveillance System

Test	Kentucky		Ohio		Pennsylvania		Virginia		West Virginia	
	App	Non-App	App	Non-App	App	Non-App	App	Non-App	App	Non-App*
Mammography in past 2 years (age 40+)	68.1	78.0	69.7	76.1	75.0	78.0	71.9	75.4	74.5	n/a
Colonoscopy/ sigmoidoscopy in past 5 years (age 50+)	66.6	62.8	40.0	48.6	43.0	48.0	55.1	64.2	53.4	n/a
Prostate-specific antigen test in past year (age 50+)	51.9	51.3	57.4	57.5	56.0	58.0	72.8	71.6	54.1	n/a
Digital rectal exam in past year (age 50+)[†]	80.1	80.2	47.4	55.3	51.0	53.0	61.0	63.0	—[‡]	n/a
Pap smear in past 3 years (age 18+, intact cervix)	78.2	85.2	80.4	84.6	83.0	87.0	84.4	87.0	83.8	n/a

* Not applicable (n/a) because all counties in West Virginia are Appalachian.
† Digital rectal exam is not an accepted cancer screening test; however, it provides additional clinical information.
‡ Insufficient data.

and evaluated. Examples include the following: (1) have members of community-based organizations lead efforts to improve cancer screening awareness and encourage preventive care; (2) use specific communication strategies (such as the media, churches, and community leaders) to disseminate accurate cancer screening information, reinforce the importance of talking to health care providers about cancer screening, and assist in changing misperceptions; (3) implement locally tested best practices to improve provider-patient communication about cancer screening; and (4) institute system-level interventions, such as chart reminder systems to initiate cancer screening and follow-up and local or mobile cancer screening units to serve the rural areas of Appalachia.

Disparities in Cancer-Related Behaviors

There are at least three types of cancer-related behaviors that may contribute to the disproportionately higher cancer incidence and mortality rates in Appalachia: tobacco use (including smoking and smokeless tobacco) and cessation; diet and physical activity, and their effect on energy and obesity; and sexual behaviors, especially those related to infection with human papillomavirus (HPV).

Tobacco Use and Cessation. Tobacco use is associated with ten anatomic sites or types of cancer, including cancers of the lung/bronchus, oral cavity/pharynx, and cervix.[28] As shown in tables 8.1 and 8.2, incidence and mortality rates of invasive cancers at these sites are generally greater among Appalachians than non-Appalachians. Tobacco smoking was found to be more prevalent than the national average in nine of the thirteen states containing Appalachian counties.[29] A recent ACCN report documented that the prevalence of cigarette smoking among both males and females aged 18 and older is greater in the Appalachian than in the non-Appalachian areas of Kentucky, Ohio, Pennsylvania, and Virginia.[30] Among rural Appalachian women residing in West Virginia, high school graduation, positive personality characteristics, and supportive spousal relationships distinguished nonsmokers from smokers.[31]

An assessment of the characteristics of rural adult tobacco users in Appalachian Ohio resulted in the following conclusions: (1) the median time to the first cigarette of the day (a measure of nicotine dependence) was low (twenty minutes), indicating a high degree of dependence; (2) the mean number of serious lifetime quit attempts (2.3) was lower than for other groups of current smokers; (3) the majority of tobacco users had not tried to quit for more than one year, with stress cited as the most common reason for resumption; (4) more than half the participants had not used any aids in previous quit attempts, but the same proportion expressed interest in using nicotine replacement in future quit attempts; (5) two-thirds reported that most or all of their friends smoked, and 48 percent identified most or all of their coworkers as smokers; and (6) only 1.6 percent reported that none of their family members smoked, and 3.4 percent said the same about their coworkers.[32]

To expand this assessment, a qualitative study was conducted to discern beliefs about tobacco use and cessation among the same rural Appalachian cohort.[33] Four focus groups revealed themes of nicotine dependence with pharmacological, psychological, social, and environmental aspects, primarily among current tobacco users. Pros and cons of tobacco use were also dominant themes among both current and former tobacco users. In addition, the importance of family and the acknowledgment of personal independence were evident. Participants' description of the addictive nature of nicotine and its pharmacological aspects indicated the need to incorporate a nicotine replacement component into tobacco treatment programs, and they cited the support of family and friends as an essential part of treatment. A preliminary study testing a tobacco cessation intervention in a rural Appalachian Ohio county suggested that a community-based intervention involving lay health advisers might be a promising cessation strategy among high-risk populations in rural Appalachia.[34] Feasibility data suggested that the intervention could be successfully implemented and that participants could be recruited and retained throughout the study. The efficacy of this tobacco cessation intervention still needs to be tested in a large-scale randomized, controlled trial. Additional information concerning the tobacco use characteristics of Appalachians can be found in the chapters on an Appalachian health lifestyle and substance abuse.

Dietary Factors, Physical Activity, and Weight Status. Both males and females are more likely to report inadequate fruit and vegetable consumption and no physical activity in the past month, as well as to have a higher prevalence of obesity in Appalachian versus non-Appalachian areas of

Kentucky, Ohio, Pennsylvania, and Virginia.[30] There has been limited research into why dietary factors, physical activity, overweight, and obesity disproportionately affect residents of Appalachia. Among low-income Appalachian women aged 40 to 64 years residing in West Virginia, primary barriers to physical activity were lack of willpower and support, but not lack of time.[35] Therefore, targeted interventions aimed at willpower and support may increase physical activity among Appalachian women. Additional information concerning the dietary characteristics of Appalachians can be found in the chapter on obesity.

Sexual Behaviors and Human Papillomavirus Infection. In most published reports concerning cancer-related disparities among residents of Appalachia, the anatomic site or type of cancer with the greatest disparities in incidence and mortality is cervical cancer.[5, 6, 8, 13, 14, 36, 37] However, tables 8.1 and 8.2 (which display the most recent incidence and mortality rates) show that disparities in colon/rectum and lung/bronchus cancers are at least as great as, if not greater than, those observed for cervical cancer. Although the development of cervical cancer depends on a complex interaction of social and behavioral factors, the strongest known risk factor is infection with human papillomavirus (HPV), a group of nearly 200 related viruses. The majority of HPV types cause no symptoms in most women; however, some HPV types can cause genital warts, and other "high-risk" types, when persistent, can lead to cancer in a minority of women.[b] Risky sexual behaviors place women at high risk for acquiring HPV. Based on more than 1,000 specimens collected from thirty-two hospitals in twenty-two countries prior to 1995, infection with HPV type 16 accounts for more than half the cases of cervical cancer and high-grade dysplasia; infection with HPV types 16, 18, 31, and 45 accounts for 80 percent of cervical cancers.[38] HPV is also associated with cancers of the anus, vagina, vulva, penis, and oral cavity/pharynx.[39]

It is possible that cervical cancer disparities in Appalachia result from differences in sexual behaviors related to the opportunity to acquire HPV infection. Evidence from the Youth Risk Behavior Surveillance System (YRBSS) suggests that the percentages of girls reporting having had sexual intercourse, early sexual intercourse, and intercourse with four or more people were generally greater in states containing Appalachian regions, and these percentages were generally greater in states with larger populations residing in Appalachian counties.[40] Compared with the median of all female students in the 2003 YRBSS, more female high school students in West Virginia reported having had sexual intercourse (54.9 versus 43.6 percent), having had sexual intercourse before age 13 (4.3 versus 3.5 percent), having had sex with four or more partners (16.6 versus 11.6 percent), and having had sex with one or more partners within the last three months (44.0 versus 34.1 percent).[40]

It is possible that risky sexual behaviors are influenced by determinants such as demographics (e.g., age), geography (e.g., remote location), acceptance of these behaviors, access to health care, socioeconomic status, and social and physical environments.[40–44] Little is known about the influence of these factors on rural Appalachian women. Determining social norms related to casual sexual relations may be important because extramarital sexual relationships, age at first intercourse, and multiple sexual partners are positively associated with HPV.[44] In addition to a higher prevalence of tobacco smoking and a lower prevalence of Pap screening, risky sexual behaviors among young Appalachian women may increase their cervical cancer risk, and this may contribute to disparities in their cervical cancer incidence and mortality rates.[45, 46]

Disparities in Access to Care

Differences in cancer incidence and mortality within Appalachia likely reflect differences in the socioeconomic and demographic characteristics of the population and variability in the access to care, especially health insurance coverage, the proportion of out-of-pocket medical expenses, and the availability of health care providers, specialists, and cancer centers.[19] Although the focus of most research pertaining to cancer health disparities in Appalachia has been on behavioral (e.g., tobacco use) or environmental (e.g., exposure to carcinogens) factors, differences in access to care cannot be discounted or ignored as a possible explanation for higher mortality rates among residents of Appalachia.

Compounding the issue of access is the fact that the distance to most cancer centers is substantial in much of rural Appalachia. One study showed that greater distance to a cancer center was associated with poorer survival among cancer patients.[47] Other studies have shown that the proportion of unstaged cancers was elevated in rural areas of Appalachia, suggesting that rural residents with cancer may not receive comprehensive diagnostic or treatment services.[8] In addition to lacking the financial resources to acquire health care, rural patients may face barriers erected by health care workers that impede their access to specialist care in urban areas.[48, 49]

The ACCN Model for Addressing Cancer Disparities in Appalachia

The Appalachian Community Cancer Network is a five-year project that includes a multidisciplinary team of collaborators from academic institutions and communities in the Appalachian counties of Kentucky, West Virginia, Ohio, Pennsylvania, New York, Maryland, and Virginia. The ACCN works to expand previous cancer control projects in Appalachia and to address cancer health disparities in the seven ACCN states. The long-term goal is to reduce cancer health disparities in Appalachia by developing, implementing, and evaluating community-based participatory research and providing appropriate training. The ACCN's objectives are to (1) build on a foundation established by previous projects and develop and maintain community partnerships to facilitate research and action to reduce cancer health disparities; (2) perform community-based participatory research, ranging from focused needs assessments to intervention research to policy assessments; (3) develop pilot research projects that focus on primary and secondary prevention of lung/bronchus, cervical, and colorectal cancers in Appalachia; (4) train researchers in community-based participatory research; (5) disseminate research findings to community and scientific partners; and (6) conduct an evaluation of the ACCN, including attention to processes, short-term impact, and achievement of outcomes.

To reach these objectives, the ACCN has formed strong relationships with both clinical and nonclinical partners. It has worked to maintain relationships with programs and facilities that provide cancer screening services and with other organizations that provide cancer-related services to those most in need—namely, the uninsured and underinsured population in the ACCN service area. The ACCN and its nonclinical partners have collaborated in successful community-based education and research activities across Central and Northern Appalachia. In partnership with the ACCN, these community organizations are working to improve the utilization of cancer screening services by conducting outreach programs to educate the local community on the importance of cancer screening and early detection, tobacco cessation, and other cancer-related issues.

One ACCN project intends to facilitate the dissemination of successful interventions and prevention activities, including smoking cessation, energy balance, and cancer screenings, to rural Appalachian populations with high rates of cancer health disparities. Another aims to test colorectal cancer screening interventions in twelve Appalachian counties in Ohio in preparation for a full-scale trial in six additional Appalachian states within the ACCN service area. In addition, ACCN partners recently conducted four regional health disparities research seminars designed to share and disseminate research findings, increase the participation of health professionals and community members in evidence-based efforts, and highlight community-based participatory research projects and evidence-based educational programs conducted by academics and community members.

Several Ohio-based projects highlight research efforts to reduce cancer among residents of Appalachia. Ohio ACCN collaborates with five community-based cancer coalitions and other organizations to increase awareness, provide education, and promote the prevention and early detection of cancer. Examples of projects conducted in Appalachian Ohio include a media campaign to increase colorectal cancer screening; a church-based physical activity program to increase walking; a workplace wellness program focused on eating a healthy diet, increasing physical activity, and screening for breast cancer; a breast cancer screening outreach project; an elementary school–based tobacco prevention program; and educational seminars on cancer survivorship, cervical cancer, and HPV.

The Ohio State University's Center for Population Health and Health Disparities (CPHHD) is focused on understanding why Appalachian Ohio has such high rates of cervical cancer incidence and mortality. Toward this end, the CPHHD conducted three related projects in clinics representing the general population of women aged 18 years and older. Community partners were organized into an advisory board and a consortium of organizations to facilitate accomplishment of the projects' goals. The overall goal of the first project was to increase the early detection of cervical cancer by increasing the proportion of Appalachian women who receive Pap smears at appropriate intervals and return for follow-up care when necessary. Women were screened for eligibility, and those in need of a Pap smear were invited to participate in a study on the effectiveness of a lay health educator in promoting Pap smear utilization and follow-up for abnormalities. From this cohort of women screened, those who smoked were invited to participate in a second project. This project tested the effectiveness of a lay health educator in promoting smoking cessation by validating cessation with saliva cotinine measurements. This study also characterized the social, behavioral, and biological aspects of tobacco consumption. A third CPHHD project examined the social, behavioral, and biological variables that might contribute to an increased risk of an abnormal Pap smear in Appalachian woman. The contribution of HPV to cervical abnormalities and their relation to individual behaviors such as smoking and sexual activity were also examined.

Summary

Cancer incidence and mortality rates are greater in the Appalachian region than in the rest of the United States. These disparities are most apparent for cancers of the cervix, colon/rectum, and lung/bronchus. Disparities in cancer stage at diagnosis have not been thoroughly analyzed and have not been evaluated with respect to unknown stage at diagnosis. Limited work suggests that among those diagnosed with the most common or screenable cancers, the proportions diagnosed at a late stage do not differ greatly. Fewer Appalachian residents report following the recommended guidelines for cancer screening. Further work is needed to understand disparities in cancer-related behaviors such as tobacco use, dietary factors, physical activity, overweight and obesity, and sexual activity. Access to care in Appalachia is problematic for numerous reasons, and poor access may contribute to higher cancer mortality rates, even in the presence of lower incidence rates. Educational attainment and income may explain some of the disparities in cancer incidence and mortality rates in Appalachia. In direct response to these findings, the ACCN is utilizing community-based research, outreach, training, and dissemination to reduce cancer disparities in Appalachia.

Further Research

Knowledge about cancer-related disparities among Appalachians will be advanced by addressing a number of issues. For instance, Appalachians face several barriers to health services related to cancer. These barriers differ, depending on whether the issue is cancer prevention, early detection, treatment, or survival. Thus, additional research is needed to assess barriers Appalachians face in each of these areas of cancer control and to identify critical barriers that influence diagnosis, completion of treatment, participation in clinical trials, and access to rehabilitation. Traditionally, cancer control has ended with treatment, but extension of cancer control activities to include rehabilitation could improve the quality of life of Appalachian cancer survivors. Many health care resources are scarce in Appalachia, with rehabilitation services being among the most difficult to obtain.

Research is needed to determine whether locally appropriate cancer prevention and control educational programs and materials are more effective in changing behaviors than commercially available programs and materials. Organizations disseminating such educational programs and materials often fail to consider the traditions, beliefs, health literacy, and support networks of local residents. In particular, given smoking's impact on the cancer-related health of Appalachians, there has been insufficient evaluation of the cost-effectiveness of community-based, nurse-managed, lay-led tobacco cessation programs.

Appalachian women have an increased risk of cervical abnormalities and HPV infection. Thus, a better understanding of HPV prevalence and of the potential interactions of immune function, tobacco use, and HPV infection is needed. In addition, more information about differences in HPV virulence, HPV types, oncogenic potential, transmission, reservoirs, and resistance between Appalachians and non-Appalachians is needed to develop effective interventions.

Coal, oil, and natural gas extraction, along with chemical manufacturing, are major industries in parts of Appalachia, resulting in increased exposure to arsenic and other carcinogens. Research is needed to better understand the influence of environmental exposures on high rates of lung and other cancers.

Policy Recommendations

Policy changes to improve the cancer-related health of Appalachians might include incorporating rehabilitation into cancer control activities. This would benefit Appalachian cancer survivors.

Based on a recent report, states collected $25.1 billion in revenue from the tobacco settlement and tobacco taxes but will spend barely 2 percent ($567.5 million) of these funds on tobacco prevention and cessation programs.[50] Policies should require states to fund tobacco prevention and treatment programs at the levels recommended by the Centers for Disease Control and Prevention. In addition, tobacco taxes should be increased, and smoke-free workplace laws should be enacted and enforced.[50]

Understanding the burden of cancer in all populations is based largely on reports from state cancer registries. Policies should support state cancer registries in Appalachia to enable them to increase their reporting rate to at least 95 percent, as recommended by the North American Association of Central Cancer Registries.

Finally, because limited resources have prevented some states with Appalachian counties from calculating and reporting incidence rates and comparing those rates in Appalachian and non-Appalachian areas, cancer incidence information from these states should routinely be reported to one central source, such as the ACCN. Incidence rates could then be monitored to identify emerging disparities in Appalachia.

Notes

a. The concept of cancer health includes not only the diagnosis and treatment of disease but also prevention efforts such as screening and education.

b. HPV types (or, more specifically, serotypes) are distinguished by a common set of antigens. Antigens (or antibody generators) are receptors present on microorganisms that determine a host's immune response.

References

1. Armstrong LR, Thompson T, Hall HI, Coughlin SS, Steele B, Rogers JD. Colorectal carcinoma mortality among Appalachian men and women, 1969–1999. *Cancer.* 2004;101:2851–2858.

2. Friedell GH, Rubio A, Maretzki A, et al. Community cancer control in a rural, underserved population: the Appalachian leadership initiative on cancer project. *J Health Care Poor Underserved.* 2001;12:5–19.

3. Friedrich MJ. Program aims to reduce cancer burden in Appalachia. *J Natl Cancer Inst.* 2002;94:1189–1190.

4. Hall HI, Rogers JD, Weir HK, Miller DS, Uhler RJ. Breast and cervical carcinoma mortality among women in the Appalachian region of the U.S., 1976–1996. *Cancer.* 2000;89:1593–1602.

5. Huang B, Wyatt SW, Tucker TC, Bottorff D, Lengerich E, Hall HI. Cancer death rates—Appalachia, 1994–1998. *MMWR Weekly.* 2002;51:527–529.

6. Hopenhayn C, Bush H, Christian A, Shelton BJ. Comparative analysis of invasive cervical cancer incidence rates in three Appalachian states. *Prev Med.* 2005;41:859–864.

7. Hopenhayn C, Jenkins TM, Petrik J. The burden of lung cancer in Kentucky. *J Ky Med Assoc.* 2003;101:15–20.

8. Lengerich EJ, Tucker TC, Powell RK, et al. Cancer incidence in Kentucky, Pennsylvania, and West Virginia: disparities in Appalachia. *J Rural Health.* 2005;21:39–47.

9. Lengerich EJ, Wyatt SW, Rubio A, et al. The Appalachia Cancer Network: cancer control research among a rural, medically underserved population. *J Rural Health.* 2004;20:181–187.

10. Singh GK, Miller BA, Hankey BF, Edwards BK. Persistent area socioeconomic disparities in U.S. incidence of cervical cancer, mortality, stage, and survival, 1975–2000. *Cancer.* 2004;101:1051–1057.

11. Singh GK, Miller BA, Hankey BF, Feuer EJ, Pickle LW. Changing area socioeconomic patterns in U.S. cancer mortality, 1950–1998. Part I—all cancers among men. *J Natl Cancer Inst.* 2002;94:904–915.

12. Spitler HD, Mayo RM, Parker VG. Patterns of breast, cervical, colorectal, and prostate cancer in the Appalachian region of South Carolina. *Ethn Dis.* 2001;11:51–59.

13. Wyatt SW, Huang B, Tucker TC, Redmond J, Hopenhayn C. Geographic trends in cervical cancer incidence and mortality in Kentucky, 1995–2000. *J Ky Med Assoc.* 2004;102:11–14.

14. Wingo PA, Tucker TC, Jamison PM, et al. Cancer in Appalachia, 2001–2003. *Cancer.* 2008;112:181–192.

15. Fisher J, Engelhardt H, Stephens J, et al. Cancer-related disparities among residents of Appalachia Ohio. *J Health Dispar Res Pract.* 2008;2(2):61–74.

16. Shell R, Tudiver F. Barriers to cancer screening by rural Appalachian primary care providers. *J Rural Health.* 2004;20:368–373.

17. Schoenberg NE, Hopenhayn C, Christian A, Knight EA, Rubio A. An in-depth and updated perspective on determinants of cervical cancer screening among Central Appalachian women. *Women Health.* 2005;42:89–105.

18. Lyttle NL, Stadelman K. Assessing awareness and knowledge of breast and cervical cancer among Appalachian women. *Prev Chronic Dis.* 2006;3:A125.

19. Hall HI, Uhler RJ, Coughlin SS, Miller DS. Breast and cervical cancer screening among Appalachian women. *Cancer Epidemiol Biomarkers Prev.* 2002;11:137–142.

20. Davis RE, Armstrong DK, Dignan M, Norling GR, Redmond J. Evaluation of educational materials on colorectal cancer screening in Appalachian Kentucky. *Prev Chronic Dis.* 2006;3:A43.

21. Leslie NS, Deiriggi P, Gross S, DuRant E, Smith C, Veshnesky JG. Knowledge, attitudes, and practices surrounding breast cancer screening in educated Appalachian women. *Oncol Nurs Forum*. 2003;30:659–667.

22. Tessaro I, Mangone C, Parkar I, Pawar V. Knowledge, barriers, and predictors of colorectal cancer screening in an Appalachian church population. *Prev Chronic Dis*. 2006;3:A123.

23. Smith RA, Cokkinides V, Brawley OW. Cancer screening in the United States, 2009: a review of current American Cancer Society guidelines and issues in cancer screening. *CA Cancer J Clin*. 2009;59:27–41.

24. Behringer B, Mabe KH, Dorgan KA, Hutson SP. Local implementation of cancer control activities in rural Appalachia, 2006. *Prev Chronic Dis*. 2009;6:A34.

25. Elnicki DM, Morris DK, Shockcor WT. Patient-perceived barriers to preventive health care among indigent, rural Appalachian patients. *Arch Intern Med*. 1995;155:421–424.

26. Hutson SP, Dorgan KA, Phillips AN, Behringer B. The mountains hold things in: the use of community research review work groups to address cancer disparities in Appalachia. *Oncol Nurs Forum*. 2007;34:1133–1139.

27. Katz ML, Wewers ME, Single N, Paskett ED. Key informants' perspectives prior to beginning a cervical cancer study in Ohio Appalachia. *Qual Health Res*. 2007;17:131–141.

28. U.S. Department of Health and Human Services. The health consequences of smoking: a report of the surgeon general. Atlanta, GA: U.S. Department of Health and Human Services, Centers for Disease Control and Prevention, National Center for Chronic Disease Prevention and Health Promotion, Office on Smoking and Health; 2004.

29. Casto BC, Sharma S, Fisher JL, Knobloch TJ, Agrawal A, Weghorst CM. Oral cancer in Appalachia. *J Health Care Poor Underserved*. 2009;20:274–285.

30. Appalachian Community Cancer Network. The cancer burden in Appalachia, 2009. Available at: http://www.accnweb.com/docs/2009/CancerBurdenAppalachia2009.pdf. Accessed April 8, 2011.

31. Song H, Fish M. Demographic and psychosocial characteristics of smokers and nonsmokers in low-socioeconomic status rural Appalachian 2-parent families in southern West Virginia. *J Rural Health*. 2006;22:83–87.

32. Wewers ME, Ahijevych KL, Chen MS, Dresbach S, Kihm KE, Kuun PA. Tobacco use characteristics among rural Ohio Appalachians. *J Community Health*. 2000;25:377–388.

33. Ahijevych K, Kuun P, Christman S, Wood T, Browning K, Wewers ME. Beliefs about tobacco among Appalachian current and former users. *Appl Nurs Res*. 2003;16:93–102.

34. Wewers ME. Tobacco cessation intervention in a rural Ohio Appalachian county. College of Public Health, The Ohio State University; 2009.

35. Rye JA, Rye SL, Tessaro I, Coffindaffer J. Perceived barriers to physical activity according to stage of change and body mass index in the West Virginia wisewoman population. *Womens Health Issues.* 2009;19(2):126–134.

36. Yabroff KR, Lawrence WF, King JC, et al. Geographic disparities in cervical cancer mortality: what are the roles of risk factor prevalence, screening, and use of recommended treatment? *J Rural Health.* 2005;21:149–157.

37. Hopenhayn C, King JB, Christian A, Huang B, Christian WJ. Variability of cervical cancer rates across 5 Appalachian states, 1998–2003. *Cancer.* 2008;113:2974–2980.

38. Bosch FX, Manos MM, Munoz N, et al. Prevalence of human papillomavirus in cervical cancer: a worldwide perspective. International Biological Study on Cervical Cancer (IBSCC) study group. *J Natl Cancer Inst.* 1995;87:796–802.

39. Watson M, Saraiya M, Ahmed F, et al. Using population-based cancer registry data to assess the burden of human papillomavirus–associated cancers in the United States: overview of methods. *Cancer.* 2008;113:2841–2854.

40. Grunbaum JA, Kann L, Kinchen S, et al. Youth risk behavior surveillance—United States, 2003. *MMWR Surveill Summ.* 2004;53:1–96.

41. Castillo MA, Tarter RE, Giancola PR, Lu S, Kirisci L, Parks S. Substance use and risky sexual behavior in female adolescents. *Drug Alcohol Depend.* 1997;44:157–166.

42. Coker AL, Hopenhayn C, DeSimone CP, Bush HM, Crofford L. Violence against women raises risk of cervical cancer. *J Womens Health (Larchmt).* 2009;18:1179–1185.

43. Luster T, Small SA. Sexual abuse history and number of sex partners among female adolescents. *Fam Plann Perspect.* 1997;29:204–211.

44. Stone KM, Karem KL, Sternberg MR, et al. Seroprevalence of human papillomavirus type 16 infection in the United States. *J Infect Dis.* 2002;186:1396–1402.

45. Paskett ED, McLaughlin JM, Reiter PL, et al. Psychosocial predictors of adherence to risk-appropriate cervical cancer screening guidelines: a cross sectional study of women in Ohio Appalachia participating in the Community Awareness Resources and Education (CARE) project. *Prev Med.* 2010;50:74–80.

46. Wewers ME, Katz M, Fickle D, Paskett ED. Risky behaviors among Ohio Appalachian adults. *Prev Chronic Dis.* 2006;3:A127.

47. Campbell NC, Elliott AM, Sharp L, Ritchie LD, Cassidy J, Little J. Rural factors and survival from cancer: analysis of Scottish cancer registrations. *Br J Cancer.* 2000;82:1863–1866.

48. Behringer B. Health care services in Appalachia. In: Couto R, Simpson NK, Harris G, eds. *Sowing Seeds in the Mountains: Community-Based Coalitions for Cancer Prevention and Control.* NIH Publication No. 94–3779 ed. Bethesda, MD: National Institutes of Health; 1994:62–80.

49. Lengerich EJ, Kluhsman BC, Bencivenga M, Allen R, Miele MB, Farace E.

Development of community plans to enhance survivorship from colorectal cancer: community-based participatory research in rural communities. *J Cancer Surviv.* 2007;1:205–211.

50. Campaign for Tobacco-Free Kids, American Heart Association, American Cancer Society Cancer Action Network, American Lung Association, Robert Wood Johnson Foundation. A broken promise to our children: the 1998 state tobacco settlement 11 years later. Washington, DC: Campaign for Tobacco-Free Kids; 2009.

9

Chronic Kidney Disease— A Hidden Illness

Barbara B. Weaner and Rebecca J. Schmidt

Many Americans are attentive to the widespread problems of heart disease, high cholesterol, and accelerating rates of obesity in the United States but are far less aware of chronic kidney disease (CKD).[1] Yet CKD (formerly called chronic renal failure) is widespread, affecting approximately one in nine adults in the United States.[2] It is estimated that 20 million American adults are currently affected by CKD, with another 20 million at risk for developing it.[2-4] Some 80,000 adults are diagnosed with CKD annually in the United States, where it is the ninth leading cause of death.[5] In addition, patients with kidney disease are often unaware that they have it, resulting in many cases going undiagnosed.[6] During the period 1988–1994, the prevalence of CKD increased 20 to 25 percent in the United States, with associated complications and high costs.[7] Since 1994 there have been yearly increases in the number of both patients beginning dialysis because of end-stage kidney disease and patients diagnosed with less severe kidney problems. The dialysis population over the age of 75 has doubled since 1997 and now totals more than 81,000 patients. Among those aged 45 to 64 years, the number of individuals with CKD has increased 82 percent in the last ten years, and CKD prevalence in those aged 20 to 44 has increased 16.5 percent.[8] Predictions are that this pattern will persist at least until 2025.[9, 10]

This chapter examines CKD in Appalachia and the efforts at West Virginia University to increase the understanding and awareness of this often hidden disease. Although increasing rates of kidney disease are fairly well documented nationally, questions about regional variations and second-ary risk factors remain largely unanswered. There is reason to believe that Appalachians may be at increased risk for this problem, although this risk has not been quantified directly. Appalachians are at risk for developing CKD partly due to the growing incidence of obesity, sedentary lifestyles, and poor nutrition, all of which increase the risk for developing the two major causes of CKD: diabetes and hypertension. Historically, portions of the Appalachian region, whether rural or urban, have been medically un-derserved and have higher rates of poverty, obesity, tobacco use, and lim-ited educational attainment.[11] The population in some areas of Appalachia is aging, due in part to the out-migration of young people and lower rates of immigration in the last half of the twentieth century.[11, 12] Thus, as a re-gion, Appalachia has multiple risk factors for developing high rates of kid-ney disease.

After examining the risk factors and prevalence of CKD in Appalachia, this chapter provides a case study in how CKD can be countered in the re-gion, concluding with research and policy recommendations.

The Hidden Nature of Kidney Disease

CKD is a silent illness for a variety of reasons. The decline in kidney func-tion is usually subtle, with few initial physical symptoms; as a result, peo-ple are often unaware that they have a problem. Significant loss of kidney function may occur before symptoms are aggravated enough to seek care. Moreover, kidney disease can result from an adverse reaction to contrast dyes used to detect problems such as heart disease. While patients and phy-sicians attend to the primary presenting problem, kidney damage may be developing without their knowledge. The chronicity and complexity of the underlying problem, coupled with the closeness with which the patient is being monitored, can influence how quickly kidney problems are detected as well as the rate of progression of kidney failure. Some conditions may necessitate the use of treatments that threaten kidney health, such as medi-cations for serious or life-threatening infections. The benefits of treating the condition outweigh the risks of not treating it, even though patients might end up with unintended long-term deficiencies in kidney function. Other issues, such as low-level environmental or occupational exposure to industrial pollution, chemicals in everyday use, poverty, lack of medical access, and poor nutritional status may be subtle but real influences on both kidney health and the treatment of kidney disease.

Kidney disease is also a silent sickness because it is not discussed. Individuals may be unaware of the existence or severity of kidney disease within their extended families, which puts them at risk. Appalachians may not discuss the severity of their illness for privacy reasons or because they do not wish to make illness the topic of conversation. They may be unaware of the diagnostic utility of a family history, waiting instead for a physician to suggest testing for kidney disease. Health care providers may not screen for CKD or comprehensively disclose the adverse kidney-related side effects of medications due to time constraints, fear of frightening their patients or deterring treatment compliance, or their own poor communication skills. A focus on short-term goals rather than long-term consequences often presents a host of barriers to CKD diagnosis and treatment.

Definition, Diagnosis, and Stages of Chronic Kidney Disease

In addition to filtering waste products from the blood, the kidneys are responsible for manufacturing hormones and enzymes that regulate and balance blood pressure, regulate acid balance in the body, and control critical salt and water balance. Other kidney hormones govern the production of red blood cells in the bone marrow and the metabolism of minerals related to the maintenance of healthy bones.

Definition. Chronic kidney disease is defined as kidney damage for greater than three months' duration, manifested by either pathological abnormalities or structural changes.[13] It can also be defined as a decline in the kidney filtration rate to less than 60 mL/minute for greater than three months.[13] The glomerular filtration rate (GFR) measures the kidney's ability to filter waste products from the blood and is considered the best measure of overall kidney function.[14] GFR in a healthy adult with normal kidney function is approximately 100 to 125 mL/minute, depending on body mass, age, gender, and race. As function declines, the kidneys are unable to carry out their metabolic and hormonal work. CKD can manifest as a decline in function or as evidence of structural damage without frank function loss.

Kidney problems are divided into two major categories: acute and chronic. Acute (rapid onset) kidney problems usually present with pain;

blood in the urine; fluid problems that manifest as swelling in the hands, feet, or face; or lung congestion causing cough or shortness of breath. Acute kidney problems are usually classified as those that persist for less than six weeks. Some acute kidney problems, if they are left untreated or persist despite treatment, may develop into CKD; others resolve completely without residual effects. By definition, chronic kidney problems are longer in duration and may or may not be symptomatic. Some kidney illnesses, such as the glomerulonephropathies, may have accompanying edema (swelling) that causes patient concern. Others, such as kidney stones, can cause severe pain and possibly urinary bleeding, alerting a patient to the problem. Inherited conditions, such as polycystic kidney disease or Alport syndrome, may be completely asymptomatic yet cause extensive loss of kidney function over time.

Diagnosis. One of the most important tools for detecting risk for CKD is a thorough medical and family history.[15, 16] The two leading causes of CKD are diabetes and hypertension. Others include inherited (genetically linked) kidney diseases, glomerulonephropathies, urologic disorders (such as kidney stones or prostate problems), urinary tract infections, autoimmune diseases, and systemic infections.[15] Advancing age and certain ethnicities (black, Hispanic, Native American, Asian, or Pacific Island heritage) place individuals at higher risk. Occupational and environmental hazards, including prolonged or heavy exposure to lead and heavy metals, hydrocarbons, grain dust, and welding fumes, also warrant close scrutiny.[17–20] In addition, the incidence of CKD is linked to poverty, lower education level, age older than 65, and history of low birth weight.[15, 21]

The simplest way to screen for CKD is a blood test for blood urea nitrogen (BUN) and creatinine (two bodily waste products) and a urinalysis to test for protein, blood, or sugar in the urine. Other tests include twenty-four-hour urine collection, X-ray, ultrasound, computed tomography (CT) scan, magnetic resonance imaging (MRI), and more extensive laboratory studies. These evaluations may be undertaken after initial screening identifies a problem, but they are not always needed to detect kidney disease.

Staging. CKD has been divided into five stages, determined by GFR.[15] GFR must be examined in a clinical context rather than relying on a single calculated blood value because of the associated age and body factors that influence the interpretation of results as well as the pattern of function. Not all kidney problems, including chronic ones, progress in severity.

In stages 1 and 2 there is near-normal blood filtration, but patients may be at risk for disease progression. Primary care focuses on risk identification, blood pressure and blood sugar control, and renal protection, such as avoiding renal-toxic medications, contrast dyes, or environmental exposure to harmful substances. Patient education is critical at this stage and should include an assessment of the patient's long-term risk and family risk factors.

In stage 3, renal filtering capacity has dropped to less than 60 percent, and other kidney functions may be compromised. For instance, there may be alterations in blood pressure control, water excretion, vitamin D metabolism, production of red blood cells, potassium excretion, and acid-base balance. These manifestations are highly variable by patient and do not necessarily follow a particular pattern or time frame.

In stage 4, kidney function is less than 30 percent, and most patients are experiencing one or more silent complications. Frequently, abnormalities are found in laboratory examinations of either blood or urine and are not perceived by the patient. For this reason, if a patient has no symptoms and is not receiving regular medical care, CKD can go unnoticed and undiagnosed even at stage 4. The patient may feel well despite severely compromised renal function.

At stage 5, kidney function has declined to less than 15 percent, and patients face the decision whether to pursue dialysis treatment or renal transplantation or opt for palliative treatment only. By this stage, almost all CKD patients report severe fatigue, and some experience nausea, intermittent vomiting, a bad taste in the mouth, aversion to meat, hiccuping, itching, restlessness at night, swelling of the extremities, shortness of breath, or cough. Often, urine production is not diminished, so patients may not associate these problems with kidney function.

Not all patients with CKD progress through all five stages. Progression is dependent on multiple factors, not all of which are clearly understood.[22] Progression may be linked to smoking, time of diagnosis, use of kidney-protective medications, or exposure to kidney-toxic medications or chemicals. Alcohol use can exacerbate kidney disease, especially in the presence of liver problems. The presence of comorbid conditions or other chronic diseases, as well as being older than 65, also impact the progression of CKD.[22] In many if not most patients, diabetes that is well controlled poses less risk of progression of CKD than uncontrolled or poorly controlled diabetes.

There is strong evidence that treatment of conditions that contribute to CKD, including elevated blood pressure, proteinuria, anemia, vitamin D deficiency, hyperphosphatemia, secondary hyperparathyroidism, hyperlipidemia, and fluid overload associated with heart disease, reduces morbidity and mortality in patients with kidney disease. Unfortunately, many people with CKD are unaware of their disease and may not seek appropriate treatment.[23–25] Early diagnosis and management of patients with CKD, followed by proactive preventive care, can positively influence the course of the disease. In some patients, progression to stage 5 CKD and the need for dialysis can be prevented. However, loss of kidney function often goes unacknowledged between patient and health care provider until the condition becomes severe or acute. Late referral is an ongoing problem, and CKD is often underrecognized by primary care physicians.

Prevalence of Chronic Kidney Disease in Appalachia

The prevalence of CKD in Appalachia is difficult to assess for a variety of reasons. There is no standardized method of data collection that measures the incidence or prevalence of CKD stages 1 to 4 in the United States. Data on CKD are extrapolated from information collected on every dialysis patient through the U.S. Renal Data System (USRDS).[8] This highly organized, very detailed database can be analyzed state by state. A regional analysis conducted in 2007 by the USRDS of 368,544 dialysis patients found that the highest adjusted rates of dialysis occurred in two regions: the southern and southeastern portions of the United States and in areas along the Mississippi River and through the Ohio Valley.[26] Although this region includes most of Appalachia, the analysis does not specifically delineate Appalachian counties as defined by the Appalachian Regional Commission. This makes separating incidence and prevalence in the 420 counties of Appalachia impossible. Patients with stage 5 disease who choose not to undergo dialysis (the majority of stage 5 patients) have not been studied.[26] The USRDS also produces an atlas that analyzes data for CKD patients in stages 1 to 4.[7] This atlas has information on blood pressure control, diabetes control, cholesterol control, and lipid control in a sample of CKD patients compared with a control group without CKD; this information can be examined by state but not by county.

Other sources of information on comorbidities are the Behavioral Risk Factor Surveillance System (BRFSS)[27] and the National Health and Nutrition Examination Survey (NHANES)[28] sponsored by the Centers for Disease Control and Prevention (CDC). The BRFSS includes a section on chronic disease indicators in which state-by-state surveys provide descriptive statistics on diabetes, nutrition, hypertension, history of stroke, heart disease, congestive heart failure, and sedentary lifestyle but not CKD. The NHANES data can be extrapolated to examine the prevalence of CKD indirectly through comorbid conditions (hypertension, diabetes, cardiovascular disease, and chronic obstructive pulmonary disease) in the surveyed population. Unfortunately, these survey data can be examined for the entire country or state by state but not by county or region, preventing an analysis by Appalachian county.

The USRDS, BRFSS, and NHANES illuminate the weaknesses in the design of CKD information gathering at the national level. County-level data are unavailable in many states due to a lack of funding and the absence of a data-collection mechanism. Personal communications with nine of the thirteen Appalachian state health bureaus to determine whether any CKD information was being collected yielded no results. As an alternative, a comparison was made of the standardized age-adjusted death rates for coronary artery disease, cerebrovascular accident, diabetes, and congestive heart disease (all CKD-related disorders) in the Appalachian and non-Appalachian counties in the thirteen Appalachian states, in the United States as a whole, and in the nation's non-Appalachian counties.[a] This analysis found the following:

- Appalachian counties in Maryland, New York, Ohio, and Pennsylvania had statistically significantly higher rates of diabetes than non-Appalachian counties. The Appalachian counties as a group had higher rates of diabetes than non-Appalachian counties in both the region and the nation. All fifty-five of West Virginia's Appalachian counties had higher diabetes-related death rates than the nation as a whole.

- Age-adjusted death rates for coronary artery disease in the Appalachian counties of Kentucky, New York, North Carolina, Ohio, Pennsylvania, Tennessee, and Virginia were significantly higher than in the states' non-Appalachian counties. The overall death rate in the Appalachian region was higher than in the non-Appalachian counties.
- Appalachian counties in Kentucky, New York, North Carolina, Ohio, Pennsylvania, Virginia, and West Virginia had higher death rates for congestive heart failure. The death rate in the Appalachian region was significantly higher than in the United States as a whole.
- The death rates for cerebrovascular events (strokes) were significantly higher in the Appalachian counties of Kentucky, Maryland, New York, North Carolina, Ohio, Pennsylvania, Tennessee, Virginia, and West Virginia than in these states' non-Appalachian counties. The death rate due to stroke in the Appalachian region was higher than in the rest of the nation.
- The regions with the highest rates of leisure-time physical inactivity were in the South and in Appalachia, where there were also high rates of diagnosed diabetes and obesity and thus a risk for CKD.[29]

Although this analysis is weakened by the lack of gender and race adjustments, which are powerful and critical factors in CKD, the results are suggestive of the potential prevalence of CKD in Appalachia, given its strong association with these comorbidities.

Elevated Risk Factors in Appalachia

Rural Appalachians often encounter shortages of medical care providers, transportation difficulties that hinder access to care, and patient-provider interactions that obstruct health care initiation and compliance.[11, 30, 31] In West Virginia, patients without the social or economic means to travel to specialists often present to medical care well past the time when medical interventions would have provided the most benefit.[32] Prior to the decentralization of nephrology clinics, patients drove up to two and a half hours one way to receive nephrology care.[32] Of particular relevance to CKD is a worldwide, nationwide, and regional shortage of nephrologists needed to care for the upsurge in patients with CKD. The number of open positions for nephrologists in the United States is already double the number of physicians in training as nephrology fellows who will be entering practice.[33, 34] The developed countries of the United States, Canada, the United Kingdom, and Australia all face dire shortages of nephrologists and are increasingly dependent on foreign-trained doctors to fill nephrology training posts.[35–38] In addition, the out-migration of young people from rural Appalachia is mirrored by the overall distribution of nephrology specialty care in the United States: most nephrologists practice in urban areas, and 48 percent practice in eight states.[39] Although these problems are not unique to Appalachia, they may be compounded in states that are considered predominantly rural.

Ecologic theory—examining how knowledge, attitudes, individual behaviors, environmental exposures, social structures, laws, and policies interact to affect both individual and community health—has yet to be applied directly to kidney health in Appalachia.[40, 41] The factors of poverty, dietary habits, and behavioral lifestyle choices (such as smoking) that already place Appalachians at risk may be compounded by environmental exposures to toxins.

Although public health research in this area is limited, Appalachians living in proximity to industrial and mining sites may be at additional risk for environmental and occupational exposures affecting kidney health.[26] Acid mine drainage, a problem at abandoned mine sites throughout Appalachia, and the more massive mountaintop removal sites may pose ongoing health risks.[42, 43] Mountaintop removal mining is associated with the increased discharge of toxic heavy metals, including arsenic, cadmium, mercury, and lead.[44, 45] All these heavy metals have been linked to possible kidney toxicity.[46–53] Mountaintop removal mining is concentrated in southern West Virginia, western Virginia, and eastern Tennessee.[54] The U.S. Geological Survey estimates that, as a result of coal mining, 109 million pounds of antimony, arsenic, beryllium, cadmium, chlorine, chromium, cobalt, lead, manganese, mercury, nickel, and selenium have contaminated streams in Appalachia. For example, all 89,431 miles of Kentucky's rivers and 228,385 acres of lakes are under advisories for mercury contamination.[55] "Hotspots" of selenium contamination have been identified along the Ohio River, the Mud River Reservoir in West Virginia, and Zeb Mountain in Tennessee.[56]

How chronic exposure to contaminated water supplies from coal slurry impoundments or underground coal slurry storage will affect the long-term health of Appalachians has yet to be determined. Additionally, massive amounts of hydrocarbons are produced in many of the chemical factories in the Ohio River Valley. Exposure to airborne toxins from these plants, as well as pollution from coal-powered electric plants in the region, may increase the health risks for residents and watershed inhabitants downstream, including an increased risk of CKD. Establishing measurable health impacts or causal relationships is difficult, however, because most of the studies on lead, cadmium, copper, tin, mercury, selenium, hydrocarbons, and solvents have examined heavy occupational exposure rather than low-grade, chronic environmental exposure. Although a few epidemiological studies have been conducted in other populations,[49, 57–60] further research is needed in Appalachia to clarify and delineate the interplay of environmental and behavioral risk factors for CKD. Limitations of such research include the insensitivity of clinical renal outcomes and the lack of uniformly accepted early markers of kidney damage from environmental heavy metal exposure.[49] The coexistence of multiple risk factors for CKD (diabetes, hypertension, gout, smoking, obesity, and coexposures to environmental risk factors such as heavy metals or hydrocarbons) in the same patients may account for the high rates of CKD in parts of Appalachia.[32] Coexposure has been demonstrated with food and smoking exposure to cadmium, increasing the effects of occupational exposure and interacting with exposure to lead.[3] Similarly, how these environmental factors are related to poor nutritional status (suggested by low albumin levels in West Virginia patients presenting with CKD) and other poverty-linked factors has yet to be elucidated.[32, 61]

Although the Appalachian Regional Commission has reported an increasing incidence of illicit drug use in Appalachia, there is scarce research on illicit drug use and CKD in the region.[62] The CDC reported that unintentional poisoning deaths more than doubled in the South (Alabama, Arkansas, Delaware, District of Columbia, Florida, Georgia, Kentucky, Louisiana, Maryland, Mississippi, North Carolina, Oklahoma, South Carolina, Tennessee, Texas, Virginia, and West Virginia), where much of Appalachia lies. The largest increases occurred in states with mostly rural populations, such as West Virginia. From 1999 to 2004, unintentional poisoning mortality increased by 550 percent in that state, compared with a national increase of 68 percent.[63] Most of the deaths (93.2 percent) were linked to opioid use, with a majority (79.3 percent) attributed to nonmedical routes of exposure, drug diversion (taking drugs prescribed to friends and family members), or multiple medication use. The combination of poverty, unemployment, and lower educational attainment was a common theme in this West Virginia cohort; the existence of this pattern in other areas of Appalachia has yet to be examined.[64]

The pathological effects of illicit drugs are complex and varied and may overlap with other coexistent risk factors in drug abusers, such as hypertension, infection with HIV or hepatitis C, poverty-induced malnutrition, or oxidative stress. Caregivers need to take thorough social histories that screen for substance abuse, and they must be aware of the association between the abuse of some substances and kidney disease.

In addition, specific parts of Appalachia may be at increased risk for CKD. For example, there is a known cluster of patients with Fabry disease, a rare genetic metabolic disorder linked with kidney disease, in southern West Virginia. Clusters of increased death rates in Appalachia, especially in eastern Kentucky, southern West Virginia, southeastern Ohio, northeastern Pennsylvania, and at the Alabama-Georgia and Alabama-Mississippi borders may have complex and interactive etiologies, including poverty, poor nutrition, limited access to care, prevalence of high-risk behavior, environmental factors, and heredity.[65, 66] It is unclear whether this may also involve some degree of CKD prevalence.

Efforts to Improve Awareness and Care

The National Institutes of Health (NIH) and the CDC have begun intervention and educational programs for primary, secondary, and tertiary prevention of kidney disease.[67] These programs focus on epidemiological disease reduction and cost containment. Primary prevention emphasizes blood sugar control, blood pressure control, and identification of risk factors (age older than 60, diabetes, hypertension, cardiovascular disease, and family history of kidney problems). Secondary prevention includes CKD education, nutritional interventions, medication interventions, and laboratory investigations based on disease states and risk factors. Tertiary prevention includes the management of specific CKD complications, including anemia, hyperparathyroidism, and hyperphosphatemia; possible renal transplantation; and possible preparation for dialysis treatment before uremic or fluid overload problems become critical. These programs are modeled after public education programs targeting hypertension and cholesterol; they are aimed at high-risk populations and primary care providers.

Similarly, efforts are under way by the National Kidney Foundation to promote kidney disease screening and to provide educational information to the public and health care providers emphasizing testing for kidney damage, identifying risk factors, and assessing level of kidney function.[68] The Kidney Disease: Improving Global Outcomes initiative also recommends targeted screening programs for high-risk patients, including those with diabetes, hypertension, HIV, or cancer; those older than 60 years; and those with family members who have kidney disease.

An Appalachian Case Study: West Virginia

West Virginia is unique among the thirteen states that have Appalachian counties because it is the only one that is entirely Appalachian. Its per capita number of patients starting dialysis each year has exceeded the national average since 1994, possibly due to the state's increasingly older, diabetic, and hypertensive population. Diabetes was recently estimated to affect 22 percent of West Virginians, compared with 7 percent nationally; hypertension affects an estimated 34 percent of the state's residents, compared with 25 percent nationally. Fifteen percent of West Virginia's population is older than 65, making West Virginia the third "oldest" state. The rural nature of West Virginia and its relatively small number of physicians (including nephrology specialists) also impact the screening and treatment of kidney disease. Thus, physicians are caring for an elderly population, an increasingly obese population (68 percent of West Virginians older than 18 years), and a population that is, in many cases, distant from care.[69]

A healthier population could optimize cost savings to private and governmental payers and positively impact the state's economy, as well as improving the overall quality of life for West Virginians. Fortunately, the West Virginia legislature (with guidance from concerned nephrologists) understands the risks of not recognizing CKD, and in 2005 it passed a resolution regarding heightened awareness of CKD. In 2007 the legislature passed a bill mandating coverage of CKD screening for persons at risk for kidney disease. The bill also acknowledged the need for better CKD education for primary health care providers, earlier diagnosis, and an enhanced ability to treat stages 1 to 4 appropriately.

To foster collaboration and collegiality among providers caring for a growing population at risk for CKD, the West Virginia Rural Nephrology Initiative was created by members of the West Virginia University (WVU) Section on Nephrology. Through partnerships and collaborations among the state government and private-practice and academic nephrologists, the West Virginia Rural Nephrology Initiative has sponsored regional outreach efforts in the form of free kidney disease screenings for patients at risk, CKD education for the lay public, and continuing medical education for primary care providers. Specifically, the initiative has accomplished the following:

- Some thirty free screening events have been conducted in West Virginia since 2006, most in conjunction with the National Kidney Foundation's Serving the Alleghenies' Kidney Early Evaluation Program (KEEP). These screenings have helped raise public awareness about the risks of CKD and the need for proactive, preventive care. Of 1,562 West Virginians screened, 63.3 percent were identified as having CKD stages 1 to 4.[70]
- In 2008 free educational packets were disseminated to individuals at risk for CKD at primary care centers, free clinics, senior centers, and public screenings. They were also distributed to pharmacists statewide for dissemination to their customers. The educational packets, designed by members of the coalition, included information about kidney disease and resources for patients and families.
- Since 2002, a number of events have been held to teach primary health care providers about CKD. These include both daylong and half-day programs dedicated to CKD education, a traveling medical education program, and an annual CKD conference to review and update practitioners' understanding of the disease. The conferences include practical diagnostic and treatment application tools for primary health care providers.

In addition, in 2004 the WVU Section on Nephrology opened the first of five off-site rural nephrology clinics, decentralizing kidney care in north-central West Virginia. Currently, 40 percent of the outpatient kidney patients at WVU are seen at these small rural clinics, which are closer to their homes. The clinics are staffed once or twice a week by nephrologists, nurse practitioners, and nurses. Preliminary data gathered between 2005 and 2008 revealed that clinic patients had similar gender and racial distributions as other kidney patients, but they came from counties with higher rates of poverty, lower rates of high school education, and fewer physicians.

The West Virginia Rural Nephrology Initiative is a model for public health awareness that could be duplicated throughout Appalachia in an effort to improve kidney health in the region. It is in harmony with the national initiatives of the NIH and the CDC for the promotion of kidney disease awareness and detection. Using data gathered in the state's rural clinics and through these projects, the vital registration office and the Bureau of Public Health in West Virginia are beginning to collect statewide data on CKD patients.

Further Research

In light of the dearth of data about CKD in the Appalachian region, significant research efforts must be undertaken to understand and appropriately address this hidden issue. Some areas that need investigation are discussed below.

The CKD risk factors that are specific to Appalachia must be better understood. Researchers should examine the relationships between CKD and exposure to low-grade environmental pollution or high occupational exposures, particularly exposure to water and air pollution associated with coal mining. In addition, nutritional status (obesity, malnutrition), substance abuse, and health beliefs and behaviors that influence nutrition, exercise, and self-care should be evaluated. Medical, anthropological, sociological, educational, and nutritional research is needed on how risk factors for CKD, especially among high-risk populations, can best be addressed.

The role of public awareness in improving CKD detection, early treatment, and outcomes requires close examination. Compared with other diseases, such as heart disease and cancer, CKD is not well known or well understood. Given the implications for primary prevention efforts, research is needed to identify effective and efficient strategies for increasing public awareness. In addition, the continuing education of primary care providers must be enhanced to increase the early diagnosis and treatment of CKD and avoid disease progression.

More effective and efficient interventions for CKD in terms of time and cost are crucial if progression to stage 5 and the need for dialysis are to be prevented. This includes interventions that align with the needs and perspectives of Appalachian patients.

Access to care, whether primary care or secondary nephrology care, is an essential element of prevention and treatment efforts, particularly in rural Appalachia. In addition to the strategic location of CKD treatment facilities, sufficient physicians and other health professionals must be available. This requires insight into what motivates new medical school graduates to choose a specialty such as nephrology, as well as how medical residents can be recruited to underserved specialties or geographic areas.

Investigation into educational initiatives that reach out to children and adolescents and their parents during health care contacts is an important research area. This will allow the process of CKD awareness and detection to begin early.

Finally, research on how to reduce obesity, inactivity, and the psychosocial stresses linked to harmful behaviors is essential to reducing the incidence and prevalence of CKD.

Policy Recommendations

Improved Access to Affordable Care. Bizzozero[39] reports that almost 48 percent of nephrologists in the United States are located in just eight states, less than half the 8,300 nephrologists in the United States are younger than 50 years, and only 60 percent report practicing clinical medicine. In the coming years, the burden of treating patients with CKD will fall more heavily on primary care providers. The importance of disseminating the Kidney Disease Outcomes Quality Initiative (KDOQI) guidelines among primary care providers cannot be underestimated if adequate patient care is to be achieved. As the U.S. population continues to age and life expectancy increases, the number of elderly who are challenged by advancing kidney disease is growing. Indeed, it is estimated that 44 percent of individuals over age 65 have some level of kidney dysfunction. Medical costs for CKD patients requiring dialysis ($75,000 per patient per year) significantly exceed the costs for CKD patients not receiving dialysis. This puts a huge strain on individuals, government payers, private insurers, public health agencies, and primary care providers. Thus, a reexamination of the payer system, access to affordable medications, preventive measures, and provider and patient education are critical policy areas if the increase in CKD is to be minimized.

Expanded Care. The responsibility for patient and provider education, early screening, and case management cannot fall on the shoulders of nephrologists and primary care providers alone. Nurses, social workers, dieticians, nutritionists, exercise physiologists, physical trainers, public educators (including gym teachers), and the media all need to participate in a regionwide effort to reduce obesity, diabetes, cardiovascular disease, sedentary lifestyle, and tobacco and drug use, all of which contribute to CKD. Policies fostering the inclusion of CKD awareness in the education of these adjunct professionals are needed to improve health outcomes in Appalachia.

Limiting Nephrotoxic Exposures. Clear policies that uphold water and air quality standards are needed to protect kidney health. This can be done on a community level, through state initiatives in agencies that oversee these regulations, or at the federal level. Policies fostering individual and collective commitments to a healthier diet, proper exercise, restriction of salt consumption, weight reduction, minimization of tobacco use, limited exposure to environmental toxins and contrast dyes, and conscientious avoidance of certain prescriptions and over-the-counter medications that threaten kidney well-being are needed to effect change.

Note

a. This analysis was conducted with help from Tom Light, statistician from the West Virginia Bureau of Public Health.

References

1. Coresh J, Byrd-Holt D, Astor BC, et al. Chronic kidney disease awareness, prevalence, and trends among U.S. adults, 1999 to 2000. *J Am Soc Nephrol.* 2005;16:180–188.

2. National Kidney Foundation: Kidney Learning System. About chronic kidney disease. Available at: http://www.kidney.org/professionals/KLS/aboutCKD .cfm. Accessed May 4, 2009.

3. Centers for Disease Control and Prevention. Notice to readers: World Kidney Day—March 13, 2008. Available at: http://www.cdc.gov/mmwr/preview/ mmwrhtml/mm5708a5.htm. Accessed October 3, 2009.

4. Coresh J, Selvin E, Stevens LA, et al. Prevalence of chronic kidney disease in the United States. *JAMA*. 2007;298:2038–2047.

5. Kung HC, Hoyert DL, Xu J, Murphy SL. Deaths: final data for 2005. *Natl Vital Stat Rep*. 2008;56:1–120.

6. Plantinga LC, Boulware LE, Coresh J, et al. Patient awareness of chronic kidney disease: trends and predictors. *Arch Intern Med*. 2008;168:2268–2275.

7. USRDS 2008 Atlas—CKD One: chronic kidney disease in the NHANES population. Available at: http://www.usrds.org/2008/view/ckd_01_nhanes.asp. Accessed September 2, 2010.

8. USRDS Coordinating Center. U.S. renal data system. Available at: http:// www.usrds.org/2008. Accessed November 24, 2009.

9. Hamer RA, El Nahas AM. The burden of chronic kidney disease. *BMJ*. 2006;332:563–564.

10. National Kidney Foundation. Chronic kidney disease. Available at: http:// www.kidney.org/kidneydisease/ckd/index.cfm. Accessed October 3, 2009.

11. Appalachian Regional Commission. The Appalachian region. Available at: http://www.arc.gov/index.do?nodeid=26. Accessed October 3, 2009.

12. Appalachian Regional Commission. The aging of Appalachia. Available at: http://aging.senate.gov/award/arc1.pdf. Accessed October 3, 2009.

13. National Kidney Foundation. KDOQI clinical practice guidelines for chronic kidney disease: evaluation, classification, and stratification. Part 4. Definition and classification of stages of chronic kidney disease. Guideline 1. Definition and stages of chronic kidney disease. Available at: http://www.kidney.org/ Professionals/Kdoqi/guidelines_ckd/p4_class_g1.htm. Accessed October 3, 2009.

14. National Kidney Foundation. KDOQI clinical practice guidelines for chronic kidney disease: evaluation, classification, and stratification. Part 5. Evaluation of laboratory measurements for clinical assessment of kidney disease. Available at: http://kidney.org/Professionals/Kdoqi/guidelines_ckd/p5_lab.htm. Accessed October 3, 2009.

15. National Kidney Foundation. KDOQI clinical practice guidelines for chronic kidney disease: evaluation, classification, and stratification. Part 4. Definition and classification of stages of chronic kidney disease. Guideline 3. Individuals at increased risk of chronic kidney disease. Available at: http://www.kidney.org/ Professionals/Kdoqi/guidelines_ckd/p4_class_g1.htm. Accessed October 3, 2009.

16. Levey AS, Schoolwerth AC, Burrows NR, et al. Comprehensive public health strategies for preventing the development, progression, and complications

of CKD: report of an expert panel convened by the Centers for Disease Control and Prevention. *Am J Kidney Dis.* 2009;53:522–535.

17. Roels HA, Hoet P, Lison D. Usefulness of biomarkers of exposure to inorganic mercury, lead, or cadmium in controlling occupational and environmental risks of nephrotoxicity. *Ren Fail.* 1999;21:251–262.

18. Weaver VM, Jaar BG. Lead related nephrotoxicity. *Up to Date.* Available at: http://www.uptodate.com/contents/lead-nephropathy-and-lead-related-nephrotoxicity. Accessed July 16, 2009.

19. Elinder C. Epidemiology and toxicity of cadmium. *Up to Date.* Available at: http://www.uptodate.com/contents/epidemiology-and-toxicity-of-cadmium. Accessed July 16, 2009.

20. Goldman RH. Arsenic exposure and poisoning. *Up to Date* 19.1. Available at: http://www.uptodate.com/contents/arsenic-exposure-and-poisoning. Accessed July 16, 2009.

21. Hossain MP, Goyder EC, Rigby JE, El Nahas M. CKD and poverty: a growing global challenge. *Am J Kidney Dis.* 2009;53:166–174.

22. McClellan WM, Flanders WD. Risk factors for progressive chronic kidney disease. *J Am Soc Nephrol.* 2003;14:S65–S70.

23. Centers for Disease Control and Prevention. An estimated 26 million adults in the United States have chronic kidney disease (CKD). Available at: http://cdc.gov/features/dschronickidneydisease/. Accessed May 4, 2009.

24. Chobanian AV, Bakris GL, Black HR, et al. The seventh report of the joint national committee on prevention, detection, evaluation, and treatment of high blood pressure: the JNC 7 report. *JAMA.* 2003;289:2560–2572.

25. Parker TF 3rd, Blantz R, Hostetter T, et al. The chronic kidney disease initiative. *J Am Soc Nephrol.* 2004;15:708–716.

26. USRDS Coordinating Center. Chapter two: incidence and prevalence. Available at: http://www.usrds.org/2009/pdf/V2_02_INC_PREV_09.PDF. Accessed October 4, 2009.

27. Centers for Disease Control and Prevention. BRFSS. Transforming information into health. Available at: http://www.cdc.gov/brfss/index.htm. Accessed May 26, 2011.

28. Centers for Disease Control and Prevention. National Health and Nutrition Examination Survey. Available at: http://www.cdc.gov/nchs/nhanes.htm. Accessed May 26, 2011.

29. Centers for Disease Control and Prevention. Physical inactivity estimates, by county. Available at: http://www.cdc.gov/Features/dsPhysicalInactivity/. Accessed February 23, 2011.

30. Tessaro I, Smith SL, Rye S. Knowledge and perceptions of diabetes in an Appalachian population. *Prev Chronic Dis.* 2005;2:A13.

31. O'Brien T, Denham SA. Diabetes care and education in rural regions. *Diabetes Educ.* 2008;34:334–347.

32. Schmidt RJ, Pellegrino BS. Low serum albumin common in rural patients with chronic kidney disease [abstract presentation]. Denver, CO: American Society of Nephrology Conference; 2010.

33. Osinski M, Wish J. Physician workforce: coming up short. Available at: http://www.nephrologyusa.com/articles/physician-workforce-coming-up-short .html. Accessed February 23, 2011.

34. Rosenberg ME. Adult nephrology fellowship training in the United States: trends and issues. *J Am Soc Nephrol.* 2007;18:1027–1033.

35. Lane CA, Brown MA. Nephrology: a specialty in need of resuscitation? *Kidney Int.* 2009;76:594–596.

36. Ad Hoc Committee on Nephrology Manpower Needs. Estimating workforce and training requirements for nephrologists through the year 2010. Executive summary. *J Am Soc Nephrol.* 1997;8(5 Suppl 9):S9–S13.

37. Neilson EG, Hull AR, Wish JB, Neylan JF, Sherman D, Suki WN. The ad hoc committee report on estimating the future workforce and training requirements for nephrology. The Ad Hoc Committee on Nephrology Manpower Needs. *J Am Soc Nephrol.* 1997;8:S1–S4.

38. Kletke PR. The changing supply of renal physicians. *Am J Kidney Dis.* 1997;29:781–792.

39. Bizzozero J. Understanding the nephrology shortage. Available at: http://www.renalbusiness.com/articles/2009/09/understanding-the-nephrologist-shortage.aspx. Accessed February 23, 2011.

40. Navarro AM, Voetsch KP, Liburd LC, Giles HW, Collins JL. Charting the future of community health promotion: recommendations from the national expert panel on community health promotion. *Prev Chronic Dis* [serial online]. 2007;4(3). Available at: http://www.cdc.gov/pcd/issues/2007/jul/07_0013.htm. Accessed July 16, 2009.

41. Smedley BD, Syme SL, Committee on Capitalizing on Social Science and Behavioral Research to Improve the Public's Health. Promoting health: intervention strategies from social and behavioral research. *Am J Health Promot.* 2001;15:149–166.

42. Hendryx M. Mortality from heart, respiratory, and kidney disease in coal mining areas of Appalachia. *Int Arch Occup Environ Health.* 2009;82:243–249.

43. Sludge Safety Project of Ohio Valley Environmental Coalition. Appalachian air quality fact sheet. Available at: http://www.sludgesafety.org/health/Air_Quality_Fact_Sheet.pdf. Accessed October 4, 2009.

44. Pond GJ, Passmore ME, Borsuk FA, Reynolds L, Rose C. Downstream effects of mountaintop removal coal mining: comparing biologic conditions using family and genus-level macroinvertebrate bioassessment tools. *J N Am Benth Soc.* 2008;27(3):717–737.

45. Stout BM. Do headwater streams recover from longwall mining impacts in

northern West Virginia? Final report. West Virginia Water Research Center; August 30, 2004.

46. Molony DA, Craig JC. Evidence-based nephrology. In: Wedeen RP, ed. *Toxic Nephropathies: Environmental Agents and Metals.* West Sussex, UK: Wiley-Blackwell; 2009:294–299.

47. Jarup L. Hazards of heavy metal contamination. *Br Med Bull.* 2003;68:167–182.

48. Jarup L, Akesson A. Current status of cadmium as an environmental health problem. *Toxicol Appl Pharmacol.* 2009;238(3):201–208.

49. Ekong EB, Jaar BG, Weaver VM. Lead-related nephrotoxicity: a review of the epidemiologic evidence. *Kidney Int.* 2006;70:2074–2084.

50. Shipper J. Arsenic in domestic well water and health in central Appalachia. *Water Air Soil Pollu.* 2005;60(1–4):327–341.

51. Carroll and Nancy Fields O'Connor Center for the Rocky Mountain West. Available at: http://www.crmw.org/. Accessed October 3, 2009.

52. Ohio Valley Educational Cooperative (OVEC). Available at: http://www.ovec.org. Accessed October 3, 2009.

53. Appalachian Voices. Available at: http://appvoices.org/. Accessed October 3, 2009.

54. National Air and Space Administration. Earth observatory: coal controversy in Appalachia. Available at: http://earthobservatory.nasa.gov/Features/Mountain topRemoval/. Accessed September 30, 2009.

55. Kentucky Department of Fish and Wildlife. Fish consumption advisories. Available at: http://www.fw.ky.gov/fishadvisory.asp. Accessed October 3, 2009.

56. Sierra Club. Toxic selenium. Available at: http://www.sierraclub.org/coal/downloads/Seleniumfactsheet.pdf. Accessed October 3, 2009.

57. Nishijo M, Morikawa Y, Nakagawa H, et al. Causes of death and renal tubular dysfunction in residents exposed to cadmium in the environment. *Occup Environ Med.* 2006;63:545–550.

58. Noonan CW, Sarasua SM, Campagna D, Kathman SJ, Lybarger JA, Mueller PW. Effects of exposure to low levels of environmental cadmium on renal biomarkers. *Environ Health Perspect.* 2002;110:151–155.

59. Navas-Acien A, Selvin E, Sharrett AR, Calderon-Aranda E, Silbergeld E, Guallar E. Lead, cadmium, smoking, and increased risk of peripheral arterial disease. *Circulation.* 2004;109:3196–3201.

60. Lin JL, Lin-Tan DT, Li YJ, Chen KH, Huang YL. Low-level environmental exposure to lead and progressive chronic kidney diseases. *Am J Med.* 2006;119:707.e1–707.e9.

61. Schmidt RJ, Pellegrino BS. Socioeconomic factors and low albumin levels in rural CKD patients [abstract presentation]. Denver, CO: American Society of Nephrology Conference; 2010.

62. Zhang Z, Infante A, Meit M, English N, Dunn M, Bowers KH. An analysis of mental health and substance abuse disparities and access to treatment services in the Appalachian region. Washington, DC: Appalachian Regional Commission; 2008. Available at: http://www.arc.gov/assets/research_reports/AnalysisofMentalHealthandSubstanceAbuseDisparities.pdf. Accessed July 16, 2009.

63. Centers for Disease Control and Prevention. Unintentional poisoning deaths—United States, 1999–2004. Available at: http://www.cdc.gov/mmwr/preview/mmwrhtml/mm5605a1.htm. Accessed February 23, 2011.

64. Hall AJ, Logan JE, Toblin RL, et al. Patterns of abuse among unintentional pharmaceutical overdose fatalities. *JAMA*. 2008;300:2613–2620.

65. Halverson JA, Ma L, Harner EJ. An analysis of disparities in health status and access to health care in the Appalachian region. Washington, DC: Appalachian Regional Commission; 2004.

66. Halverson JA, Bischak G. Underlying socioeconomic factors influencing health disparities in the Appalachian region. Washington, DC: Appalachian Regional Commission; 2008.

67. U.S. Department of Health and Human Services, Public Health Service. Progress review—chronic kidney disease. Available at: http://www.healthypeople.gov/2010/Data/2010prog/focus04/2002fa04.htm. Accessed May 1, 2009.

68. National Kidney Foundation. KEEP. Available at: http://www.kidney.org/news/keep/KEEPabout.cfm. Accessed May 1, 2009.

69. West Virginia Department of Health and Human Resources. 2006 West Virginia behavioral risk factor survey report. Available at: http://www.wvdhhr.org/bph/hsc/statserv/Pub.asp?ID=103. Accessed May 1, 2009.

70. National Kidney Foundation. KEEP screening data for West Virginia. Personal communication.

10

Trauma

*Levi D. Procter, Andrew C. Bernard, Paul A. Kearney,
and Julia F. Costich*

This chapter addresses the problem of injury in rural areas of Appalachia, including the role of trauma systems in caring for the injured and the inadequacies of these systems in rural areas. Because systems for collecting data on injury are fragmented and limited in scope, the precise analysis of injury data in Appalachia remains impossible, even in the twenty-first century. Therefore, injury data from three Appalachian states are used as a surrogate for other rural areas in Appalachia. This chapter outlines specific deficiencies and concludes with recommendations for future research and policy initiatives.

Epidemiology

Trauma is the number-one cause of death in the first four decades of life in developed countries. Nearly 9 million people worldwide are injured annually, 300,000 of whom suffer permanent disability.[1] Unintentional injury (UI) is the term for injury that is not caused by the human intent to harm oneself or another person.[2] UI accounts for more than 100,000 deaths in the United States each year and is the fourth leading cause of death in all age groups.[1, 3, 4] Major traumatic injury and death are much more common for men than for women, with men representing approximately two-thirds of the total population injured. Motor vehicle crashes (MVCs) are the leading cause of UI, accounting for more than 1 million injuries worldwide annually. Falls are the second most common cause of UI in those aged 45 to 75 years and the leading cause of unintentional death in persons older than 75 years, followed by poisoning, drowning, and burns.[1] In 2005 fatal and nonfatal UIs resulted in $625 billion in U.S. health care costs.

Injury in Rural America

Rural populations across the United States have significantly worse outcomes from UIs than their urban counterparts. Only 30 percent of the U.S. population lives in rural areas, but nearly 70 percent of injury-related deaths occur there.[5, 6] In rural America a pedestrian struck by an automobile is three to four times more likely to die than one injured in an urban area,[7] and the risk of death from MVCs is fifteen times as high.[8] The likelihood of death from UIs in rural areas is inversely proportional to population density.[9–12]

In addition, injured rural patients are typically older and frequently die at the scene with lesser degrees of injury.[13] Rutledge and coworkers[13] found that injured rural patients who survived at least twenty-four hours were older, had more comorbidities, had less overall injury, and were more likely to die from multiple organ system failure when compared with similarly matched urban patients.

In rural areas lacking trauma systems, UI-related deaths are distributed in a trimodal pattern—immediate, early, and late—which is also the basis for trauma system design.[14] The first sixty minutes after injury—the "golden hour" of trauma—account for the highest number of deaths.[15, 16] In the classic statement by Dr. R. Adams Cowley, "there is a golden hour between life and death. If you are critically injured you have less than 60 minutes to survive. You might not die right then; it may be three days or two weeks later—but something has happened in your body that is irreparable."[16] Some 45 to 50 percent of those severely injured die immediately or very soon after injury.[14, 17] The early mode is between one and four hours after injury, representing some 24 percent of deaths, and the late mode includes deaths occurring more than one week after injury due to multiple organ failure.[14, 17] Late deaths now account for only 7.6 percent of all trauma deaths in areas with established trauma systems, reflecting improvements in critical care and resuscitation.[17]

Immediate deaths point to the need for better trauma prevention initiatives and education. Improvements in prevention are critical to lessening injury severity and mortality. For instance, trauma prevention programs that focus on safe workplaces, use of seat belts, alcohol and substance abuse deterrence, proper helmet usage, and firearm safety offer the greatest potential benefit in terms of preventing immediate deaths. The severely injured who do not die immediately represent a sizable injured population for whom appropriate trauma care, if delivered quickly and efficiently, can provide significant benefit.

Epidemiology in Three Rural Appalachian Areas

Death certificate data provide the most comprehensive surveillance of fatal injuries from a geographic perspective. For example, the Kentucky Injury Prevention and Research Center receives cause-of-death information from the National Center for Health Statistics, part of the Centers for Disease Control and Prevention. UI is a significant cause of death and morbidity within the fifty-four Appalachian counties in Kentucky. The most common cause of injury-related death is MVC, followed by falls.[18] Death due to MVC is inversely proportional to population density in the community of injury.[9] For the period 1999–2006, the fatality rate for Appalachian Kentucky counties was 69.7 percent higher for MVCs, 24.8 percent higher for other causes of injury, and 37.8 percent higher overall than for non-Appalachian Kentucky counties (table 10.1).[19, 20] Children in Appalachian Kentucky counties have an even higher rate of trauma-related death than do other rural Kentucky children.[21]

Similarly, death certificate data from the Tennessee Department of Health for 2005 and 2006 indicated elevated injury rates in the state's fifty-two Appalachian counties. On average, MVC death rates for the Appalachian counties were 73.7 percent higher, while death rates from other

Table 10.1. State Death Rates for Motor Vehicle Collisions in Appalachian versus Non-Appalachian Counties	
State	**Percentage Higher in Appalachian vs. Non-Appalachian Counties**
Kentucky	69.7
Tennessee	73.7
West Virginia*	46.8
* Because West Virginia is entirely Appalachian, the non-Appalachian comparison was based on the national rate.	

trauma were 79.7 percent higher than for the non-Appalachian counties (table 10.1). In West Virginia, which is entirely Appalachian, the motor vehicle–related death rate in 2005 was 23.4 per 100,000 population, or 46.8 percent higher than the 15.94 per 100,000 national rate. In West Virginia, traumatic injuries from other causes had a 36.3 per 100,000 death rate.

High-Risk Injuries Specific to Appalachia

In addition to experiencing elevated death rates from the types of trauma that are common across the United States, residents of Appalachia engage in certain occupational and recreational activities that expose them to a high risk of injury. Three that deserve special attention are underground coal mining, logging, and all-terrain vehicle (ATV) use.

Coal Mining. Coal mining has a large economic impact in Appalachia, and despite safety improvements, it remains one of the nation's most hazardous occupations. In 2002 mining had the highest reported mortality rate of any occupation,[22] with Appalachian coal miners suffering higher age-adjusted mortality in direct proportion to the density of coal mines.[23] In 2007 coal mining injuries killed 27 Americans, including 9 in Kentucky and West Virginia; it permanently disabled an additional 45, of whom 28 were in the same two states.[24] These figures are near the averages for the previous five years. For bituminous coal miners, the rate of injury requiring days away from work or a job change was among the highest of all occupations, at 4.9 per 100,000 employees, well above the private industry average of 4.4 per 100,000.[25]

Mining activity waxes and wanes with the economy, so consistent injury prevention initiatives are challenging to sustain. Regulatory efforts have had only mixed success, and the continuing presence of owner-operated, unregulated mines elevates the risk of injury even further. Appalachian communities bear the long-term burden of supporting the large number of disabled former miners. The presence of a disproportionate population of unemployed, permanently disabled workers makes communities less attractive to new businesses and imposes a burden of caregiving that diverts resources from other uses. The chronic pain that often accompanies disability from a mining-related injury is an important factor in the epidemic of prescription drug abuse in the region.[26]

Logging. Logging takes a disproportionate toll in terms of injury where the terrain is rough and production is less mechanized, as in Appalachia.[27, 28]

In 2007 logging workers were second only to fishermen in the rate of fatal occupational injuries.[25] The impact of nonfatal logging injuries can only be guessed because relatively few Appalachian residents are directly employed by logging companies; however, a substantial (and unknown) number work as independent contractors and are unlikely to appear in analyses based on worker compensation data. West Virginia has one of the highest logging fatality rates even though it accounts for only 2 percent of the total logging workforce, surpassing fatalities in the mining and construction industries.[29]

All-Terrain Vehicles. The popularity of ATVs in rural America is well known, as is their association with serious injury and death.[30] In Kentucky, ATV-related injuries were responsible for 279 hospitalizations and 46 deaths in 2006 alone. ATVs present an unusually complex regulatory problem because the majority of sales take place between private parties rather than through dealerships, and much use occurs where it is unlikely to be subject to surveillance by law enforcement. Anecdotally, illegal ATV use may not result in pursuit by law enforcement officers because of the potentially deadly consequences of prompting the rider to increase vehicle speed. Although all states with Appalachian counties have some form of ATV law on the books, the effectiveness of these laws can clearly be questioned in light of continued increases in ATV-related injury and death. Several Appalachian states have attempted to lure tourist revenue by creating ATV trails. Such sites have a clear advantage over less organized ATV use because safety measures such as helmets, appropriately sized equipment for younger riders, and safe riding environments can be enforced.

Trauma Systems and Rural America

Trauma is a disease with identifiable causes and profound financial, social, personal, and psychological impacts. Successful management of traumatic injuries requires prompt and efficient transport, evaluation, and treatment of injuries. These fundamental concepts are the basis of a trauma system. A trauma system is defined as "an organized approach to acutely injured patients in a defined geographical area that provides full and optimal care and that is integrated with the local or regional emergency medical service (EMS) system" (p. 57).[31] Trauma systems are designed to deliver cost-effective care from prehospital to rehabilitation. The regionalization of trauma care allows the most appropriate utilization of health care resources to deliver the most efficient care. In addition to providing acute trauma care, a trauma system has the responsibility to educate health care providers who encounter these patients, identify trauma-related risk factors, and prevent injury. Injury is largely preventable through education, engineering, enforcement, and other well-documented strategies. Planning for the entire range of disasters—including industrial calamity, extreme weather conditions, and terrorism—provides regions with the skill sets and resource stewardship to provide optimal trauma care in all circumstances.

Research demonstrates that in states or regions with trauma systems, the odds of injury-related death are 15 to 20 percent lower than in places without such systems.[32] Quality of care in formally verified facilities is substantially better.[32] Formal protocols for prehospital and hospital care are a fundamental component of trauma systems and lead to improved patient outcomes. Trauma systems benefit public health within a community by lowering MVC-related mortality rates by 17 percent.[32] Despite these documented benefits of trauma systems, fifteen states have no formal trauma system, and three of them are rural states.[32] Other states have trauma systems that are inadequately funded or lack the necessary capacity. Trauma centers in Appalachia are located primarily in urban population centers. The region is so vast that although a state may have one or more trauma centers, large populations still live far from a verified center. The distance and time from a trauma center significantly affect the care of traumatically injured patients in rural areas. Locating the injured may be difficult, and it is compounded by poor road systems and treacherous terrain that make the pickup and transport of these patients exceedingly difficult. Often these localities lack sufficient ambulances to cover their own territories and are required to serve adjacent counties simultaneously. Urban trauma centers adjacent to rural areas bear the burden of caring for these injured patients. A well-designed regional trauma system can help eliminate the delay in transfer and lift the burden of care off adjacent urban trauma centers.

Rural Disparities in Trauma Education for Providers

Knowledge and techniques in trauma care have improved significantly over the past three decades. A common framework for trauma care, Advanced Trauma Life Support (ATLS), originated in 1979 and has been taught worldwide in more than fifty countries to more than 1 million doctors.[33] ATLS uses a standardized approach for all trauma patients and emphasizes early transfer when the patient's needs exceed local capabilities. ATLS improves outcome, decreases resource utilization, and expedites care.[33] Unfortunately, more than thirty years after its inception, ATLS education is not yet universal among emergency department physicians, and fewer ATLS-trained physicians practice in rural areas than in urban areas.[34, 35] Similar to ATLS is the Trauma Nursing Core Course (TNCC) developed by the Emergency Nurses Association. TNCC teaches core concepts plus technical skills to nurses who provide trauma care, but like ATLS, TNCC courses and TNCC-trained nurses are centered in urban areas.

To address the outcome discrepancy between rural and urban trauma victims, the Rural Trauma Subcommittee of the American College of Surgeons Committee on Trauma developed the Rural Trauma Team Development Course (RTTDC). The goal of the RTTDC is to ensure that hospitals respond to trauma victims in an organized manner, establish priorities, and, when appropriate, transfer without delay. The RTTDC is an adjunct to ATLS and is not intended to replace it. Data emerge daily regarding ways to improve trauma and critical care; however, the institution of better practices in rural areas lags far behind.

These educational initiatives serve to standardize care of the injured regardless of setting. Adherence to the basic principles of life-sustaining care and expeditious transport is critical to rural trauma care. Courses such as ATLS, TNCC, and RTTDC serve to educate the entire team involved in the care of traumatically injured patients, including paramedics, nurses, physicians, and hospital administrators. Such across-the-board education is the only way to instill the basic principles of trauma care and standardize care through protocols that are applied to every patient every time.

Rural Emergency Department Staffing

The staffing of rural emergency departments varies significantly. Typical staffing consists of physician assistants (PAs), nurses, nurse practitioners (NPs), and doctors of medicine (MDs) or doctors of osteopathy (DOs) who are either members of the hospital medical staff or contracted through emergency medical groups to staff the emergency department.[36] There is no consistency with regard to which staff members are available at any time. For example, a staff MD or DO may cover the daytime shift, while a PA or NP covers the night shift and a contracted emergency room physician covers the weekend. There are many other potential combinations that are often in a state of flux.

The experience of each staff member in these rural emergency departments varies as well. Some are trained emergency physicians; others may be family practitioners or internists. Nearly all physicians, NPs, and PAs in these locations are current in their Advanced Cardiac Life Support (ACLS) training; however, very few have ATLS or Pediatric Advanced Life Support (PALS) training. Also, few hospitals have programs that teach staff members to work as a team, such as the RTTDC. In a survey of rural hospitals, more than half had nurses with trauma training through the TNCC. Finally, rural emergency departments lack protocols for trauma care, although the majority of them have protocols for managing patients with chest pain that improve outcomes.[36]

Delays in Transferring Rural Trauma Victims

Even with the best trauma care, injuries incurred in rural areas are often more severe and have poorer outcomes, including higher mortality rates, than those occurring in urban areas.[37] One national analysis found that smaller rural counties had even higher rates of death due to trauma than larger rural counties, where trauma death rates were 27 percent higher than in urban counties.[38] In rural areas, access to critical resources, such as well-designed and well-maintained roadways, efficient communication systems, and economic resources, is limited.[39, 40] Rural citizens are also more likely to drive under the influence of alcohol[41] and less likely to wear seat belts.[2, 41–43]

Roadways that lack modern safety features and are inadequately maintained lead to both injury and logistical problems in rural areas. The discovery of accident scenes on rural roadways is often delayed because of sparse traffic, vision obscured by hilly terrain, and decreased availability of emergency contact devices such as cellular phones.[44, 45] After a trauma victim is found, securing and transporting the patient can be difficult. All these factors can delay trauma care and elevate death rates compared with urban areas.[45]

Patients who are severely injured far from trauma centers may require helicopter transport, which has its own hazards. Not uncommonly, patients travel by ground ambulance to helicopter landing areas for transport to a higher level of care. Safely placing a patient on a helicopter can take a significant amount of time, further delaying emergency care. In an ideal trauma system, injured patients are taken to the closest center that can manage their level of injury severity. Without protocols and regional trauma systems, an injured patient may simply be taken to the closest hospital, or the ambulance may bypass a center that could stabilize and resuscitate the patient prior to transfer to the most appropriate center.

In Central Appalachia there is often just one ambulance to serve several adjacent counties. Multiple simultaneous victims in different counties can create a triage nightmare for these ambulance crews. Not all ambulance services can provide advanced life support, which means that the severely injured may receive only basic life support. Appalachian trauma systems can help alleviate this problem by creating protocols for these situations whereby care is delivered to achieve the most benefit, congruent with the available resources.

Transfer of trauma victims to definitive care is essential, regardless of the injury site, but it is crucial in rural trauma settings. For example, in 2008 the average time from patient arrival at a community hospital to arrival at the level I trauma center in Lexington, Kentucky, was 5.8 hours, far in excess of the golden hour. Among the reasons for transfer delay are a lack of understanding of priorities owing to educational deficiencies and the absence of standardized trauma training. The performance and interpretation of diagnostic studies prior to transfer can increase delays. A study by the University of Kentucky Trauma Program indicated that up to 25 percent of emergency physicians obtain imaging studies to reduce the liability risk, even if doing so delays the transfer of injured patients.[46] Approximately 33 percent of respondents indicated that imaging is performed because of perceived requirements of the receiving center. However, a delay in definitive care for trauma, especially in patients who are hemorrhaging, worsens outcome. Only rudimentary testing is needed before the transfer of severely injured patients. The adage taught in the RTTDC is, "If the imaging won't change what care is provided at the sending facility, then it can be obviated." The sooner a severely injured trauma patient is evaluated at a definitive care institution, the better the outcome.

There is also a significant disparity in pediatric trauma care in both urban and rural areas across the United States. The Institute of Medicine reports: "Only six percent of U.S. emergency departments have all the supplies necessary for handling pediatric emergencies, and only about half of the departments had even 85 percent of the essential supplies." Further, it notes that about 90 percent of the children who did not survive their traumatic injuries died before reaching the hospital.[47]

Further Research

Addressing the problem of injury in rural Appalachia requires a multifaceted approach based on effective prevention, prompt transportation to appropriate evaluation and treatment services, well-designed trauma systems located in the right geographic areas, and properly trained personnel. The design and implementation of this approach will require an enhanced body of research knowledge. Some important questions that need to be answered are the following:

- How can successful injury prevention initiatives and related population health activities in the Appalachian region be translated and disseminated to other areas?
- What strategies and policies have enabled state and local governments to provide adequate emergency medical services for rural areas in Appalachia with excessive rates of traumatic injury and death?
- How can smaller hospitals serving predominantly rural areas in Appalachia be equipped in a cost-effective manner to stabilize trauma patients when immediate transfer to definitive care is not practical?
- What trauma system design features in rural Appalachia are associated with reduced fatality rates and other improvements in patient outcomes?
- What types of analyses are needed to develop a comprehensive description of Appalachian trauma issues, and what data elements are missing?

Policy Recommendations

The impact of trauma in Appalachia is underappreciated. Appalachian trauma care is generally underdeveloped and lacks organization; it is fragmented, understaffed, and underfunded. Trauma systems have resulted in improved outcomes and quality of care for trauma patients, highlighting the need for local-area trauma systems in Appalachia. Recommendations for reducing the disease burden from trauma include the following:

- Increase policy makers' awareness of the need for regional trauma systems in Appalachia. Effective trauma systems in other parts of the country have reduced the incidence and severity of trauma-related death and disability, but they require considerable initial investment. Data registries, facility construction, transport arrangements, health care providers, and other critical components are often lacking in Appalachia and cannot be supported by the local tax base alone.
- The three pillars of injury prevention—education, engineering, and enforcement—have been inadequately deployed in the Appalachian region and must be accorded greater attention if the burden of trauma is to be reduced.
- State policy must provide unambiguous direction to elements of local and regional trauma care systems in Appalachia to ensure transfer protocols that connect patients with definitive care as quickly as possible.

References

1. Fraser V, Burd L, Liebson E, Lipschik G, Peterson CM. Trauma, accident, and injury. In: *Diseases and Disorders.* Tarrytown, NY: Marshall Cavendish; 2007:855–860.

2. Zwerling C, Merchant JA, Nordstrom DL, et al. Risk factors for injury in rural Iowa: round one of the Keokuk County rural health study. *Am J Prev Med.* 2001;20:230–233.

3. Fingerhut LA, Warner M. Injury chartbook, health, United States, 1996–97. Hyattsville, MD: National Center for Health Statistics; 1997.

4. Centers for Disease Control and Prevention. CDC—injury—WISQARS (Web-based Injury Statistics Query and Reporting System). Available at: http://www.cdc.gov/injury/wisqars/. Accessed October 5, 2009.

5. Rogers FB, Shackford SR, Osler TM, Vane DW, Davis JH. Rural trauma: the challenge for the next decade. *J Trauma.* 1999;47:802–821.

6. Wayne R. Rural trauma management. *Am J Surg.* 1989;157:463–466.

7. Muelleman RL, Walker RA, Edney JA. Motor vehicle deaths: a rural epidemic. *J Trauma.* 1993;35:717–719.

8. Maio RF, Green PE, Becker MP, Burney RE, Compton C. Rural motor vehicle crash mortality: the role of crash severity and medical resources. *Accid Anal Prev.* 1992;24:631–642.

9. Baker SP, Whitfield RA, O'Neill B. Geographic variations in mortality from motor vehicle crashes. *N Engl J Med.* 1987;316:1384–1387.

10. Peek-Asa C, Zwerling C, Stallones L. Acute traumatic injuries in rural populations. *Am J Public Health.* 2004;94:1689–1693.

11. Rutledge R, Fakhry SM, Baker CC, et al. A population-based study of the association of medical manpower with county trauma death rates in the United States. *Ann Surg.* 1994;219:547–563; discussion 563–567.

12. Eberhardt MS, Ingram DD, Makuc DM, et al. Urban and rural health chartbook, health, United States, 2001. Hyattsville, MD: National Center for Health Statistics; 2001.

13. Rutledge R, Smith CY, Azizkhank RG. A population-based multivariate analysis of the association of county demographic and medical system factors with per capita pediatric trauma death rates in North Carolina. *Ann Surg.* 1994;219:205–210.

14. Trunkey DD. Trauma: accidental and intentional injuries account for more years of life lost in the U.S. than cancer and heart disease. Among the prescribed remedies are improved preventive efforts, speedier surgery and further research. *Sci Am.* 1983;249:28–35.

15. Lerner EB, Moscati RM. The golden hour: scientific fact or medical "urban legend"? *Acad Emerg Med.* 2001;8:758–760.

16. Golden hour (medicine). Available at: http://www.lumrix.net/health/Golden_hour_(medicine).html. Accessed May 6, 2011.

17. Demetriades D, Kimbrell B, Salim A, et al. Trauma deaths in a mature urban trauma system: is "trimodal" distribution a valid concept? *J Am Coll Surg.* 2005;201:343–348.

18. Rinker CF, Schmitz GD. Rural trauma. In: Feliciano DV, Mattox KL, Moore EE, eds. *Trauma.* 6th ed. New York, NY: McGraw-Hill; 2008:157–167.

19. Baker SP, Whitfield RA, O'Neill B. County mapping of injury mortality. *J Trauma.* 1988;28:741–745.

20. Kearney PA, Stallones L, Swartz C, Barker DE, Johnson SB. Unintentional injury death rates in rural Appalachia. *J Trauma.* 1990;30:1524–1532.

21. Svenson JE, Stapczynski JS, Nypaver M, Calhoun R. Development of a statewide trauma system: classification of levels of care available to injured patients. *J Ky Med Assoc.* 1996;94:63–69.

22. Research and Statistics Department. Injury facts. Itasca, IL: National Safety Council; 2002.

23. Hendryx M, Ahern MM. Mortality in Appalachian coal mining regions: the value of statistical life lost. *Public Health Rep.* 2009;124:541–550.

24. Mine Safety and Health Agency. Injury experience in coal mining, 2007. Washington, DC: U.S. Department of Labor; 2007. Available at: http://www.msha.gov/Stats/Part50/Yearly%20IR's/2007/2007-Coal-IR.pdf. Accessed September 9, 2010.

25. Census of fatal occupational injuries summary, 2009. Available at: http://www.bls.gov/news.release/cfoi.nr0.htm. Accessed September 2, 2010.

26. Hughes AA, Bogdan GM, Dart RC. Active surveillance of abused and misused prescription opioids using poison center data: a pilot study and descriptive comparison. *Clin Toxicol (Phila).* 2007;45:144–151.

27. Helmkamp JC, Derk SJ. Nonfatal logging-related injuries in West Virginia. *J Occup Environ Med.* 1999;41:967–972.

28. Mujuru P, Helmkamp JC, Mutambudzi M, Hu W, Bell JL. Evaluating the impact of an intervention to reduce injuries among loggers in West Virginia, 1999–2007. *J Agric Saf Health.* 2009;15:75–88.

29. Bell JL, Helmkamp JC. Non-fatal injuries in the West Virginia logging industry: using workers' compensation claims to assess risk from 1995 through 2001. *Am J Ind Med.* 2003;44:502–509.

30. David J. Part III. Report on all-terrain vehicle–related deaths, January 1, 1985–December 31, 1996. Bethesda, MD: U.S. Consumer Product Safety Commission; 1998.

31. Hoyt DB, Coimbra R, Potenza BM. Trauma systems, triage, and transport. In: Feliciano DV, Mattox KL, Moore EE, eds. *Trauma.* 6th ed. New York, NY: McGraw-Hill; 2008:57–81.

32. MacKenzie EJ, Hoyt DB, Sacra JC, et al. National inventory of hospital trauma centers. *JAMA.* 2003;289:1515–1522.

33. American College of Surgeons. ATLS. *Advanced Trauma Life Support for Doctors.* 8th ed. Chicago, IL: American College of Surgeons; 2002.

34. Esposito TJ, Copass MK, Maier RV. Analysis of surgical participation in the Advanced Trauma Life Support course: what are the goals and are we meeting them? *Arch Surg.* 1992;127:721–725; discussion 726.

35. Helmkamp JC. All-terrain vehicle–related deaths among the West Virginia elderly, 1985 to 1998. *Am J Public Health.* 1999;89:1263–1264.

36. Casey M, Wholey D, Moscovice I. Rural emergency department staffing: potential implications for the quality of emergency care provided in rural areas. Minneapolis, MN: The Upper Midwest Rural Health Research Center; 2007.

37. Svenson JE, Spurlock C, Nypaver M. Factors associated with the higher traumatic death rate among rural children. *Ann Emerg Med.* 1996;27:625–632.

38. Coben JH, Tiesman HM, Bossarte RM, Furbee PM. Rural-urban differences in injury hospitalizations in the U.S., 2004. *Am J Prev Med.* 2009;36:49–55.

39. Graham JD. Injuries from traffic crashes: meeting the challenge. *Annu Rev Public Health.* 1993;14:515–543.

40. Karlaftis MG, Golias I. Effects of road geometry and traffic volumes on rural roadway accident rates. *Accid Anal Prev.* 2002;34:357–365.

41. Blatt J, Furman SM. Residence location of drivers involved in fatal crashes. *Accid Anal Prev.* 1998;30:705–711.

42. Baker DR, Clarke SR, Brandt EN Jr. An analysis of factors associated with seat belt use: prevention opportunities for the medical community. *J Okla State Med Assoc.* 2000;93:496–500.

43. Lundell JA. Motor vehicle occupant safety in a rural state. *Tex J Rural Health.* 2003;21(4):2–10.

44. Rogers FB, Shackford SR, Hoyt DB, et al. Trauma deaths in a mature urban vs rural trauma system: a comparison. *Arch Surg.* 1997;132:376–381; discussion 381–382.

45. Grossman DC, Kim A, Macdonald SC, Klein P, Copass MK, Maier RV. Urban-rural differences in prehospital care of major trauma. *J Trauma.* 1997;42:723–729.

46. Lee CY, Bernard AC, Fryman L, et al. Imaging may delay transfer of rural trauma victims: a survey of referring physicians. *J Trauma.* 2008;65:1359–1363.

47. Vane DW, Shackford SR. Epidemiology of rural traumatic death in children: a population-based study. *J Trauma.* 1995;38:867–870.

11

Mental Health

Susan E. Keefe and Lisa Curtin

Appalachia presents striking challenges for the field of mental health. Multiple social and economic stressors, including high rates of unemployment and poverty, low levels of education and health insurance coverage, long travel distances to services, few institutional resources, and cultural differences,[a] create the conditions for a high prevalence of mental and emotional problems. Yet some types of mental health services tend to be unavailable in the region and, if available, underutilized.

This chapter argues that mental health researchers and practitioners must be familiar with both biomedical and ethnomedical models to create and deliver appropriate mental health services for Appalachians. Medical anthropologists use the term *ethnomedicine* to refer to the beliefs and practices related to health, illness, and healing among ethnic groups. Ethnomedical systems are based on ethnic groups' assumptions about the nature of health, the causes of illness, the classification of illnesses and relevant symptoms, diagnostic practices and the treatment of illness, and the appropriate delivery of health care services. Ethnomedical systems vary widely in their conception of these basic attributes. This chapter assumes that Appalachians have their own ethnomedical beliefs and practices that often differ from those embodied in the biomedical system—that is, the Western scientific medical system developed over the past 200 years.

Taking their assumptions from biomedicine, mental health professionals generally believe that there are universally detectable mental diseases that are treatable with standardized medications or psychotherapy protocols. Concepts of what is normal and what is pathological may be treated as fixed absolutes that can be universally applied. Assessment instruments may be considered "culture free" and are used to measure the incidence and prevalence of mental diseases around the world. Universal scientific techniques are sought for the diagnosis and treatment of these mental diseases that are thought to be grounded in organic and biological or genetic processes, measures, and outcomes. It is often difficult for mental health professionals trained in these biomedical assumptions to understand and make sense of Appalachian ethnomedicine.

Taking into consideration both the biomedical and ethnomedical perspectives, this chapter examines the current literature in five topical areas: (1) the prevalence of mental illness in Appalachia; (2) social, cultural, economic, and ecological stressors affecting Appalachians' mental health; (3) local knowledge about mental health and mental illness and strategies for coping with adversity; (4) indigenous help-seeking behavior; and (5) mental health services in the region. Recommendations for research and policy development are presented in the concluding sections.

Prevalence of Mental Illness

Mental illness is identified as a health risk both nationally[1] and worldwide.[2] Diagnosis of a mental illness typically relies on meeting the criteria for specific symptoms and functional impairment,[3] as defined in the fourth edition of the *Diagnostic and Statistical Manual of Mental Disorders (DSM-IV)*.[4] During any one-year period, nearly one-quarter of the U.S. population experiences a mental illness or a mental illness that co-occurs with substance abuse. The most common disorders are specific phobias, social phobias, and major depression[5]; the majority of individuals with a mental illness fail to receive professional care.[2]

In a study funded by the Appalachian Regional Commission (ARC),[b] Zhang and colleagues[6] found that Appalachian residents aged 12 years and older reported a greater prevalence of serious psychological distress (SPD) compared with age-matched non-Appalachian residents (13.5 versus 11.6 percent). In addition, Appalachians reported a significantly higher prevalence of major depressive episodes (MDEs) during a one-year period compared with non-Appalachians (8.2 versus 7.6 percent). Although depression and substance abuse frequently co-occur[7] due to self-medication (abuse of substances to cope with depression), chronic substance use (sleep, mood, and appetite disturbances caused by alcohol abuse), or independent comorbidity, the greater prevalence of MDEs among Appalachian residents was independent of this co-occurrence. The highest prevalence rates for MDEs (10.6 percent) and SPD (16.1 percent) occurred in the economically distressed Central Appalachian coal mining region. Prevalence rates in the other Appalachian subregions were 8 percent for MDEs and 12.7 percent for SPD in Southern Appalachia, and 7.9 percent for MDEs and 13.8 percent for SPD in Northern Appalachia.[6]

Locally conducted studies in Appalachia[8–12] and in rural areas[13] also found high rates of depression among residents. The Appalachian region is more rural than the rest of the United States: 42 percent of its residents live in rural areas, compared with 20 to 25 percent of the national population. This suggests that comparisons with the rural mental health literature are appropriate. For example, a large-scale cross-sectional study using face-to-face interviews estimated that 2.6 million adults living in the rural United States suffer from depression; the unadjusted prevalence rate of depression was higher among rural residents than among urban residents.[13] Investigations conducted in rural Appalachia also suggest relatively high levels of depression. Rates of depression are generally higher among women than men, and rates of depression among women in rural Appalachia have been consistently high.[8–12] However, a large telephone interview survey of men in rural West Virginia found that their rate of depressive symptoms was greater than the national average,[10] suggesting that rates of major depression may be higher as well. Rather than assessing symptoms of depression and conducting geography-based comparisons, Keefe and Parsons[11] compared depressive symptoms reported by native and nonnative respondents living in a rural Appalachian county in western North Carolina. Using a telephone survey of health behaviors and symptoms, they found that 21 percent of native Appalachian participants reported depressive symptoms, compared with 9 percent of nonnative participants.

High rates of depression and psychological distress among Appalachians are likely related to a multitude of economic stressors. In addition, concerns about stigma and confidentiality, as well as the acceptance of adversity, may limit their likelihood of seeking professional help. Thus, Appalachians may pursue mental health services later in the course of their illness, resulting in greater impairment and distress.

Nationally, major depression and other mental illnesses are associated with approximately 90 percent of suicides.[14] Rates of suicide are approximately three times higher among men than women, are highest for men aged 65 and older, and are higher in rural than urban areas.[15–18] Halverson and colleagues[19] found that Appalachian residents are at risk for suicide; the highest rates were among men aged 35 and older, and suicide rates were higher in the Central and Southern subregions than in the Northern subregion. Variability was apparent, with relatively higher suicide rates among individuals aged 65 and older in counties in western Virginia and northeastern Alabama.

High rates of depression and psychological distress are risk factors for suicide among Appalachians. In addition, changing socioeconomics and demographics, ready access to firearms, longer travel distances to services, and use of services later in the course of mental illnesses may explain higher suicide rates in rural areas than in urban areas. However, it is also possible that there are rural-urban differences in listing suicide in death reports.[17]

Epidemiological studies of childhood mental illnesses lag behind adult studies due to assessment difficulties and the importance of the developmental context in children. The Great Smoky Mountains Study,[20, 21] however, assessed youths aged 9, 11, and 13 (oversampled for Cherokee Indian participants) in Appalachian counties of North Carolina using telephone interviews and, for a subset of participants, parent and child interviews. This longitudinal study found that approximately 20 percent of the children in the interview sample met the criteria for a *DSM* disorder during the prior three months. The most common problems were anxiety disorders, enuresis, tic disorders, conduct disorders, oppositional defiant disorders, and hyperactivity. Psychiatric disorders were more common among boys than girls. Comparisons between Appalachian children under the age of 12 and children in the rest of the country are lacking.

In addition to documented higher rates of psychological distress, depression, and suicide in Appalachia relative to the rest of the United States, there are indications of other mental health problems. For example, abuse of prescription opiates and synthetics and corresponding admission rates for treatment are higher in Appalachia, particularly in the coalfields, compared with non-Appalachian areas.[6] Another area of concern is intimate partner violence, although quantitative studies comparing rates in

Appalachian and non-Appalachian areas could not be found. There is evidence that addressing intimate partner violence may be complicated due to geographic isolation and family values in Appalachia.[22]

Military veterans, who are vulnerable to adjustment problems, depression, and post-traumatic stress, often have difficulty accessing treatment when they return home to rural areas.[23] According to a newspaper report of the West Virginia Returning Soldiers Study, significantly more soldiers returning to rural West Virginia suffered from mental health problems (56 percent), primarily symptoms of post-traumatic stress disorder and depression, compared with those returning to urban West Virginia (32 percent) and to bases outside West Virginia (34 percent).[24] In addition, West Virginia National Guard members were more likely than active-duty soldiers to report symptoms of post-traumatic stress disorder and depression, potentially owing to the strain of multiple and unpredictable deployments.[24]

Stressors Related to Mental Health Problems

Mental health is not merely the absence of mental illness. The Centers for Disease Control and Prevention (CDC) includes personal, social, professional, and physical functioning, as well as the ability to cope with stressors, as constituent elements of mental health.[25] Social, economic, and ecological stressors are experienced by many Appalachian residents at high rates,[26, 27] and such stressors are associated with the onset and maintenance of mental health problems.[28]

Overall, Appalachia experiences higher rates of poverty, lower median household income, and lower levels of educational attainment than the United States as a whole.[27] In addition, worker displacement (loss of work due to positions being abolished or business or plant closures) is a potent economic stressor in Appalachia. For example, although rates of worker displacement between 2001 and 2003 were similar in Appalachia and the rest of the country, Appalachians were more likely to be displaced from long-term jobs (twenty- versus ten-year average tenure), to be older, to lack a high school diploma, and to still be out of work by 2004.[29]

An inverse relationship between socioeconomic status and mental illness has long been documented among adults.[28, 30] Similarly, a higher percentage of children living in poverty have mental health problems.[31, 32]

Mental illness among youths in the Great Smoky Mountains Study was associated with poverty and other risk factors, including family history of mental illness, multiple residential moves, and parenting styles (e.g., lack of warmth, harsh discipline). Although black children had higher overall rates of poverty compared with white children, poverty did not increase the risk of psychiatric disorders (beyond that related to other risk factors) among black children, but it did increase the risk among white children.[20, 21] It is not clear whether socioeconomic stress triggers mental illness, mental illness results in lower socioeconomic attainment due to impaired functioning, or mental illness and socioeconomic status have no causal relationship. The empirical evidence, however, indicates that socioeconomic stressors can directly impact the development or expression of mental illnesses.[28]

In turn, socioeconomic realities such as insurance coverage often dictate access to mental health and substance abuse services. Halverson and colleagues[19] noted that, overall, Appalachian and non-Appalachian regions had similar access to public or private health insurance coverage, with the lowest rates of coverage experienced by white residents in eastern Kentucky. However, a recent comparison of access to mental health and substance abuse treatment found that 67 percent of hospital stays in Appalachia were covered by Medicaid or Medicare, compared with 57 percent outside of Appalachia.[6] Also, rates of private insurance coverage were lower in Appalachian than in non-Appalachian counties. Disparities in expected payments by private insurance for hospital stays were noted in economically distressed counties (Appalachian 11.9 percent; non-Appalachian 19.3 percent), competitive counties (Appalachian 17.9 percent; non-Appalachian 33.9 percent), and attainment counties (Appalachian 32.7 percent; non-Appalachian 39.7 percent).[c] Further, it is likely that high out-of-pocket copayments and deductibles prevent many Appalachians from utilizing private insurance coverage even if they have it. Indeed, Huttlinger and colleagues[9] found that 35 percent of their study participants from the coalfields of southwestern Virginia who had insurance had difficulty affording copayments and deductibles.

Stressful life events, including but not limited to economic stressors, are also associated with greater psychological distress[33] and the onset of mental illnesses such as depression.[34] For example, Appalachian women entering the workforce is likely a stressful adjustment for families, given women's traditional domestic role.[35] In addition, Appalachians who migrate, typically to urban areas for employment, may experience a loss of social support and loss of meaning, leading to distress and depression.[36] Indeed, Halperin and Reiter-Purtill[37] found that Appalachian migrants living in the Cincinnati area who presented for treatment had more severe "nerves" and greater economic stressors than Appalachians living and seeking treatment in rural Appalachia. Appalachians may also experience stress associated with real or perceived prejudices and inequalities,[38] which in turn may increase their psychological distress, similar to that experienced by ethnic minorities.[39]

Lack of availability, accessibility, and acceptability of services may contribute to psychological distress and mental illnesses. Indeed, many barriers to mental health and substance abuse services were noted in qualitative case studies of six Appalachian counties by Zhang and colleagues.[6] Concerns about stigma, privacy and confidentiality, transportation, limited payment options and facility choices, and cultural or family barriers were identified as interfering with the utilization of mental health services. Not surprisingly, health disparities are greatest in rural Appalachia, and the identified barriers to treatment are similar to those noted in the rural United States in general.[18, 40, 41]

Interestingly, Zhang and colleagues[6] found that over a one-year period, Appalachians were more likely than non-Appalachians to use intensive outpatient mental health and substance abuse treatment, as well as prescription medication treatment. However, client perception of treatment, objective quality of treatment, and level of participation (e.g., dropout rates, filling of prescriptions) are unknown. Appalachians were also more likely to access services via the emergency room and private physicians, particularly in distressed counties and in coal mining regions, than were non-Appalachians. Despite the utilization of available services for substance abuse and mental health problems, access to inpatient and residential treatment was less common in Appalachian counties than in non-Appalachian counties. This suggests that Appalachians with severe mental health and substance abuse problems may not receive adequate outpatient treatment or timely access to inpatient services, resulting in the increased use of emergency services. Thus, it is possible that despite the utilization of outpatient services, mental health and substance abuse problems escalate because services are less than acceptable, not readily accessible, ineffective, or not available. This interpretation is consistent with findings that rural residents often seek treatment later in the course of their illness, when symptoms cause greater impairment and require more costly and intensive interventions.[18]

In summary, stressors experienced by Appalachians likely contribute to higher risk for and higher rates of psychological distress and some mental illnesses. Socioeconomic stressors, including lower average income and educational attainment and higher rates of poverty and underemployment, increase the risk of mental illness and decrease access to treatment. In addition, economic stressors, such as women entering the workforce and the migration of family members, may threaten the traditional structure of Appalachian families and communities and the supports they rely on. These stressors appear to jeopardize mental health.

Local Knowledge about Mental Illness

Local knowledge refers to the ethnomedical meanings and explanations Appalachian people ascribe to symptoms of and treatments for mental illness. As Hill and Fraser[42] point out, local knowledge about illness and local health-seeking practices are important factors in the development of appropriate and acceptable mental health service delivery programs.

The analyses in this section are based on qualitative studies of rural, mostly white Appalachians. However, studies of rural black and American Indian populations in Appalachia, as well as urban Appalachians show many similarities.[37, 42–44] Although there is no indication that significant differences exist based on social class, it should be noted that these studies tend to be limited to lower-class, working-class, and lower-middle-class people and, as such, are representative of the rural Appalachian population as a whole. There have been no studies to date of the mental health beliefs of urban or college-educated native Appalachians. Local knowledge about mental health in Appalachia is shaped by three attributes: a belief in God, a collective identity, and coping strategies anchored in everyday lifeways.

Health and Healing Come from God. For many rural Appalachians, health and well-being come from God.[43, 45–47] Religious beliefs and practices give life meaning and are integral to everyday life. Prayer and faith are important for life and thus for health management as well—both the prevention of illness and healing. Some rural Appalachians say that prayer, hymn singing, reading the Bible, and attending church services relax them and give them a feeling of peaceful serenity.[43] They "turn their worries over to Jesus." In other words, God is the source of their feelings of well-being, and in times of pain and discomfort, the Lord gives believers enormous comfort and strength and the courage to handle adversity.[46] Scholars often gloss these beliefs with the term *fatalism,* which is deterministic and pejorative.[d] Many of these same beliefs are held by mainstream Americans, who would never be called fatalistic. Most scholars who have done in-depth ethnographic research emphasize that Appalachians are neither passive nor apathetic in their health beliefs and behavior.[44, 45, 48–51] They do, however, have a distinctive approach to health care. As Anglin[52] points out, what health professionals describe as fatalism may simply be rural Appalachians' pragmatic assessment of their risk for a given disease or the likelihood of health care accessibility and affordability.

Rural Appalachians do not divide health and illness into physical versus mental problems, as does Western biomedicine.[42, 43, 46] Like many rural residents, rural Appalachians integrate health, religion, and morality, considering a wider range of causes of health problems and a wider range of treatment options than biomedicine does. Rural Appalachians may conceptualize sickness as having multiple causes, including natural causes, such as environmental toxins and bacteria, and supernatural causes, such as chastening by God or satanic forces.[45] They also acknowledge the effects of socioeconomic problems, such as poverty and the decline of their rural communities due to globalization, and social discord, such as family problems and spousal abuse, on their health and well-being.[22, 42, 53] Their recognition of the psychological impact of stress in their lives is evident in the use of local ethnomedical terms to label certain complaints, such as feeling "weak and dizzy" or having a bad case of "nerves."[53, 54] Appalachians are concerned about the high rate of depression and the devastation caused by alcoholism and substance abuse in their communities.[9, 42, 55] But their understanding of the cause of mental illness is often rooted in their own and others' behavior rather than biological etiology, and they view cause and cure more holistically, blurring the mind-body distinction.[42, 45] As a result, they often make moral judgments about pathological behavior, recommending punishment rather than mental health care.[56] This is one reason Appalachians are less likely than non-Appalachians to enter the mental health system through individual or self-referral.[57] More often, Appalachians are referred to mental health services by their physicians or other agencies and services.

Rural Appalachians are described as taking a practical and pragmatic approach to life, recognizing that disease, accidents, and other hardships will always be present.[44, 48, 58] Like rural people everywhere, they display an ethic of endurance in response to physical and psychological hardships.[47, 48] For Appalachians, belief in God and belief in modern medicine are not mutually exclusive, and their religious beliefs are not a barrier to seeking health care. Although rural Appalachian people generally believe that God is in control of things, they also see God working through human beings, including medical practitioners and the medications they prescribe. They appreciate it when health care providers acknowledge and incorporate their spiritual needs. They are grateful when nurses pray with them and read them scriptures; they may also want their doctors to talk about spirituality and pray with them, especially before operations.[46]

There are no in-depth ethnographic or qualitative studies of rural or urban Appalachian beliefs about mental illness and its causes in general. However, it can be assumed that mental illness is not regarded as a separate class of illness. Physical, mental, emotional, and spiritual problems are considered within the religious perspective that circumscribes most Appalachians' view of the world. Some problems, such as alcoholism, may be regarded as sins.[35] Yet there is evidence that rural Appalachians see the individual's personality as fixed by God and changeable only by him; they are therefore fairly tolerant of a wide range of behaviors.[42, 56] The ethic of independence in rural Appalachia requires that people not impose on others, so they often avoid problematic individuals and situations rather than intervene. Problems and conflicts are dealt with by "getting right with God." As a result, conflict becomes inner conflict first and foremost, and the only real remedy comes from within, from an individual's spiritual relationship with God. Getting "saved" is often the recommended route to improving mental health.

Collectivism as Opposed to Individualism. It is helpful to explore another difference between Appalachian and non-Appalachian behavior that

Triandis[59] describes as collectivism versus individualism. Whereas non-Appalachians might best be characterized as individualistic, rural Appalachian communities often fit the collectivist pattern, in which people are connected as kin, friends, and neighbors who rely on reciprocal exchange to meet their social and economic needs. In collectivist groups, individuals tend to think of themselves as interdependent rather than independent, and they are more interested in knowing about others than in self-knowing. This conflicts with Western psychotherapy, in which self-reflection and self-change are encouraged and expected, and the inability to describe and discuss the self independent of others and of situations is a symptom of psychopathology. In collectivist societies, the self is defined by in-group relationships, and if change is needed, the best option is to change the self to fit the situation rather than vice versa. The focus is on one's obligation to a small group of people with whom one has close relationships, as opposed to individual rights in casual relations with strangers. Emotions in collectivist societies tend to be other-focused (e.g., empathy) rather than self-focused (e.g., anger). In these societies, shame is more common than guilt, encouraging secrecy and silence in social arenas.

In a study of battered women, Fiene[22] found that rural Appalachian women are reluctant to disclose their victimization even to close family members. Battering becomes a secret that protects the core of the woman's identity as a good wife and mother by hiding information that would expose her to shame and the negative opinion of others. The women Fiene interviewed received little support from their batterers' relatives or even their own families. Furthermore, some family members counseled the women not to leave their partners because it would be against God's word (that a wife should obey her husband). In a study of family alcohol problems among female nursing assistants and licensed practical nurses in a regional medical center in eastern Tennessee, Howell and Fiene[35] found acceptance of both the biomedical disease model and the ethnomedical "religious sin" model of alcoholism. They also found that these women followed a strategy of "keeping family secrets" and were reluctant to acknowledge family alcohol problems publicly. Based on these findings, Howell and Fiene recommended that, rather than promoting provider-defined definitions of alcoholism and treatment, employee assistance programs should make self-help books and referral lists available. When consulted by employees, these programs should ensure that counseling is available with a neutral and confidential "outsider" not tied to community social networks. Clearly, therapeutic intervention in Appalachia must be sensitive to the social pressures that may be imposed by collectivist beliefs.

In collectivist societies, emotional problems are more likely to be experienced as bodily symptoms.[60] Studies of depression, for example, in non-Western and collective societies find that somatization, or the expression of personal and social distress in an idiom of bodily complaints and help seeking, is relatively common. There is some evidence that rural Appalachians are less likely to experience depression as a mood disorder and more likely to experience it as a relationship disorder with somatic rather than emotional symptoms. In this case, family support therapies as opposed to individual psychotherapy might be more beneficial for rural Appalachian clients.

Rates of depression appear to be higher among Appalachians than non-Appalachians,[6, 9, 11, 61–63] and researchers have noted a tendency for rural Appalachians to experience mental illness through somatization.[37, 47, 63] For example, Keefe and colleagues[63] found that rural Appalachian women scored significantly higher than national norms on a scale measuring somatic complaints, while men had elevated, but not statistically significantly higher, scores. Somatization commonly leads rural Appalachians with mental health problems to seek help from primary care physicians or, in times of crisis, emergency rooms rather than from mental health professionals.[6]

Coping Strategies. Rural Appalachians have coping strategies that help them respond to hardships and difficulties. Certainly, their extensive kinship networks and their strong religious beliefs and practices are fundamental to their ability to meet life's challenges. Self-reliance is a strong value, and researchers have found that rural Appalachians tend to avoid agencies and institutions in general.[50, 64] For example, they resist institutionalizing family members for any reason.[65] There is also the tendency to emphasize pragmatism, common sense, determination, and perseverance.[51, 52, 58, 66] Living in the present and focusing on the problem at hand are common strategies. In a study of elderly rural Appalachian women, Hayes[50] found that living in the moment helped them overcome the uncertainty of the future and maintain their health. This entailed keeping a positive attitude, not dwelling on problems, and taking one day at a time. Denham found that rural Appalachian families tend to project contentment and thankfulness: "Their lifeways demonstrated a peaceful acceptance, caring for the troubles of today, but not prematurely fretting over tomorrow's woes" (p. 304).[49] Studies of rural Appalachian women note that they have positive self-evaluations and value their own competencies, even if they are not recognized by others.[49, 50, 66] Perhaps most significantly, rural Appalachians value action, activity, and working. In her study of elderly women, Hayes[50] found that being physically active by working in the home and the garden was a primary strategy for maintaining health. The rural lower-class Appalachian women that Fiene[66] studied were completely absorbed by the details of daily life, especially child care, which they saw as a lifelong task. In the studies by Hayes and Fiene, the home was an important place for women to connect with nature, carry out their roles as wives and mothers, and find solitude. Mothers in rural Appalachian families are central in caring for family members and making health care decisions, which simultaneously contributes to their self-esteem.[49, 67]

These coping strategies also reveal the weak points in rural Appalachian life, where difficulties might become unbearable and veer out of control. Stress points include the following: individuals in spiritual crisis, individuals with family or marital discord, individuals without a permanent place to call home, families in which the mother-child relationship has broken down, migrants who lack local support networks, and disabled or physically ill individuals who cannot work. Limited research suggests that depression rates for rural Appalachian men are relatively high compared with national rates.[10, 68] Recent social and economic changes have threatened male status in the mountains, suggesting that men, who are expected to be the heads of their households, might have particular difficulty adjusting to social change and maintaining their health and self-esteem in contemporary society.[47]

Help-Seeking Strategies

Researchers have noted that rural Appalachians often find it difficult to ask for help. Instead, they may wait for others to anticipate their needs and volunteer to fulfill them.[50, 69] This works well in a communal society where people tend to be personally knowledgeable about and sensitive to the situations of others. It is difficult, but not impossible, for agencies to fill a similar role; this is more likely to occur in small, community-based agencies whose personnel are intimately connected to residents' support networks.[69] In general, however, rural Appalachians tend to avoid institutional help.

A more common help-seeking strategy is to turn to family and friends for advice and assistance, especially for help with nursing care, child care, or transportation to appointments.[22, 42, 53, 54, 62, 64] Keefe[70] describes the strength of these natural support systems in rural Appalachian communities. An exception involves problems that might elicit negative attitudes, such as alcohol abuse or spouse battering, which would be considered family secrets. A number of other symptoms of mental illness might fall into this category, including child abuse, juvenile misbehavior, substance abuse, sexual deviancy, addictions such as gambling and excessive spending, and irrational and violent behavior. These kinds of behavioral symptoms provoke strong moral judgments and are not likely to be adequately addressed by the natural support systems in rural Appalachian communities. Another area in which natural support systems fall short is dealing with devastating family crises that require significant material and social resources, such as caring for a handicapped child.[71]

The other common help-seeking strategy among rural Appalachians is to turn to religious resources.[42–45, 48, 53, 72, 73] Especially important are individual rituals such as prayer and Bible reading. Church pastors are not commonly asked for assistance. Pastors are often community members without special theological training, and rather than keeping family secrets, they may use the pulpit to criticize the behavior of congregants during services. Among rural Appalachians, the support of the religious community as a whole is sought when dealing with sickness because group prayer is believed to be more powerful in reaching God.

Although church congregations sometimes honor prayer requests that reveal few details about sensitive problems, more often, when such a request concerns a medical problem, it includes specific information about the illness, the treatment required (such as hospitalization or surgery), and the name of the ill person and his or her relationship to the petitioner.[45] This information circulates throughout the congregation, and prayer is often followed up with personal hospital visits, food, cards, and other expressions of sympathy and support. Simpson and King[74] suggest that religion-health partnerships offer an opportunity for improving health promotion in rural Appalachian communities. But they also acknowledge the difficulty of working with independent mountain churches that lack a mainline hierarchy. Moreover, some churches may not approve of worldly efforts involving social change.

Because rural Appalachians may experience depression and anxiety as physical illnesses with somatic symptoms, they often end up in a primary care physician's office for diagnosis and treatment. Their concept of illness includes a broad range of ethnomedical complaints that have no biomedical counterparts, creating misunderstandings in doctor-patient interactions and resulting in stress, noncompliance, and misdiagnosis, as well as extraneous tests and laboratory workups. In a study of patients in an outreach clinic in rural Virginia, Nations and colleagues[54] found that 45 percent of their sample presented with at least one ethnomedical problem, with a total of fourteen different folk illnesses identified by respondents. None of these ethnomedical problems were recorded by physicians on the patients' medical charts, whereas 76 percent of the biomedical complaints were recorded. The authors concluded that the physicians attended to the biomedical disease symptoms but not the underlying cultural meaning and human significance of the problems.

There is little information on the extent to which Appalachians are referred to mental health services by primary care physicians. Given many doctors' reluctance to give mental health referrals, the difference between the biomedical and ethnomedical paradigms, and the perceived stigma of mental illness, it is unlikely that primary care doctors make many referrals that result in consultations with mental health professionals. In a study of more than 4,000 mental health and detoxification center intakes of native Appalachians at a western North Carolina agency, Keefe[57] found that only 20 percent had been referred by physicians.

There has been considerable study of the syndrome of "nerves" in rural Appalachia, an ethnomedical affliction that can affect help-seeking behavior. The condition is characterized by a range of symptoms, including feelings of nervousness, anger, impatience, fearfulness, and depression, as well as physical agitation and restlessness, insomnia, and crying. Various somatic complaints are also mentioned, including gastrointestinal disturbances, weight loss, increased heart rate, elevated blood pressure, chest pain, head-aches, breathing difficulty, and blackouts. Severe cases of nerves often result in hospitalization or attempted suicide.[37, 53] While physicians often equate nerves with biomedical diagnoses such as depression and anxiety,[75, 76] Van Schaik[77] argues that both critical and interpretive analyses are better at revealing the meaning of the illness. Those suffering from nerves are of-ten overwhelmed by poverty, family difficulties (especially with children), alcoholism in the family, grief over the death of family members, or the far-reaching demands of family life. The accumulated distress of all these things results in symptoms or acute episodes of nerves. Physicians validate the illness and provide "nerve pills," shots, or hospitalization, but the so-cial causes are rarely addressed. For rural Appalachians, the condition of nerves provides an interpretive framework for constructing an illness re-ality that takes into account the source of distress and makes sense of the symptoms. Critical theory, according to Van Schaik, goes further than in-terpretive analysis in acknowledging that these meanings are shaped by re-lationships of power based in the material conditions of existence. In this sense, economic inequality and domination in rural Appalachia—which developed as a peripheral region to provide labor and natural resources to the core of the country—have consequences in shaping the meaning and understanding of people's behavior. The medicalization of rural Appala-chians' lived experience conceals these other interpretations of the source of suffering.

Mental Health Services

It appears that rural Appalachians benefit little from currently available mental health services. Certainly, the fact that many are uninsured or un-derinsured for mental illness and are unable to afford mental health care accounts for some of this lack of benefit. Studies also suggest that the Ap-palachian population is unaware of the existence of many mental health services.[9, 64] Moreover, availability does not necessarily result in utilization of services. For example, in a study of Cherokee and white youths in west-ern North Carolina, Costello and associates[78] found that professional men-tal health services went unused by families with disturbed children both on the reservation (where the Indian Health Service provides low-cost treat-ment) and off it.

Clearly, accessibility and affordability are only part of the problem. As discussed earlier in this chapter, nothing in the rural Appalachian ethnomedical understanding of illness would lead these people to seek help from a mental health agency. Indeed, Huttlinger and colleagues[9] found that the majority of their participants reported coping with depression "at home" rather than seeking professional help. In addition, there is a lack of public health knowledge among rural Appalachian people.[44, 58, 65] For example, in a survey of more than 1,000 adults living in rural West Virginia, Muntaner and Barnett[10] found that a sizable proportion of those who self-reported good mental health also reported depressive symptoms, suggesting that many are unaware of the current guidelines for a medical diagnosis of depression. As a result, rural Appalachians tend to be directed into the mental health system through social institutions such as law enforcement and school systems rather than through self-referral.[57]

There is also evidence that the organization and delivery of mental health services discourage service utilization by Appalachians. Typically located in large urban centers, mental health services are often organized in a bureaucratic manner that fails to provide the informal and personal interaction that makes Appalachians comfortable.[50, 69] Psychotherapy may be unsuccessful because it emphasizes individual rather than family treatment, promotes insight rather than the resolution of relationship problems, and directly confronts emotions and feelings rather than relying on more symbolic, metaphorical, and ritualized healing techniques.[68, 79–83] Mental health professionals who are not Appalachian natives may harbor prejudices against Appalachians, blaming their beliefs for treatment failures.[58, 84] Furthermore, as MacDonald[69] points out, rural Appalachians are likely to express dissatisfaction with services by choosing not to return, while providers may assume that such clients are unmotivated and irresponsible "no-shows." One study found that a personal reminder call from the therapist significantly increased appointment keeping at rural Appalachian mental health centers.[85]

Keefe[86] has called for improvement in the cultural competency of mental health professionals working in Appalachia. Mental health agencies in the region should include the client's birthplace on intake forms, allowing the identification of native Appalachian versus non-Appalachian clients.[57] In addition, alternative models of mental health service delivery should be considered. Glisson and Schoenwald,[87] for example, offer a model of successful children's mental health treatment that includes home-based therapy and the creation of community alliances to support service delivery. Similarly, McInnis-Dittrich[83] describes a home-based mental health intervention for elderly Appalachian women that builds on natural helper networks of family and friends. School mental health programs also offer an effective community-based model for rural Appalachian children displaying disruptive behavior,[88] and such programs have a broad potential to address a variety of mental health problems experienced by children and adolescents.[89] The development of church-health partnerships offers another community-based route for addressing mental health needs.[74]

The National Advisory Committee on Rural Health and Human Services[90] suggests that rural communities consider the integration of behavioral health care and primary health care to address barriers of access and stigma and to more fully integrate health services. Because rural Appalachians generally present to their primary care physicians or to the emergency room for mental health needs,[6] the integration of mental health and primary care services holds promise for meeting mental health needs. Access to mental health care in the context of general medical care may alleviate some concerns about stigma and confidentiality in rural Appalachia (where, for example, a person's car might be seen parked outside the mental health center). If this approach is taken, physicians and health care practitioners in hospitals would benefit from training in awareness of local ethnomedical beliefs and practices.

Rural Appalachian residents may find integrated mental health services, peer paraprofessional services (e.g., Vet to Vet),[91] guided self-help (e.g., books),[92] and telehealth (e.g., virtual visits via videophone or the Internet)[93] appealing alternatives to traditional mental health services. Telehealth is a promising and potentially nonstigmatizing way to provide mental health services to individuals who live far from treatment sites or lack transportation but have access to telephones or the Internet. Focus groups conducted separately with primary care physicians and depressed patients in rural Nebraska revealed that participants perceived telehealth as a viable solution to the problem of treatment access. Although participants expressed concerns about the potentially impersonal nature of the contact and implications for the therapeutic relationship, they proposed solutions such as an initial in-person meeting.[94] Assessment and intervention techniques would need to be practiced and evaluated to determine their appropriateness in rural Appalachia.[68] It is possible that these suggested changes in the delivery of mental health services may increase utilization rates and successful treatment among rural Appalachian patients.

Further Research

Additional research is required to enhance an understanding of the mental health issues in Appalachia and to develop and implement cost-effective solutions to those issues. For example, research is needed on the ethnomedical system in Appalachia with regard to mental health beliefs and practices. Since most of the research thus far has emphasized rural populations, an important issue is the impact of social class and rural or urban residence on Appalachian mental health beliefs and practices. Mental health research on ethnic minorities in Appalachia is needed to understand diversity in the region.

More population-based studies are needed to provide a better description of the epidemiology of mental illnesses experienced by the people of Appalachia. For example, the most recent large-scale comparison of rural Appalachia to the rest of the United States addressed only rates of depression and psychological distress; it did not compare rates of anxiety disorders or other common mental illnesses.[6]

Given the ethnomedical differences in Appalachians' conceptions of mental health, mental health agencies and professionals must develop and evaluate more culturally competent assessments of psychological distress and mental illness, and they must gear their provision of therapeutic services toward Appalachians. Given the inadequate delivery of mental health services in the region, more research is needed to examine the costs and outcomes of various mental health services delivery models. For example, what is the relative effectiveness of home-based models versus telehealth models versus urban mental health centers in Appalachia? Community-based participatory research involving community members in all parts of the research process is a promising way to utilize local data, increase community participation, and potentially increase meaningful mental health outcomes.[95]

Policy Recommendations

Without adequate policies and plans, mental health in Appalachia will be addressed in an inefficient and fragmented manner. Comprehensive mental health policies should include a broad spectrum of actions, including the following:

- Intake forms at mental health services should include a question about birthplace to allow comparisons of Appalachian natives and non-Appalachians.[57] Identifying both state and county or city would allow clients to be classified according to the counties designated by the Appalachian Regional Commission.
- Integrated models of service delivery, including both primary care physicians and mental health professionals, should be developed, especially for rural areas of Appalachia. These models are critical, given Appalachians' tendency to consult primary care physicians for mental health problems.
- Mental health services must be decentralized to deliver adequate services to rural areas. New models are needed, perhaps relying on outreach psychiatric social workers and nurses.
- Greater attention must be given to public mental health education in Appalachia. The dissemination of information through trusted interpersonal networks rather than through anonymous public media announcements would be especially effective.
- Policies that address the economics of mental health and the lack of inexpensive insurance coverage for mental health services are needed. The current system of organizing and financing mental health services imposes an enormous emotional and financial burden on persons with mental health disorders and their families.

Notes

a. The term *cultural differences* refers to beliefs, values, moral frameworks, worldview, and meaning.

b. The Appalachian Regional Commission contracted with the National Opinion Research Center at the University of Chicago and East Tennessee State University to examine mental health, substance abuse, and treatment access disparities in the Appalachian region relative to the rest of the nation.[6] The investigators also explored differences within the Appalachian subregions (Southern, Central, and Northern) and among economic development levels (distressed, at-risk, transitional, competitive, and attainment counties). Qualitative case studies in the form of focus groups were conducted in six Appalachian counties to provide a methodology for local data collection and analysis and to contextualize the secondary data analysis findings. Public access data on mental health and substance abuse diagnoses and treatment were analyzed, such as the 2002–2005 National Survey on Drug Use and Health (NSDUH). The NSDUH is the largest national survey of noninstitutionalized U.S. citizens aged 12 and older. The investigators used in-person computer-assisted structured interviews using *DSM-IV* criteria[4] and individual self-report assessments to gather national and state-level estimates of drug use and related variables. The NSDUH was not designed to assess the prevalence of all mental illnesses, assess the entire Appalachian region, or provide regional estimates. Thus, Zhang and colleagues[6] suggest interpreting their secondary analyses and findings with caution.

c. The percentages are based on 2004 data from a reanalysis of the Healthcare Cost and Utilization Project, which was designed to be representative of U.S. hospital utilization. However, the data are limited to thirty-seven states and ten of thirteen Appalachian states, and they exclude long-term-care and psychiatric hospitals.

d. Much of the previous research on Appalachian mental health tended to be judgmental and theoretically suspect, largely employing the dated "culture of poverty" paradigm that blames victims for their problems. More recent research often repeats the same cultural stereotypes, simply counseling the withholding of judgment on questionable cultural values such as fatalism and traditionalism (e.g., compare Ball,[96] Goshen,[97] and Polansky and associates[98] with Hansen and Resick,[65] Helton,[99] MacAvoy and Lippman,[100] Purnell and Paulanka,[101] and Yelton and Nielson[102]).

References

1. Center for Mental Health Services, Manderscheid RW, Berry JT, eds. Mental health, United States, 2004. DHHS Publication No. [SMA]-06-4195. Rockville, MD: Substance Abuse and Mental Health Services Administration; 2006.

2. Demyttenaere K, Bruffaerts R, Posada-Villa J, et al. Prevalence, severity, and unmet need for treatment of mental disorders in the World Health Organization world mental health surveys. *JAMA.* 2004;291:2581–2590.

3. World Health Organization. The ICD-10 classification of mental and behavioural disorders: clinical descriptions and diagnostic guidelines. Geneva, Switzerland: World Health Organization; 1992.

4. American Psychiatric Association. *Diagnostic and Statistical Manual of*

Mental Disorders: Text Revision, 4th ed. Washington, DC: American Psychiatric Association; 2000.

5. Kessler RC, Chiu WT, Colpe L, et al. The prevalence and correlates of serious mental illness (SMI) in the National Comorbidity Survey Replication (NCS-R). In: Center for Mental Health Services, Manderscheid RW, Berry JT, eds. Mental health, United States, 2004. DHHS Publication No. [SMA]-06-4195. Rockville, MD: Substance Abuse and Mental Health Services Administration; 2006.

6. Zhang Z, Infante A, Meit M, English N, Dunn M, Bowers KH. An analysis of mental health and substance abuse disparities and access to treatment services in the Appalachian region. Washington, DC: Appalachian Regional Commission; 2008. Available at: http://www.arc.gov/assets/research_reports/AnalysisofMentalHealthandSubstanceAbuseDisparities.pdf. Accessed September 7, 2011.

7. Kessler RC. The epidemiology of dual diagnosis. *Biol Psychiatry.* 2004;56:730–737.

8. Hauenstein EJ, Peddada SD. Prevalence of major depressive episodes in rural women using primary care. *J Health Care Poor Underserved.* 2007;18:185–202.

9. Huttlinger K, Schaller-Ayers J, Lawson T. Health care in Appalachia: a population-based approach. *Public Health Nurs.* 2004;21:103–110.

10. Muntaner C, Barnett E. Depressive symptoms in rural West Virginia: labor market and health services correlates. *J Health Care Poor Underserved.* 2000;11:284–300.

11. Keefe SE, Parsons P. Health and life-style indicators in a rural Appalachian county: implications for health-care practice. In: Keefe SE, ed. *Appalachian Cultural Competency: A Guide for Medical, Mental Health, and Social Service Professionals.* Knoxville, TN: University of Tennessee Press; 2005:183–195.

12. Simmons LA, Huddleston-Casas C, Berry AA. Low-income rural women and depression: factors associated with self-reporting. *Am J Health Behav.* 2007;31:657–666.

13. Probst JC, Laditka SB, Moore CG, Harun N, Powell MP, Baxley EG. Rural-urban differences in depression prevalence: implications for family medicine. *Fam Med.* 2006;38:653–660.

14. Moscicki EK. Epidemiology of completed and attempted suicide: toward a framework for prevention. *Clin Neurosci Res.* 2001;1(5):310–323.

15. Hauenstein EJ, Petterson S, Merwin E, Rovnyak V, Heise B, Wagner D. Rurality, gender, and mental health treatment. *Fam Community Health.* 2006;29:169–185.

16. Rost K, Fortney J, Fischer E, Smith J. Use, quality, and outcomes of care for mental health: the rural perspective. *Med Care Res Rev.* 2002;59:231–265; discussion 266–271.

17. Singh GK, Siahpush M. Increasing rural-urban gradients in U.S. suicide mortality, 1970–1997. *Am J Public Health.* 2002;92:1161–1167.

18. Wagenfeld MO, Murray JD, Mohatt DF, DeBruyn JC. Mental health and rural America, 1994–2005: an overview and annotated bibliography. NIH Publication No. 94-3500. Washington, DC: Department of Health and Human Services, U.S. Public Health Service; 1994.

19. Halverson JA, Ma L, Harner EJ. An analysis of disparities in health status and access to health care in the Appalachian region. Washington, DC: Appalachian Regional Commission; 2004.

20. Costello EJ, Angold A, Burns BJ, et al. The Great Smoky Mountains Study of youth: goals, design, methods, and the prevalence of *DSM-III-R* disorders. *Arch Gen Psychiatry.* 1996;53:1129–1136.

21. Costello EJ, Farmer EM, Angold A, Burns BJ, Erkanli A. Psychiatric disorders among American Indian and white youth in Appalachia: the Great Smoky Mountains Study. *Am J Public Health.* 1997;87:827–832.

22. Fiene JI. Battered women: keeping the secret. *Affilia.* 1995;10:179–193.

23. U.S. Department of Veterans Affairs. About rural veterans. Available at: www.ruralhealth.va.gov/page.cfm?pg=2. Accessed August 16, 2009.

24. Eyre E. Recent rural vets at high risk. *Charleston Gazette,* November 11, 2008.

25. U.S. Department of Health and Human Services. Mental health: a report of the surgeon general—executive summary. Rockville, MD: U.S. Department of Health and Human Services, Substance Abuse and Mental Health Services Administration, Center for Mental Health Services, National Institutes of Health, National Institute of Mental Health; 1999.

26. Stevenson E, Shannon L, Walker R, Mateyoke-Scriverner A, Logan TK, Cole J, eds. Kentucky women in substance abuse treatment: rural Appalachia. KTOS in-Focus No. 1(2). Lexington, KY: Center on Drug and Alcohol Research, University of Kentucky; 2008.

27. Ziliak JP. Human capital and the challenge of persistent poverty in Appalachia. Cleveland, OH: Federal Reserve Bank of Cleveland; 2007.

28. Hudson CG. Socioeconomic status and mental illness: tests of the social causation and selection hypotheses. *Am J Orthopsychiatry.* 2005;75:3–18.

29. Herzenberg S, Price M, Wial H. Displacement in Appalachia and the non-Appalachian United States 2001–2003: findings based on five displaced worker surveys. Harrisburg, PA: Keystone Research Center; 2005.

30. Faris REL, Dunham HW. *Mental Disorders in Urban Areas: An Ecological Study of Schizophrenia and Other Psychoses.* Chicago, IL: University of Chicago Press; 1939.

31. Bourdon KH, Goodman R, Rae DS, Simpson G, Koretz DS. The strengths and difficulties questionnaire: U.S. normative data and psychometric properties. *J Am Acad Child Adolesc Psychiatry.* 2005;44:557–564.

32. Wadsworth ME, Raviv T, Reinhard C, Wolff B, Santiago CD, Einhorn L. An

indirect effects model of the association between poverty and child functioning: the role of children's poverty-related stress. *J Loss Trauma.* 2008;13:156–185.

33. Ensel WM, Lin N. The life stress paradigm and psychological distress. *J Health Soc Behav.* 1991;32:321–341.

34. Lewinsohn PM, Allen NB, Seeley JR, Gotlib IH. First onset versus recurrence of depression: differential processes of psychosocial risk. *J Abnorm Psychol.* 1999;108:483–489.

35. Howell BJ, Fiene JI. Designing employee assistance programs for Appalachian working-class women: the alcohol and stress research project. In: Keefe SE, ed. *Appalachian Cultural Competency: A Guide for Medical, Mental Health, and Social Service Professionals.* Knoxville, TN: University of Tennessee Press; 2005:247–266.

36. Lantz JE, Harper K. Network intervention, existential depression, and the relocated Appalachian family. *Conventional Family Therapy.* 1989;11:213–223.

37. Halperin RH, Reiter-Purtill J. "Nerves" in rural and urban Appalachia. In: Keefe SE, ed. *Appalachian Cultural Competency: A Guide for Medical, Mental Health, and Social Service Professionals.* Knoxville, TN: University of Tennessee Press; 2005:265–284.

38. Smith KB, Bylund RA. Cognitive maps of class, racial, and rural Appalachian inequalities among rural Appalachians. *Rural Sociol.* 1983;48:253–270.

39. Al-Issa I, Tousignant M. *Ethnicity, Immigration, and Psychopathology.* New York, NY: Plenum Press; 1997.

40. Stamm BH. Essays from the field. In: Stamm BH, ed. *Rural Behavioral Health Care.* Washington, DC: American Psychological Association; 2003.

41. New Freedom Commission on Mental Health. Subcommittee on rural issues: background paper. Publication No. SMA 04–3890. Rockville, MD: Department of Health and Human Services; 2004.

42. Hill CE, Fraser GJ. Local knowledge and rural mental health reform. *Community Ment Health J.* 1995;31:553–568.

43. Arcury TA, Quandt SA, McDonald J, Bell RA. Faith and health self-management of rural older adults. *J Cross Cult Gerontol.* 2000;15:55–74.

44. Coyne CA, Demian-Popescu C, Friend D. Social and cultural factors influencing health in southern West Virginia: a qualitative study. *Prev Chronic Dis.* 2006;3:A124.

45. Keefe SE. Religious healing in southern Appalachian communities. In: Ray C, ed. *Southern Heritage on Display: Public Ritual and Ethnic Diversity within Southern Regionalism.* Tuscaloosa, AL: University of Alabama Press; 2003:144–166.

46. Lowry LW, Conco D. Exploring the meaning of spirituality with aging adults in Appalachia. *J Holist Nurs.* 2002;20:388–402.

47. Horton CF. Women have headaches, men have backaches: patterns of illness in an Appalachian community. *Soc Sci Med.* 1984;19:647–654.

48. Cavender AP, Beck SH. Generational change, folk medicine, and medical self-care in a rural Appalachian community. *Hum Organ.* 1995;54:129–142.

49. Denham SA. Family health in a rural Appalachian Ohio county. *Journal of Appalachian Studies.* 1996;2(2):299–310.

50. Hayes PA. Home is where their health is: rethinking perspectives of informal and formal care by older rural Appalachian women who live alone. *Qual Health Res.* 2006;16:282–297.

51. Stephens CC. Culturally relevant preventive health care for southern Appalachian women. In: Keefe SE, ed. *Appalachian Cultural Competency: A Guide for Medical, Mental Health, and Social Service Professionals.* Knoxville, TN: University of Tennessee Press; 2005:197–217.

52. Anglin MK. Activists and advocates as actors in health care. In: Couto RA, Simpson NK, Harris G, eds. *Sowing Seeds in the Mountains: Community-Based Coalitions for Cancer Prevention and Control.* Bethesda, MD: National Cancer Institute, Rural Appalachia Leadership Initiative on Cancer; 1994:179–193.

53. Van Schaik E. The social context of "nerves" in eastern Kentucky. In: Keefe SE, ed. *Appalachian Mental Health.* Lexington, KY: University Press of Kentucky; 1988:81–100.

54. Nations MK, Camino LA, Walker FB. "Hidden" popular illnesses in primary care: residents' recognition and clinical implications. *Cult Med Psychiatry.* 1985;9:223–240.

55. Plaut T, Landis S, Trevor JP. Community coalition building in the Madison County health project. In: Keefe SE, ed. *Participatory Development in Appalachia: Cultural Identity, Community, and Sustainability.* Knoxville, TN: University of Tennessee Press; 2009:231–246.

56. Flaskerud JH. Perceptions of problematic behavior by Appalachians, mental health professionals, and lay non-Appalachians. *Nurs Res.* 1980;29:140–149.

57. Keefe SE. An exploratory study of mental health service utilization by Appalachians and non-Appalachians. In: Keefe SE, ed. *Appalachian Mental Health,* Lexington, KY: University Press of Kentucky; 1988:145–158.

58. Rosswurm MA, Dent DM, Armstrong-Persily C, Woodburn P, Davis B. Illness experiences and health recovery behaviors of patients in southern Appalachia. *West J Nurs Res.* 1996;18:441–459.

59. Triandis HC. Collectivism and individualism as cultural syndromes. *Cross-Cult Res.* 1993;27:155–180.

60. Kleinman A, Kleinman J. Somatization: the interconnections of Chinese society among culture, depressive experiences, and the meanings of pain. In: Kleinman A, Good B, eds. *Culture and Depression: Studies in the Anthropology and Cross-Cultural Psychiatry of Affect and Disorder.* Berkeley, CA: University of California Press; 1985:429–490.

61. de Groot M, Doyle T, Hockman E, et al. Depression among type 2 diabetes rural Appalachian clinic attendees. *Diabetes Care.* 2007;30:1602–1604.

62. Greenlee R, Lantz J. Family coping strategies and the rural Appalachian working poor. *Contemp Fam Ther.* 1993;15:121–137.

63. Keefe SE, Hastrup JL, Thomas SN. Psychological testing in rural Appalachia. In: Keefe SE, ed. *Appalachian Cultural Competency: A Guide for Medical, Mental Health, and Social Service Professionals.* Knoxville, TN: University of Tennessee Press; 2005:285–297.

64. Behringer B, Friedell GH. Appalachia: where place matters in health. *Prev Chronic Dis.* 2006;3:A113.

65. Hansen MM, Resick LK. Health beliefs, health care, and rural Appalachian subcultures from an ethnographic perspective. *Fam Community Health.* 1990;13:1–10.

66. Fiene JI. The construction of self by rural low-status Appalachian women. *Affilia.* 1991;6:45–60.

67. Denham SA, Meyer MG, Toborg MA, Mande MJ. Providing health education to Appalachia populations. *Holist Nurs Pract.* 2004;18:293–301.

68. Keefe SE. Introduction. In: Keefe SE, ed. *Appalachian Cultural Competency: A Guide for Medical, Mental Health, and Social Service Professionals.* Knoxville, TN: University of Tennessee Press; 2005:2–26.

69. MacDonald FF. A case study of insider-outsider dynamics in rural community development. *Human Services in the Rural Environment.* 1990;14:15–20.

70. Keefe SE. Southern Appalachia: analytical models, social services, and native support systems. *Am J Community Psychol.* 1986;14:479–498.

71. Dunst CJ, Trivette CM, Cross AH. Social support networks of families with handicapped children. In: Keefe SE, ed. *Appalachian Mental Health.* Lexington, KY: University Press of Kentucky; 1988:101–121.

72. Barish R, Snyder AE. Use of complementary and alternative healthcare practices among persons served by a remote area medical clinic. *Fam Community Health.* 2008;31:221–227.

73. Arcury TA, Preisser JS, Gesler WM, Sherman JE. Complementary and alternative medicine use among rural residents in western North Carolina. *Complementary Health Practice Review.* 2004;9:93–102.

74. Simpson MR, King MG. "God brought all these churches together": issues in developing religion-health partnerships in an Appalachian community. *Public Health Nurs.* 1999;16:41–49.

75. Ludwig AM. "Nerves": a sociomedical diagnosis . . . of sorts. *Am J Psychother.* 1982;36:350–357.

76. Ludwig AM, Forrester RL. Nerves, but not mentally. *J Clin Psychiatry.* 1982;43:187–190.

77. Van Schaik E. Paradigms underlying the study of nerves as a popular illness term in eastern Kentucky. *Med Anthropol.* 1989;11:15–28.

78. Costello EJ, Farmer EMZ, Angold A. Same place, different children: white and American Indian children in the Appalachian mountains. In: Cohen P,

Slomkowski C, Robbins LN, eds. *Historical and Geographical Influences on Psychopathology*. Mahwah, NJ: Lawrence Erlbaum; 1999:279–298.

79. Cole C. Appalachian family therapy. In: Keefe SE, ed. *Appalachian Mental Health*. Lexington, KY: University Press of Kentucky; 1988:175–187.

80. Keefe SE, Greene S. Mental health therapy for Appalachian clients. In: Keefe SE, ed. *Appalachian Cultural Competency: A Guide for Medical, Mental Health, and Social Service Professionals*. Knoxville, TN: University of Tennessee Press; 2005:301–314.

81. Lantz J. Existential family treatment with an urban-Appalachian adolescent. *J Family Psychotherapy*. 1995;6:15–27.

82. Lemon SD, NewField NA, Dobbins JE. Culturally sensitive family therapy in Appalachia. *J Systemic Therapies*. 1993;12:8–26.

83. McInnis-Dittrich K. An empowerment oriented mental health intervention with elderly Appalachian women: the women's club. *J Women Aging*. 1997;9:91–105.

84. Sovine ML. Mental health professionals in Appalachia. In: Keefe SE, ed. *Appalachian Mental Health*. Lexington, KY: University Press of Kentucky; 1988:223–239.

85. Shoffner J, Staudt M, Marcus S, Kapp S. Using telephone reminders to increase attendance at psychiatric appointments: findings of a pilot study in rural Appalachia. *Psychiatr Serv*. 2007;58:872–875.

86. Keefe SE. *Appalachian Cultural Competency: A Guide for Medical, Mental Health, and Social Service Professionals*. 1st ed. Knoxville, TN: University of Tennessee Press; 2005.

87. Glisson C, Schoenwald SK. The ARC organizational and community intervention strategy for implementing evidence-based children's mental health treatments. *Ment Health Serv Res*. 2005;7:243–259.

88. Owens JS, Murphy CE, Richerson L, Girio EL, Himawan LK. Science to practice in underserved communities: the effectiveness of school mental health programming. *J Clin Child Adolesc Psychol*. 2008;37:434–447.

89. Michael KD, Renkert LE, Wandler J, Stamey T. Cultivating a new harvest: rationale and preliminary results from a growing interdisciplinary rural school mental health program. *Advances in School Mental Health Promotion*. 2009;2(2):40–50.

90. The National Advisory Committee on Rural Health and Human Services. The 2004 report to the secretary: rural health and human services issues. Washington, DC: National Advisory Committee on Rural Health and Human Services; 2004. Available at: http://www.hrsa.gov/advisorycommittees/rural/2004secreport .pdf. Accessed September 7, 2011.

91. Resnick SG, Rosenheck RA. Integrating peer-provided services: a quasi-experimental study of recovery orientation, confidence, and empowerment. *Psychiatr Serv*. 2008;59:1307–1314.

92. den Boer PC, Wiersma D, Van den Bosch RJ. Why is self-help neglected in the treatment of emotional disorders? A meta-analysis. *Psychol Med.* 2004;34:959–971.

93. Graham MA. Telepsychiatry in Appalachia. *Am Behav Sci.* 1996;39:602–615.

94. Swinton JJ, Robinson WD, Bischoff RJ. Telehealth and rural depression: physician and patient perspectives. *Fam Syst Health.* 2009;27:172–182.

95. Jones KM, Gray AH, Paleo J, Braden CJ, Lesser J. Community and scholars unifying for recovery. *Issues Ment Health Nurs.* 2008;29:495–503.

96. Ball RA. A poverty case: the analgesic subculture of the southern Appalachians. *Am Sociol Rev.* 1968;33:885–895.

97. Goshen CE. Characterological deterrents to economic progress in people of Appalachia. *South Med J.* 1970;63:1053–1061.

98. Polansky NA, Borgman RD, De Saix C. *Roots of Futility.* 1st ed. San Francisco, CA: Jossey-Bass; 1972.

99. Helton LR. Folk medicine and health beliefs: an Appalachian perspective. *J Cult Divers.* 1996;3(4):123–128.

100. MacAvoy S, Lippman DT. Teaching culturally competent care: nursing students experience rural Appalachia. *J Transcult Nurs.* 2001;12:221–227.

101. Purnell LD, Paulanka BJ. People of Appalachian heritage. In: Purnell LD, Paulanka BJ, eds. *Guide to Culturally Competent Health Care.* Philadelphia, PA: F. A. Davis; 2005:46–58.

102. Yelton D, Nielson C. Understanding Appalachian values—implications for occupational therapists. *Occupational Therapy in Mental Health.* 1991;11(2/3):173–195.

12

Substance Abuse

Michael S. Dunn, Bruce A. Behringer,
and Kristine Harper Bowers

Substance abuse has become a major health concern in Appalachia. In pockets of rural Appalachia, poor economic prospects, high unemployment rates, limited transportation networks, long distances to medical facilities, and a scarcity of treatment facilities and service organizations influence a community's ability to cope with the production, distribution, and use of drugs, illicit and otherwise. Data for the region indicate that the substances of choice include alcohol, tobacco, prescription drugs, methamphetamine, marijuana, and newer versions of drugs as they become available.[1,2] Anecdotal evidence also indicates the presence of rolling addictions in Appalachia, such as from OxyContin to hydrocodone to Acomplia.[3,4]

This chapter explores substance abuse in rural Appalachia, including its prevalence and health consequences, influencing factors, community responses, and prevention and treatment. It concludes with suggestions for further research and policy development. Throughout the discussion, the term *substance abuse* refers to overindulgence in and dependence on drugs (e.g., alcohol, tobacco, prescription drugs, marijuana, methamphetamine) that may have harmful consequences.

Prevalence and Health Effects of Abused Substances

Alcohol. Appalachians have a long history of producing and consuming alcohol, which remains the region's most abused legal substance. Today, the market for moonshine (illicitly distilled liquor) has declined because safe, legal alcohol can be produced at a similar cost and is available commercially.[5] It has been suggested that most of the moonshine made today is consumed by the distiller, sold to connoisseurs of artisanal whiskey, or purveyed to naïve tourists looking for the "essence of hillbilly culture."[6] Moonshine has also declined in use due to negative health consequences. For example, four adults in Atlanta in 2000 were treated for moonshine-related lead poisoning caused by the tubing used to build the still.[7]

Among adolescents, the rate of alcohol abuse in rural Appalachia is typically higher than in urban areas. This may be the result of greater tolerance for alcohol use or because drinking is considered normal everyday behavior.[8] One study found that 36 percent of rural adolescents thought that binge drinking (consuming more than five drinks on an occasion) was a risky behavior, compared with 39 percent of urban adolescents. Similar results were found among young adults and adults. This suggests that perceptions play a significant role in the use and abuse of alcohol by adolescents in Appalachia.[9]

Among adults, the heavy use of alcohol and binge drinking are lower in Appalachia than nationally. One study found that among Appalachian adults who used alcohol, fewer reported heavy use and binge drinking during the past year compared with adults living in non-Appalachian areas. Additionally, this study found that alcohol treatment was lower in Appalachia than in the nation as a whole.[10]

Tobacco. Tobacco use in the form of cigarette smoking is the most preventable cause of premature morbidity and mortality, yet a significant number of adolescents and adults engage in this behavior. Cigarette smoking is more prevalent among rural Appalachians compared with the general U.S. population.[11] One study found that a greater percentage of current adult smokers lived in Ohio's Appalachian counties than in the state's non-Appalachian counties (31.5 versus 26.1 percent).[12] Another study conducted in West Virginia found similar results.[13]

In general, Appalachia has high rates of cancer associated with tobacco use. Several studies have found that the incidence and death rates for all cancers are higher in Appalachia than in the rest of the United States.[14-16] In particular, lung cancer rates for males and females were 25 and 8 percent higher, respectively, than for rest of the country.[16]

A study was conducted in the coalfield region of Appalachia to determine perceptions of tobacco use and the role of the family. It found that both adults and adolescents agreed that rural Appalachian adolescents typically begin to experiment with smoking between the ages of 11 and 13. Additionally, the modeling of family behavior influences adolescent smoking behavior. This study also found that the use of smokeless tobacco is prevalent among underground coal miners because they are not allowed to smoke in the mines.[17]

Prescription Drugs. Nonmedical use of prescription drugs is reportedly the primary form of substance abuse in some areas of Appalachia.[18, 19] Among people in eastern Kentucky who are arrested for DUI, more are found to have prescription drugs in their systems than alcohol.[20] A study conducted in the Appalachian coalfields of Kentucky found that on a per capita basis, drugstores, hospitals, and other legal outlets received more prescriptions for painkillers than did the rest of the nation.[21] Some of these drugs are then sold on the street, where the profit margin is significant. As enforcement efforts have increased in this area, a "pipeline" has developed, originating in Florida, to supply prescription painkillers in Kentucky, Tennessee, Virginia, and beyond, as evidenced by the number of drug dealers from rural Appalachian states arrested in Florida and charged with prescription drug fraud and drug trafficking.[22, 23]

OxyContin is the most widely abused prescription drug in Central Appalachia and is linked to criminal activities such as robbery, theft, assault, and prescription drug fraud. County sheriffs report a noticeable uptick in property crimes with direct links to prescription drug abuse, with the perpetrators seeking either the actual drugs or funds to purchase drugs. Other synthetic opioids used to treat chronic pain are also widely abused,[a] with deleterious social and physical consequences such as hormonal changes (decreased fertility), immune suppression, associative or adaptive tolerance, desensitization or hypersensitivity to pain, respiratory depression, psychosis, and death.[20]

Studying health disparities in the Appalachian coalfields, Zhang and colleagues[10] found that hospital admission rates for the abuse of prescription opiates and synthetic opiates were higher in Appalachia than in the rest of the nation. In focus group interviews, the researchers found that key community stakeholders attribute prescription drug abuse to the relatively easy access to these drugs through family, friends, and drug dealers. The drugs are often acquired or stolen from family members first; once those sources are depleted, the user seeks other means of obtaining the drugs on the street.[10] It has been reported that nationwide, the sale of hydrocodone is highest in rural areas of West Virginia, Kentucky, and Tennessee.[24] Another study in the Appalachian region of Tennessee found that admission rates for the treatment of prescription drug abuse increased significantly, from 8.36 percent to 19.07 percent, between 1998 and 2002.[25] This increase may be related to the easy access to prescription drugs.

Prescription drug abuse can have serious consequences, including death. More than 340 individuals died from overdoses related to synthetic narcotics in eastern Kentucky during a sixteen-month period from 2003 to 2004.[26] Additionally, 485 people died in Kentucky in 2008 from overdoses of prescription drugs. According to medical examiners' reports, the drugs most commonly implicated in those deaths included methadone, oxycodone, alprazolam, morphine, diazepam, and fentanyl. The number of deaths from these drugs was higher than the number of deaths associated with cocaine and heroin combined.[27]

Methamphetamine. Methamphetamine (meth) is a large part of the substance abuse problem in Appalachia. Clients in treatment for methamphetamine abuse increased from 3.5 to 6.27 percent over a five-year period in Appalachian Tennessee.[25] Although another study conducted in Central Appalachia found that admission rates for treatment of methamphetamine abuse were lower than in the rest of the nation, the region's usage rates are rising faster than the nation's.[10] As another indicator of the problem, Tennessee had more seizures of meth labs (539) than any other state in the southeastern United States in 2007.[28] In eastern Kentucky, 377 meth labs were seized in 2005. However, as law enforcement reduced the number of meth labs in the state, trafficking in the drug increased from new sources, such as rogue foreign and domestic precursor chemical companies and mobile labs run by independent small manufacturers.[29]

Methamphetamine is widely accessible because the precursor ingredients are readily available, home manufacture is easy, and the costs of ingredients and production are low.[28, 30] Meth is typically produced in clandestine labs in private homes, garages, and motel rooms.[10] Although reports from Tennessee indicated a decrease in meth lab seizures between 2003 and 2008, there has been an increase in the use of alternative means of production, such as the "shake and bake" method, which does not require heating of the materials and can be done in a soda bottle in any location.[b]

Methamphetamine production itself is a danger to health. Due to the chemicals used, people in and around the area can be exposed to toxins through air emissions, spills, fires, and explosions.[31] Reports indicate that nearly 20 to 30 percent of meth labs are discovered because of fires and explosions, which often result in serious burns or death. Home labs in particular are a serious health threat to children. Individuals who use meth are subject to health consequences, including extreme weight loss, oral health problems such as "meth mouth," and psychological disturbances such as anxiety, confusion, mood disturbances, and violent behavior. Long-term chronic abuse can cause a variety of psychotic manifestations, including paranoia, hallucinations, and delusions.[32]

Marijuana. The federal Appalachian high intensity drug trafficking area (HIDTA) encompasses sixty-seven counties in eastern Kentucky, eastern Tennessee, and southern West Virginia (map 12.1). This area, third in the nation for marijuana cultivation, is known as the "Marijuana Belt" because its soils and temperatures are ideal for growing marijuana.[29] The proximity of a number of large national forests allows marijuana cultivation sites to be hidden in a broad expanse of this remote area. Cultivation often occurs on these public lands because even if the illegal plants are detected, attributing ownership of them is difficult, allowing growers to avoid the seizure of personal property. Once the plants are harvested and processed, the drug is transported across state lines. In fact, most marijuana produced in-state is exported.[29]

As shown in table 12.1, large amounts of illegal drugs are seized in the Appalachian HIDTA. For instance, more than 2,000 kilograms of commercial-grade marijuana, 1,150 kilograms of hydroponic marijuana, 209 kilograms of powder cocaine, and 9 kilograms of methamphetamine were seized in 2007. The states differ in terms of the amount and type of drugs seized. For example, more methamphetamine was seized in Tennessee than in West Virginia and Kentucky combined.

The abuse of any legal or illegal drug can have devastating consequences for individuals, families, and communities, including criminal prosecution, co-occurring mental issues, lifetime disability, and death. One study conducted in Kentucky found that more than 2,600 drug-related deaths were reported in a two-year period, with 1,300 of these deaths occurring in eastern Kentucky.[33] Drug-related deaths in this mountainous region

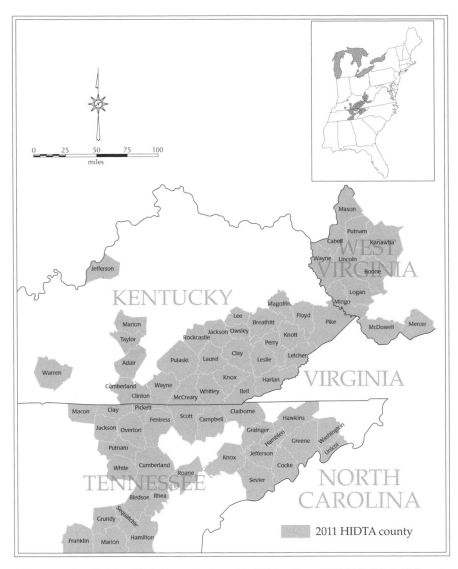

Map 12.1. Appalachian High-Intensity Drug Trafficking Area (HIDTA). (Dick Gilbreath, University of Kentucky Cartography Lab)

Table 12.1. Appalachian HIDTA Drug Seizures (in Kilograms), 2007

State	Powder Cocaine	Crack Cocaine	Ice Methamphetamine	Powder Methamphetamine	Commercial-Grade Marijuana	Hydroponic Marijuana	Heroin	Oxycodone (Dosage Units)	Hydrocodone (Dosage Units)
Kentucky	2.20	1.24	1.63	0.18	648.27	910.04	0.02	11,331	14,282
Tennessee	197.82	2.52	7.41	4.27	1,265.00	2.27	4.00	1,069	1,475
West Virginia	9.66	2.52	0.00	0.39	169.82	237.79	0.04	5,945	3,458
Total	209.68	6.28	9.04	4.84	2,083.09	1,150.10	4.06	18,345	19,215

Source: National Drug Intelligence Center, 2008.

occurred at four times the rate in the rest of the state, indicating that treatment is either not used or not readily available.[33] Another study found that of 129 drug-related deaths in the Appalachian HIDTA, 104 involved prescription drugs, cocaine, methamphetamine, or a combination thereof.[28]

In addition, substance abuse can lead to a breakdown of the family as a social support structure. When families protect addictive behaviors or when family ties are broken because of addiction, interpersonal systems break apart, and family dissolution can create social crises in the community. Zhang and colleagues[10] found that addiction in Appalachia is long lasting, extending over generations in some cases.

Factors Influencing Substance Abuse

Substance abuse in rural Appalachia is influenced by a number of critical factors. A large-scale study sponsored by the Appalachian Regional Commission (ARC) identified key economic, generational, and recreational factors affecting mental health and substance abuse in the region.[10]

Economic Factors. Economic stressors, such as the loss of community infrastructure, personal income, and worthwhile employment, have become common in rural Appalachian communities experiencing generational poverty and low rates of employment. These harsh socioeconomic conditions can lead to depression and substance abuse, a common response to the loss of economic viability. The availability of fulfilling employment and greater wealth relative to prior generations is considered a deterrent to substance abuse by community stakeholders. This perception underscores the fact that both substance abuse and the tolerance of abuse are rising in communities that have experienced economic losses due to plant closures, layoffs, and a dearth of well-paying jobs.[10] Some individuals who lose their jobs seek alternative occupations, such as cultivating marijuana or cooking meth, while many others are prompted to use illegal substances as a result.[34] Some stakeholders participating in the ARC study reported an unemployable workforce in their communities due to alcohol and other addictions. As employers leave communities (or are not willing to locate in them) because of a poorly prepared workforce, economic development is further constricted. Lack of job opportunities contributes to stress, depression, anxiety, and other mental health issues among workers, often resulting in drug use to cope with emotional problems.

Zhang and colleagues[10] found that the type of employment available in rural Appalachia may add to problems of substance abuse as well as being affected by it. Where employment opportunities exist, the workforce is often concentrated in industries requiring heavy physical labor such as mining, timber, and construction. These occupations involve long hours and dangerous work.[35] In some cases, doctors may dispense prescription painkillers to keep workers employed, production up, and paychecks flowing to families. An unintended consequence of this practice may be addiction to prescription drugs.[34] A certain level of pain relief has become socially acceptable, with the institution of medically mandated pain assessments in recent years.[36] Prescription drug addiction among Appalachian workers affects not only that individual but also those who work with the addict, and it sets a precedent for tolerating drug use in the workplace.[10]

Generational Factors. The focus groups conducted by Zhang and colleagues[10] indicate that substance abuse is a modeled behavior in much of Appalachia. The norms of a family or community may promote the use and abuse of various substances. Children who mimic the behavior of significant others or caregivers, and children without regular supervision, are more likely to begin using alcohol and other drugs.[37, 38] Parents and family members who use alcohol and drugs may set this behavior as a standard for their children.[37, 39] For example, some prescription drug users grew up in families where substance abuse was both a means of controlling the home environment and a recreational norm.[40] Research shows that if children have these negative role models, their behaviors may disrupt schools and destroy the traditional social fabrics of communities.[10]

Recreational Factors. Boredom and lack of recreational activities are other reasons for substance abuse. Some rural Appalachian communities lack the resources to provide recreational activities for their youths, who may turn to substance abuse to reduce boredom and achieve a sense of belonging. Appalachian communities offering broader educational opportunities, more after-school programs (including sports and music), more community involvement by adults, and greater awareness of the consequences of substance abuse were less likely to report high levels of substance abuse.[10]

Community Response to Substance Abuse

Local perceptions of alcohol, tobacco, and other drug use play a significant role in determining whether and what type of community action occurs. Multiple studies have assessed how Appalachian communities feel about drug use and addiction, as well as the perceived impact of such behavior on the community.[1, 9, 41] In general, these studies found that communities see alcohol and illicit drug use as their greatest problem; they maintain that substance abuse is widespread and on the increase, particularly among adolescents. In one study, 47 percent of residents indicated that alcohol was the biggest problem, and 43 percent cited illegal drugs, followed by tobacco (8 percent) and prescription drugs (2 percent).[9] Community members believe that substance abuse impacts every family and has the potential to destroy the community through increased unemployment and criminal activity. They believe that alcohol use by teens increases traffic accidents and criminal activity and, along with smoking, leads to the use of other drugs. Community leaders also assert that substance abuse is often the result of self-medication used as a coping mechanism for underlying issues such as depression or deeper psychological trauma. They acknowledge the need for some type of intervention but admit they do not know how to solve the problem. Some community members advocate more prevention programs for adolescents[9]; others see the lack of treatment options as an obstacle to preventing substance abuse and its consequences in rural Appalachia. Unless more facilities for recovery and reentry become available, many believe that controlling substance abuse will be difficult.[41]

Drug-related crime is also an issue in rural Appalachia. Individuals steal prescriptions from family and friends and rob their neighbors to fund their drug habits. In Tazewell, Virginia, robberies, thefts, and burglaries increased by 48 percent in a five-year period as a result of drug abusers seeking drugs and money.[42] Consequently, a community's perception of its safety and welfare, as well as its way of life, is gravely impacted.

Substance Abuse Treatment

Substance abuse treatment is most effective when it is initiated by the abuser. Although the problem is individual in nature, it affects one's family, friends, and community. Eventually, a personal commitment to stop using drugs is needed, and typically, most abusers need drug treatment. Some factors affecting drug treatment in Appalachia include stigma, cost, personal preferences, and access to and availability of treatment centers.

Mental Health Stigma and Denial. The ARC study found that the stigma attached to seeking mental health services prevents many addicts from getting treatment.[10] Also, community stakeholders cited parental denial of children's mental health needs and multigenerational acceptance of mental health and substance abuse problems as barriers to treatment. Generational addiction may be the default behavior. Some rural Appalachians avoid treatment even if services are available because they fear being observed and judged by others or because the family views professional counseling as a sign of personal or moral failure. This causes some people suffering from depression and other disorders to use alcohol and drugs to cope with their emotional or physical pain.

Costs and Personal Preferences. A significant number of Appalachian residents have no insurance or only limited insurance, which prevents them from seeking or receiving services. Alternatively, some rural Appalachians may avoid seeking professional help for health problems, including substance abuse, because they do not want to be "beholden." Regardless of the illegality or the degree of personal and family disruption their drug use causes, some rural Appalachians would rather self-medicate to relieve their pain, depression, or other health problems because it avoids the perceived embarrassment of seeking the assistance of a professional health care provider.[43] People's behaviors are directly influenced by their beliefs, so patients who fear that a health care provider may take advantage of them or reveal their problems to the community may be reluctant to seek help.[44] Conversely, participants in a focus group reported that being able to care for oneself and one's family is of the utmost importance. The family is often the primary arena of decision making in rural Appalachia, acting as a resource for problem solving and assistance; community or church affiliation is often secondary to the family unit. Family problems are considered private, and social services agencies are regarded as an unreliable replacement for the family circle. This attitude may influence an individual's decision to seek outside help. Substance abuse is often not recognized as a harmful behavior until an adverse personal experience, criminal activity, emotional response, or other detrimental outcome reveals the extent of the addiction and its consequences for the lives of others.[1,2] Seeking the help of social services may be a last resort in response to such a crisis.[45]

Access and Availability. Lack of transportation often prevents people in rural Appalachia from receiving community-based services. Treatment centers may be more than an hour's drive from home. Individuals willing to seek help and who have the resources to obtain treatment may still find it difficult to make the trip to a treatment facility. Working individuals may not have the time to travel to the treatment center or participate in recovery groups. As a result, they may suffer in pain or continue their addictive habits.[10]

Due to the scarcity of treatment facilities in rural Appalachia, community-based health care services are limited. A study conducted by Project HOPE found few treatment options among the most distressed counties in Appalachia.[46] Only 8 percent of distressed Appalachian counties had substance abuse treatment services, and 20 percent of these counties had hospital-affiliated mental health services. The ARC study found that access to inpatient treatment and nonhospital residential treatment for substance abuse or mental health issues was less common in Appalachia than elsewhere. Specifically, a smaller proportion of Appalachians who sought treatment in an inpatient facility was able to obtain services compared with those outside the region.[10] Community stakeholders observed that their individual counties lacked adequate mental health services, and inpatient treatment facilities were not nearby or not readily available. In addition, the scope of services was limited; treatment was often provided by counselors, psychologists, or psychiatrists who practiced in the county for only a day or two each week. The lack of a residential treatment facility was the most commonly cited medical service gap, and those in crisis often had to leave the region to obtain help. As a result, the ARC study concluded that people in Appalachia had difficulty obtaining inpatient and long-term residential treatment due to the existence of fewer residential treatment facilities. This implies that most individuals in need of inpatient or residential treatment have to either struggle with their addiction or seek care far from home.

Conversely, the ARC study found that, over a one-year period, a greater proportion of adults in Appalachia received outpatient mental health treatment compared with the rest of the nation. Treatment facilities in the region were more likely to accept payment from governmental sources such as Medicaid or to have sliding payment scales. However, the number of patient contacts did not address the key issues of accessibility, availability, and quality of care.

Substance Abuse Prevention Programs

Because of the region's heterogeneity, a one-size-fits-all approach is unlikely to be effective in addressing substance abuse in rural Appalachia. A number of interventions have been employed, but community-based initiatives appear to be the most successful, at least in the Appalachian coalfields.

Community coalitions help residents mobilize resources and organize activities to improve the health and welfare of their community.[47, 48] By bringing together various stakeholder groups such as local government, law enforcement, education, health agencies, churches, nonprofits, businesses, and private citizens, coalitions can identify, plan, and initiate public health programs that would not be possible through a single agency.[49–52] The successful community-based initiatives described below illustrate the effectiveness of this approach.

Coalition on Appalachian Substance Abuse Policy (CASAP). Formed in response to the growing problem of substance abuse in Central Appalachia, this coalition of representatives from Kentucky, Tennessee, Virginia, West Virginia, and Ohio involves public officials, local communities, and treatment professionals. CASAP's mission is to "seek change in public policy, increase human and financial resources, develop educational materials, and provide a forum for knowledge exchange to address substance abuse in Appalachia to decrease the destructive impact of substance abuse on personal, community and economic development."[36] It seeks to prevent substance abuse by (1) increasing communication among Appalachian communities, addressing substance abuse and health problems, and identifying common interests and concerns; (2) providing information to increase the understanding of how substance abuse affects economic development and overall well-being; (3) developing and using locally appropriate data-collection strategies; (4) exploring national and statewide policies to better identify Appalachian-specific substance abuse problems; (5) identifying resources for addressing substance abuse problems; and (6) proposing policies to solve those problems. This primarily grant-funded nonprofit organization cannot claim a decrease in substance abuse, but it makes the topic a priority among community coalitions, state agencies, and providers in the core Appalachian states.[36]

Strong Through Our Plan (STOP). This community-based organization, developed in Gilbert, West Virginia, "is committed to a high quality of life free of the impact of substance abuse and its adverse affects through service and mobilization of our communities."[53] The coalition was formed as a result of growing problems related to the use of OxyContin and other prescription drugs in the community. In Gilbert, once known as "Pillbert," the STOP agenda focuses on attacking problems associated with nonmedical prescription drug use, such as crime and addiction. STOP's intervention efforts include education, supply and demand reduction, alternative youth activities, rehabilitation, public relations, and political action. The education intervention sponsors workshops for parents and adolescents and invites speakers to cover different aspects of substance abuse and addiction. The supply and demand intervention involves speakers from pharmaceutical companies addressing the issue of OxyContin addiction. The coalition's proactive stance has had some positive results, and STOP activities have now spread to multiple communities in West Virginia.[53] The power of STOP is based on the premise that "a committed community is frequently the best, sometimes the only, remedy to a serious, life threatening drug problem in Appalachia."[18]

Appalachian Regional Commission (ARC). This federal development agency is a funding source for local coalitions. In March 2006 the ARC and the federal Office of Rural Health Policy awarded $161,000 to East Tennessee State University's College of Public and Allied Health for a training conference to arm community coalitions with the knowledge and tools needed to address substance abuse and its symptoms in their communities. Twenty-six local coalitions from Alabama, Kentucky, South Carolina, Tennessee, Virginia, and West Virginia attended the conference and were awarded seed money in the form of small challenge grants to fight substance abuse in their respective communities. Their progress was evaluated after six months and after two years. Coalition activities included (1) educating law enforcement and emergency personnel about evidence collection and record keeping using the drug-endangered children protocol; (2) purchasing and distributing educational materials about methamphetamine and substance abuse to youth and community groups; (3) purchasing media airtime to implement community awareness programs; (4) developing educational materials about methamphetamine production for use by hotel and motel owners and managers, real estate agents, and property managers; (5) designing and implementing training modules for those seeking jobs in public transportation and for coal miners that included basic information about alcohol and other drug use, appropriate screening techniques, the risks and impact of drug use, and sources of help; (6) teaching about substance abuse prevention at health fairs; (7) mapping current local prevention programs and activities; and (8) completing a gap analysis of preferred drug prevention activities.

On follow-up, the results of these twenty-six local coalitions seemed applicable to many southeastern Appalachian communities dealing with substance abuse. The majority of the teams perceived a threat to the health and welfare of their communities as a result of substance abuse, although many barriers hindered the full implementation of community plans. Lack of volunteer manpower, time for training, and money were the most frequently cited barriers to action by the community teams, although time seemed to be a greater barrier than money.[c]

Operation UNITE. A nonprofit foundation in Kentucky, UNITE works to rid communities of illegal drugs through investigation, treatment coordination, support for families and friends of addicts, and community education. UNITE's goal is to "educate and activate individuals, by developing and empowering community coalitions, to no longer accept or tolerate the drug culture."[54] Launched in 2003, UNITE has engaged in counterdrug initiatives, public education about the dangers of substance abuse, and treatment coordination for substance abusers. UNITE coordinates more than thirty local coalitions involving over 8,000 volunteers who are responsible for creating antidrug programs and events in their counties. Through these efforts, local coalitions are able to spread the word regarding the dangers of substance abuse and offer prevention activities. The majority of adolescents in Kentucky are receiving drug education through UNITE. UNITE also provides treatment vouchers to individuals who cannot afford residential drug treatment, and since 2005, more than 1,500 men, women, and children in eastern Kentucky have received drug treatment through these vouchers. Addicts who otherwise would not have received care are resuming drug-free lives. Communities have become more livable, with less criminal activity. Local health and welfare systems show less strain because former addicts are more likely to be employable and become productive members of the community. UNITE groups also assist local, state, and federal law enforcement agencies by providing supplementary drug detection equipment to help build strong cases against drug dealers. As a result, UNITE's counterdrug initiatives have a 97 percent conviction rate.[54] Additionally, between 2003 and 2004, UNITE seized over $1.6 million worth of drugs and saw the street supply of OxyContin decrease to 10 percent of all prescription drugs seized.[55]

Further Research

To advance an understanding of the issues surrounding substance abuse in the Appalachian region, a number of additional research questions must be addressed, including the following.

What role does theory play in explaining regional characteristics and substance abuse behaviors in rural Appalachia? To date, there has been limited theory-based research that analyzes the interpersonal factors related to substance abuse in Appalachia. Research in this area could explore the beliefs and behaviors associated with substance abuse. For example, determining the role of significant others in substance use behaviors and behavioral control could be useful in the design of preventive interventions.

What community characteristics contribute to a reduction in substance abuse in Appalachia? The salience of community factors such as norms, resources, volunteer involvement, and community awareness related to substance abuse is an area that needs to be clarified.

What is the relationship between a community's resources and its addiction rates, as well as its success in preventing substance abuse? Identifying Appalachian best practices can help determine which components of coalition organization, community education, and intervention are most effective in preventing substance use and abuse.

What influence do employment options have on one's self-esteem, and how does this affect the initiation or escalation of substance abuse? Research should explore the effect of repetitive, low-paying jobs on mental health and substance abuse. Exploring how traditional types of work, such as coal mining and trucking, and contemporary occupations, such as jobs in computer call centers and service industries, relate to the prevalence or prevention of substance abuse is another path for researchers.

What are the financial or other incentives underlying the current volume of painkillers prescribed by doctors? Do the financial incentives associated with the patient's work environment or the nature of the job play a role? What incentives does a physician have to prescribe more painkillers than might be considered medically necessary? Researchers should explore the decision-making processes among workers, managers, and prescribers to gain a better understanding of the factors involved in choosing to treat pain with medication and not pursue alternative methods of pain relief. This information would be helpful in the development of educational materials about the dangers and consequences of using medication as the sole mechanism for pain relief.

The relationship between substance abuse and economic conditions in Appalachian communities needs to be explored. Does substance abuse result in an unemployable workforce, or do high rates of underemployment or unemployment lead to substance abuse? Are both these dynamics at work simultaneously? What effects does this have on the community? Health promotion efforts in the workplace as well as more testing, treatment, and recovery programs could result in increased productivity. It would be useful to conduct cost-benefit analyses to determine the direct impact of health promotion efforts, as well as pinpoint and clarify relevant issues in the work environment.

What are the most commonly used inpatient, outpatient, and residential treatment options, and how effective are they in treating addiction in rural Appalachia? What factors hinder the seeking of treatment? More needs to be known about appropriate and place-based substance abuse treatment options in Appalachia. First, barriers to treatment must be identified, and effective ways of overcoming these barriers and sufficient supports must be developed. The stigma associated with treatment and recovery needs to be explored and dissipated to ensure appropriate treatment referrals for substance abusers. Second, reasons for the scarcity of residential treatment facilities in the region must be identified. Appalachia lacks a sufficient number and variety of residential treatment options, and as a result, many individuals receive only outpatient care. Why is it that more options do not exist?

Policy Recommendations

The well-documented problem of substance abuse in rural Appalachia can be addressed through the implementation of policy initiatives such as the following.

Local, state, and federal government policies should be analyzed for effectiveness. Identifying and disseminating the policies that are most effective in halting drug use, diversion, and distribution would help other communities adopt uniform and consistent structures. A list of best practices for policy initiatives could be developed based on this information.

More facilities are needed in the region to provide treatment, counseling, and recovery services. Regional and federal support and funding are needed to make this a reality. Policies that create reimbursement mechanisms that reach across state borders and that employ more trained counselors would also address treatment issues in Appalachia. Free or reduced-cost community-based mental health and substance abuse treatment services should be a priority in the region. The development of a comprehensive service delivery infrastructure in rural communities—one that is responsible and responsive to the needs of substance abusers—would be of great value in reducing substance abuse.

Policies promoting community capacity building and mobilization in Appalachia should be developed as a means of preventing substance abuse. Schools, local government, law enforcement, health agencies, youth, and concerned citizens should be included in community antidrug coalitions. Diversity among coalition members increases the breadth of community interest and resources, produces more "buy-in," and brings different temperaments, talents, and convictions to the table. The entire community needs to be involved and committed to effect positive change, and the participation of many community sectors increases the likelihood of change.

It has been suggested that legalizing drugs would decrease criminal activity and reduce overcrowding in prisons. In 2008 there were 500,000 nonviolent drug offenders in prisons and jails and more than 1.8 million drug arrests.[56] As a result, the U.S. government is paying billions of dollars annually to house nonviolent individuals. Additionally, the societal costs of alcohol and tobacco use are significantly higher than the costs of illegal drug use. In the mid-1990s alcohol- and tobacco-related consequences were estimated at $86 billion and $65 billion, respectively, compared with $58 billion for illegal drug use, including enforcement and incarceration.[57] As such, the issue of legality should be explored to determine what type of policy might be satisfactory to all involved—that is, those for and against legalization.

Policies related to law enforcement and the use of federal land to cultivate illegal drugs are required. The Appalachian mountains are an ideal place to grow marijuana and to produce methamphetamine because of the rural geography and low population density. This area is difficult to patrol, and due to the downsizing of police forces as a result of economic issues, the situation may only get worse.[20] A better use of resources should be explored to eradicate the illegal production of drugs on federal land.

Drug courts, which are designed to be an alternative to the traditional court system, are lacking in Appalachia.[58] Through drug courts, nonviolent substance abuse offenders are entered into a comprehensive program of supervision, substance abuse treatment, and drug testing instead of the jail or prison system.[59] These programs have proved to be successful. A study conducted in Kentucky found that two years after completing a drug court program, only 20 percent of participants had been convicted of a new felony, compared with 57 percent of non–drug court participants. Additionally, Kentucky saves roughly $2 million a year by not having to incarcerate eligible drug court participants.[60] As such, drug courts seem to be an effective means of reducing drug-related offenses.

Notes

a. Narcotic drugs include natural opiates such as morphine and codeine, semisynthetic opioids (opiate-like drugs) such as hydrocodone and oxycodone (OxyContin), and fully synthetic opioids such as methadone. Each of these substances has a legitimate medical use but can be abused by nonprescription use, overuse, or illicit trading in pills or prescriptions. Methamphetamine is a medical stimulant used to treat exogenous obesity or attention-deficit hyperactivity disorder. It is subject to abuse by nonscientific production methods, inappropriate dosages, and high frequency of use.

b. The "shake and bake" method is a "cold cook" process that produces small amounts of methamphetamine by combining easily procured ingredients in a plastic soda bottle with pseudoephedrine in an amount that falls below legal reporting requirements. This method is faster and more mobile than those requiring open-flame heating and distillation over several days. Although the risk of fire is diminished, explosions can be more intense, and producers may discard the environmentally hazardous two-liter bottles along roadsides and in common waste containers, putting the public in danger.

c. This work was supported by a grant from the ARC (grant no. CO-15197-302-2005). The federal Office of Rural Health Policy also contributed support through the ARC.

References

1. Behringer B, Jessee R, Dunn M, Bowers K. Focus on rural substance abuse in Appalachia. *Rural Roads.* 2007;5:6–10.

2. Behringer B, Friedell GH. Appalachia: where place matters in health. *Prev Chronic Dis.* 2006;3:A113.

3. Associated Press. Hydrocodone use, legal and not, quietly growing. *Charleston Gazette,* August 5, 2007. Available at: www.wvgazette.com/section/news/2007080427. Accessed June 10, 2009.

4. Breen T. After OxyContin scare, Appalachian addicts turn to hydrocodone. *Lexington Herald-Leader,* June 20, 2009. Available at: www.kentucky.com/181/story/103054.html. Accessed September 10, 2009.

5. WhiskeyWise. Moonshine whiskey—illegal whiskey production in the USA. Available at: http://www.whiskeywise.com/Moonshine-Whiskey.html. Accessed September 2, 2010.

6. Alford R. Stills in the hills: moonshine enjoys new popularity as colorful history attracts tourists. *Victoria Advocate,* January 11, 2004. Available at: http://news.google.com/newspapers?nid=861&dat=20040111&id=EJwMAAAAIBAJ&sjid=4GEDAAAAIBAJ&pg=4473,2556824. Accessed June 1, 2009.

7. Yee D. Study: moonshine common in urban Atlanta. Available at: www.kentucky.com/mid/kentucky/news/breaking_news/6642544.htm. Accessed June 1, 2009.

8. Carsey Institute. Building knowledge for rural America's families and communities in the 21st century. *Reports on Rural America.* 2006;2(1).

9. Brushy Fork Institute. Mountain. *Promise.* 2004;14:12–15.

10. Zhang Z, Infante A, Meit M, English N, Dunn M, Bowers KH. An analysis of mental health and substance abuse disparities and access to treatment services in the Appalachian region. Washington, DC: Appalachian Regional Commission; 2008. Available at: http://www.arc.gov/assets/research_reports/AnalysisofMentalHealthandSubstanceAbuseDisparities.pdf. Accessed April 5, 2009.

11. Centers for Disease Control and Prevention. Cigarette smoking among adults—United States, 2004. *MMWR Morb Mortal Wkly Rep.* 2004;54(44):1121–1124.

12. Ohio Department of Health. Cancer incidence and mortality among Ohio residents, 1999–2003. Columbus, OH: Cancer Incidence Surveillance System, Ohio Department of Health, Ohio State University; 2005.

13. Thoenen E. Health risks: the Appalachian lifestyle. Charleston, WV: West Virginia Department of Health and Human Resources, Health Statistics Center; 1995.

14. Centers for Disease Control and Prevention. Cancer death rates—Appalachia, 1994–1998. *MMWR Morb Mortal Wkly Rep.* 2002;51:527–529.

15. Hall HI, Rogers JD, Weir HK, Miller DS, Uhler RJ. Breast and cervical carcinoma mortality among women in the Appalachian region of the U.S., 1976–1996. *Cancer.* 2000;89:1593–1602.

16. Wingo PA, Tucker TC, Jamison PM, et al. Cancer in Appalachia, 2001–2003. *Cancer.* 2008;112:181–192.

17. Meyer MG, Toborg MA, Denham SA, Mande MJ. Cultural perspectives concerning adolescent use of tobacco and alcohol in the Appalachian Mountain region. *J Rural Health.* 2008;24:67–74.

18. Appalachian Regional Commission. Substance abuse in Appalachia. Washington, DC: Appalachian Regional Commission; 2009. Available at: http://www.arc.gov/index.do?nodeId=1750. Accessed April 5, 2009.

19. Drug Enforcement Administration. OxyContin: pharmaceutical diversion. Drug intelligence brief. Arlington, VA: Drug Enforcement Administration; 2002.

20. Friends of Narconon. Kentucky factsheet. Available at: http://www.friendsofnarconon.org/drug_distribution_in_the_United_States/Kentucky_drug_facts_Kentucky_factsheet. Accessed August 29, 2011.

21. Johnson L. Eastern Kentucky, painkiller capital. *Lexington Herald-Leader,* January 19, 2003.

22. Yohe R. Prescription pill pushers flying into the tri-state. Available at: www.wsaz.com/newsohio/headlines/36351344.html. Accessed May 20, 1009.

23. Ludlow R. Troopers snare narcotics that roll into Portsmouth. *Columbus Dispatch,* December 14, 2008:B5.

24. Bass F. Pain medicine use has nearly doubled. Available at: www.bcbs.com/news/national/ap-pain-medicine-use-has-nearly-doubled.html. Accessed April 5, 2009.

25. Satish K. Substance abuse trends in Tennessee's Appalachian region (1998–2002). SAT report, vol. 1, no. 2:1–4. Memphis, TN: Institute for Substance Abuse Treatment Evaluation (I-SATE), University of Memphis; 2004. Available at: http://www.drugscience.org/Archive/bcr2/cashcrops.html. Accessed March 3, 2009.

26. Maimon A. Methadone abuse hits Kentucky hard. Available at: www.breathittonline.com/news/cod/info.html. Accessed February 15, 2009.

27. Potter M. Prescription drug abuse ravages state's youth. Available at: http://www.msnbc.msn.com/id/31707246/ns/health-addictions. Accessed September 2, 2010.

28. National Drug Intelligence Center. Appalachia high intensity drug trafficking area drug market analysis 2007. Available at: http://www.justice.gov/ndic/pubs27/23935/index.htm. Accessed September 2, 2010.

29. Drug Enforcement Administration. DEA briefs and background, drugs and drug abuse, state factsheets, Kentucky. Available at: http://www.usdoi.gov/dea/pubs/state_factsheets/kentucky.html. Accessed February 17, 2009.

30. National Drug Intelligence Center. Kentucky drug threat assessment: methamphetamine. Available at: http://www.usdoj.gov/ndic.pub1.htm. Accessed February 17, 2009.

31. Centers for Disease Control and Prevention. Acute public health consequences of methamphetamine laboratories. *MMWR Morb Mortal Wkly Rep.* 2005;54:356–359.

32. National Institute on Drug Abuse. Methamphetamine—InfoFacts. Available at: http://www.nida.nih.gov/InfoFacts/methamphetamine.html. Accessed September 2, 2010.

33. Matthews D. Appalachian substance abuse strategic initiative. Final report. Washington, DC: Appalachian Regional Commission; 2002.

34. National Drug Intelligence Center. Appalachia high intensity drug trafficking area drug market analysis 2008. Available at: http://www.justice.gov/ndic/pubs27/27483/index.htm. Accessed September 2, 2010.

35. Schaefer W. OxyContin called likely to spread: Appalachian economy tied to painkiller abuse. *Cincinnati Enquirer,* February 10, 2001:B11.

36. Coalition on Appalachian Substance Abuse Policy. Overview of substance abuse in Appalachia. Available at: http://cdar.uky.edu/casap/overview.html. Accessed February 22, 2011.

37. Bahr SJ, Hoffmann JP, Yang X. Parental and peer influences on the risk of adolescent drug use. *J Prim Prev.* 2005;26:529–551.

38. Allen M, Donohue WA, Griffin A, Ryan D, Turner MM. Comparing the influence of parents and peers on the choice to use drugs. *Crim Justice Behav.* 2003;30:163–186.

39. Fulkerson JA, Pasch KE, Perry CL, Komro K. Relationships between alcohol-related informal social control, parental monitoring and adolescent problem behaviors among racially diverse urban youth. *J Community Health.* 2008;33:425–433.

40. Manchikanti L, Pampati V, Damron KS, Beyer CD, Barnhill RC, Fellows B. Prevalence of prescription drug abuse and dependency in patients with chronic pain in western Kentucky. *J Ky Med Assoc.* 2003;101:511–517.

41. Dunn M, Behringer B. Evaluation of a community approach to address substance abuse, including methamphetamine in Appalachia. Johnson City, TN: Office of Rural and Community Health and Community Partnership, East Tennessee State University; 2007.

42. Bowman R. Prescription for crime. *Time,* March 21, 2005. Available at:

www.time.com/time/magazine/article/0,9171,1039712,00.html?promoid=rss_
nation. Accessed September 2, 2010.

43. Behringer B, Friedell GH, Dorgan KA, et al. Understanding the challenges of reducing cancer in Appalachia: addressing a place-based health disparity population. *Californian J Health Promot.* 2007;5:40–49.

44. Glanz K, Rimer BK, Lewis FM. *Health Behavior and Health Education: Theory, Research, and Practice.* 3rd ed. San Francisco, CA: Jossey-Bass; 2002.

45. Coyne CA, Demian-Popescu C, Friend D. Social and cultural factors influencing health in southern West Virginia: a qualitative study. *Prev Chronic Dis.* 2006;3:A124.

46. Stensland J, Mueller C, Sutton J. An analysis of the financial conditions of health care institutions in the Appalachian region and their economic impacts. Washington, DC: Appalachian Regional Commission; 2002. Available at: http://www.arc.gov/researchreports.asp?F_CATEGORY=13. Accessed March 5, 2007.

47. Provan KG, Nakama L, Veazie MA, Teufel-Shone NI, Huddleston C. Building community capacity around chronic disease services through a collaborative interorganizational network. *Health Educ Behav.* 2003;30:646–662.

48. Wolff T. The future of community coalition building. *Am J Community Psychol.* 2001;29:263–268.

49. Hawkins DJ, Catalano RF, Arthur MW. Promoting science-based prevention in communities. *Addict Behav.* 2002;27:951–976.

50. Shortell SM, Zukoski AP, Alexander JA, et al. Evaluating partnerships for community health improvement: tracking the footprints. *J Health Polit Policy Law.* 2002;27:49–91.

51. Hasnain-Wynia R, Margolin FS, Bazzoli GJ. Models for community health partnerships. *Health Forum J.* 2001;44:29–33.

52. Kurland J, Zeder J. Coalition-building: the promise of government. *Am J Community Psychol.* 2001;29:285–291.

53. Strong Through Our Plan (STOP). About us. Available at: http://stopcoalition.org/abutus.aspx. Accessed February 11, 2009.

54. Operation UNITE. About UNITE. Available at: http://www.operationunite.org/index.php. Accessed September 2, 2010.

55. Rosenberg D. Kentucky's pain: three years into OxyContin abuse, the casualties continue. But there's hope where it all began. Available at: www.newsweek.com/id/150118. Accessed April 20, 2009.

56. Nadelman EA. Let's end drug prohibition. *Wall Street Journal,* December 5, 2008:A21.

57. DuPont RL, Voth EA. Drug legalization, harm reduction, and drug policy. *Ann Intern Med.* 1995;123:461–465.

58. McVay DA, ed. *Drug War Facts.* 6th ed. Lancaster, PA: Common Sense for Drug Policy; 2009.

59. U.S. Department of Justice. Defining drug courts: the key components.

Available at: http://www.ncjrs.gov/pdffiles1/bja/205621.pdf. Accessed April 20, 2009.

60. Kentucky Mountain News. Drug news. Available at: http://www.breathittonline.com/news/cod/drugs2.html. Accessed September 2, 2010.

13

Oral Health

Daniel W. McNeil, Richard J. Crout, and Mary L. Marazita

Oral health is a sentinel marker of overall health status. In Appalachia, it serves as a mirror reflecting health and well-being in the region. Whereas *dental health* involves a singular focus on dentition (teeth), *oral health* is a more comprehensive concept that includes the well-being of the oral cavity and areas of the head and neck, including aspects of function and appearance. Important health factors related to oral health but not typically considered part of dental health include diet, tobacco use, psychological functioning, pregnancy, cardiovascular disease, and head and neck cancer. Like other areas of health, oral health is not simply the absence of disease[1]; given the importance of the mouth in various consumptive and social arenas, oral health implies functioning that allows a high quality of life. Social aspects such as the smile and the facial structure are included in oral health, as is psychosocial development[2]; the enjoyment of foods that require biting and chewing, such as raw fruits and vegetables; and ongoing self-care behaviors that prevent disease, such as toothbrushing and flossing.

Stereotypical views of Appalachians include images of people with broken teeth, missing teeth resulting in gaping holes in the dentition, or completely absent teeth.[3] Although some scientific data support the extent of edentulism (toothlessness) in Appalachian states,[4] the understanding of the antecedents of and solutions to oral health problems is in its infancy. There is a growing public awareness of oral health problems in Appalachia, as evidenced by reports in the popular press, such as the comprehensive newspaper series "The State of Decay" in West Virginia.[5] In an attempt to transcend stereotypes about toothlessness and "fatalism," this chapter broadly examines oral health in Appalachia, presents findings from research conducted at the Center for Oral Health Research in Appalachia, and discusses research and policy needs to promote better oral health among Appalachians.

Oral Health and Disease

Many of the environmental and behavioral factors associated with oral health in Appalachia are observed in other rural areas as well. The determinants of oral health vary across the region, given that Appalachia spans thirteen states, each of which has its own policies, laws, and social and environmental influences. Among other factors, including psychosocial ones,[6] state laws governing dentistry and dental hygiene differ considerably, as does the public funding of dental services for low-income residents through Medicaid.

Although caries (cavities) is the most common chronic disease in childhood,[1] numerous other oral conditions are important to health status throughout life. Consideration of the complete range of diseases is beyond the scope of this chapter, but the most common disorders are addressed in terms of their relation to Appalachia.

Edentulism. Edentulism in the adult population is a major problem in the region. Adults in some parts of Appalachia (e.g., West Virginia and eastern Kentucky) have lost more teeth than their peers in other states,[4] and more West Virginians over age 65 have lost six or more teeth (66 percent) than their counterparts in any other state or jurisdiction. Complete tooth loss in West Virginia is the highest in the nation for those older than 65 (38 percent) and is twice the national average.[4]

Tooth loss may be considered the unfortunate end point of progressive oral disease so extreme that there is no proper foundation for the teeth. Tooth loss, however, may also occur through extraction due to caries so extensive that a tooth is no longer vital, or it may be caused by trauma related to accidents or injuries. In some population groups in Appalachia and elsewhere, extracting natural teeth is regarded as a viable health choice because of the belief that it will prevent future pain or other dental problems.[7] Although lore suggests that having a tooth extracted (or the complete absence of teeth) is preferable to keeping a tooth (or teeth), missing teeth actually set the stage for other oral problems. Historically, marital dowries were sometimes given to couples for full mouth extractions and the construction and fitting of upper and lower dentures.[8] Even today, patients at dental clinics sometimes choose extraction even when the natural tooth could be saved, or they request the extraction of other teeth near a diseased tooth. The idea is that once the mouth is numbed, nearby teeth should be removed for practicality's sake, given the expectation that all of one's teeth will ultimately be extracted. There are also socioeconomic antecedents and implications, in that extraction is typically less expensive and fear-inducing than other treatments such as root canal therapy.[9] Although Appalachians (like people elsewhere) view the loss of teeth, particularly visible ones, negatively, missing dentition may be an unfortunate consequence of economic and social circumstances. Attention to oral health may be superseded by more pressing financial needs for food, transportation, and other health care, among other necessities.[7]

Loss of permanent teeth can negatively affect not just appearance but also oral health. Teeth adjacent to the open space become mobile, allowing food to be trapped and affecting how the teeth fit together. The lack of natural teeth affects nutrition and, ultimately, weight and cholesterol levels, as fresh fruits and vegetables may be less likely dietary choices. Joshipura and colleagues[10] observed a significantly lower intake of vegetables, fiber, and carotenoids and a higher intake of cholesterol and saturated fat in a cohort of edentulous men compared with a control sample of men with twenty-five or more teeth. Hung and associates[11] longitudinally evaluated men aged forty to seventy-five from 1986 to 1994. The loss of five or more teeth in this cohort was associated with a less healthy diet. Any tooth loss was associated with the consumption of fewer apples, pears, and raw carrots. These findings have strong implications for the overall health of Appalachians, given the high prevalence of tooth loss in some areas.[4]

Periodontal Disease. One of the primary causes of tooth loss is periodontal disease, which affects the gingivae (gums). Periodontal conditions range from gum inflammation (gingivitis) to serious pathology resulting in major damage to the soft tissue and bones (upper and lower jawbones) that support the teeth. The more severe type, periodontitis, is the presence of gingival inflammation at sites where the connective tissue fibers have become detached from the outside covering of the root. Periodontal disease can be a precursor to tooth loss because, with compromised gingivae, there is no proper foundation for the tooth. Infection and inflammation also lead to the loss of tooth-supporting bone.[12] In advanced cases, teeth are lost. Moreover, evidence has linked periodontal disease to heart attack, stroke, diabetes, hypertension, adverse pregnancy outcome,[13–15] and cognitive dysfunction.[16] Many of these health problems are known to occur more frequently in Appalachia than elsewhere.[17]

Periodontal disease leading to tooth loss has a number of possible antecedents, primarily related to lifestyle. The factors associated with an increased risk for periodontitis and more severe disease are poor oral hygiene, tobacco use, type 1 and type 2 diabetes, stress, depression, poor nutrition, obesity, and physical inactivity.[18] Many of these issues affect Appalachian populations. Use of tobacco—either smoking or using smokeless products—imparts a greater risk for periodontal disease. Individuals who smoke cigarettes and pipes have a much greater loss of supporting bone than nonsmokers in international studies.[19–21] In addition, periodontal disease is more severe and more prevalent in patients with both type 1 and type 2 diabetes mellitus.[22] This issue is a critical one, given that type 2 diabetes is more prevalent in Appalachia than in other parts of the United States.[23] Patients with type 2 diabetes and periodontitis have a faster rate of supporting bone loss than those without diabetes.[24]

Poor oral hygiene is also closely associated with periodontal disease. Some forms of periodontal disease, however, appear to be biologically determined, related to genetic predisposition or other diseases. Certain oral pathogens are part of a causative chain that can lead to periodontal disease, recession of the gums, and bone loss, but the broader question is how these pathogens became colonized and grow. Possible explanations include poor oral hygiene, insult to the tissues from tobacco use, genetic predisposition, or other factors.

Caries. Along with tooth loss, caries accounts for most of the public's focus on oral health. Caries is an infectious disease that can affect both the primary dentition ("baby teeth") and the permanent dentition; it can occur at any time during the life span, although it typically begins in childhood.[25] Caries is the most common chronic childhood disease, being five times more prevalent than asthma and seven times more prevalent than hay fever.[1] Yet it is underrecognized in terms of its health and psychosocial impact. The 2000 surgeon general's report on oral health indicated that 80 percent of caries in the United States was found in 20 percent of the population, with ethnic and racial groups at increased risk.[1] Historically[26] and currently, residents of Appalachia are more affected by caries and other oral diseases than many other groups in the nation. Within Appalachia, particular parts of the region or specific population groups may be especially affected by caries.

Toothbrushing, flossing, and other oral hygiene behaviors are associated with the prevention of caries. Social factors can either predispose individuals to caries or protect them from caries and other oral diseases. Poor and disadvantaged groups are disproportionately affected by caries, and contributing factors include fluoride use and diet.[25] Risk for caries can be conceptualized in three domains: the social arena, the oral environment, and microbiological factors.[27] The social arena includes socioeconomic status, education, and income, all of which are known to be lower in portions of Appalachia than elsewhere in the country.[28]

Historically, the fluoridation of public water supplies heralded a tremendous decrease in caries nationally and internationally. In Appalachia, however, large numbers of residents depend on private water supplies such as wells and cisterns.[29] Although it is possible to use fluoride supplements in private water supplies, doing so represents an additional time and cost burden, making it less likely to occur. Water quality from private water supplies is also an issue in some parts of Appalachia because wells and other sources may be contaminated with pollutants due to the lack of sanitary sewage disposal, mountaintop removal and other mining, and various industrial activities. Bottled water can be used, but most brands either are not fluoridated or contain insufficient fluoride levels to provide a health benefit.[30] Although bottled water with added fluoride is sold, its availability in all areas is uncertain; using it also demands extra time in identification and selection and likely entails extra cost.

Diet has a major impact on caries. Liquids and other foods that are high in sugar predispose one to caries. Consumption of soft drinks and other sugary beverages and foods is implicated in dental erosion—the acidic etching away of enamel and dentine.[31] Dietary practices in Appalachia are likely factors in the region's elevated rate of caries.[32] For example, a high rate of soft drink consumption, particularly Mountain Dew, among young people has been implicated as a dietary and behavioral factor associated with rampant caries.[33, 34] National media attention was focused on this issue when ABC's *20/20* reported on Mountain Dew usage among youths in eastern Kentucky.[35] In addition to sociocultural factors, giving soft drinks or juice drinks to young children may be a function of poor water quality or the unavailability of clean drinking water.

Oral Cancers. The prevalence of oral cancers is higher than the national average in half the Appalachian states, with greater associated mortality in ten of the thirteen states.[36] The high rate of tobacco use in Appalachia,[37] including "spit" or smokeless tobacco, suggests a greater propensity to develop oral cancers, although other factors, such as alcohol consumption, may interact with tobacco use to affect risk. Among those who use spit or smokeless tobacco, pouches can form between the gingivae and cheek tissue, providing a place for pathological changes to occur. There is an association between spit or smokeless tobacco use and the development of oral cancers, although data from West Virginia[38] revealed no increased incidence or mortality from such use. It was suggested, however, that the low rate of alcohol consumption in the state may be involved, as alcohol is known to interact synergistically with tobacco to produce ill effects.

There are a number of other biopsychosocial determinants of oral cancers. For example, ill-fitting dentures that produce oral sores are associated with an increased risk of developing oral cancers.[39] It is important for individuals with dentures to have periodic oral health exams,[39] but the rate of annual dental visits for adults in Appalachia is lower than the national average[4] and much lower than is typically recommended. Given the high rate of edentulism in Appalachia, one might presume a high rate of denture use, which could be associated with an increased risk for oral cancers. Such a conclusion would be speculative, however, although some data do exist on edentulism and denture use in Appalachia. In one sample of community-dwelling adults aged 73 to 95 in Appalachian Pennsylvania, 44.7 percent had full dentures, 28.9 percent had partial dentures, and 26.4 percent had no dentures; some of those in the last group were dentate, and others were edentulous but without dentures.[40] A study of adults aged 65 and older in Kentucky found that nearly half (46.7 percent) were edentulous, and 89.5 percent of those individuals had dentures.[41] Of the elders considered dentate, about half (51.5 percent) had some sort of prosthetic aid for missing dentition (e.g., fixed or removable partial dentures).

Other Oral Conditions and Diseases. In addition to periodontitis, caries, and oral cancers, there are numerous other oral conditions that may be affected by environmental and behavioral factors in Appalachia. Drug use has become a critical element affecting oral health in Appalachia. In particular, methamphetamine (meth) production and use have greatly increased in rural parts of the United States since the 1990s.[42] Small communities and rural areas such as those found in Appalachia have been particularly affected.[43] The use of methamphetamine is associated with a constellation of oral health problems referred to as "meth mouth,"[44] including dry mouth (xerostomia),[45] rampant decay (caries), and grinding of the teeth (bruxism). Methamphetamine stimulates the central nervous system and results in physical overactivity and hyperthermia, which leads to excessive perspiration, reduced salivary flow, and, ultimately, a sensation of dryness.[46] Rather than drinking water, methamphetamine users often crave sugar and typically drink large quantities of nondiet soft drinks.[47] Without the protective buffering effects of saliva, caries is often widespread in methamphetamine users.[45] Methamphetamine use also increases motor activity, inducing excessive chewing, grinding, or clenching, which contributes to the destruction of already compromised dentition.[48] As such, dentists, dental hygienists, and dental assistants may be the first health professionals to interact with a methamphetamine abuser due to the pain and oral dysfunction associated with meth mouth.

In a comprehensive view, oral health can affect and be affected by a variety of lifestyle issues, health behaviors, and diseases. Tobacco is an important factor in Appalachia, both as a harmful substance and as an agricultural and economic force.[49] Given that the rate of tobacco use is higher in at least some parts of the region[37] than in the general U.S. population, there are implications for the incidence of various forms of cancer, including but not limited to oral cancer. Diet, nutrition, and food availability (food insecurity) are concerns in many places in Appalachia,[50] and they broadly affect a variety of health aspects, including prenatal development. The condition of the teeth, gums, and oral cavity affects one's food choices and one's quality of life.[11] Diet and nutrition, in turn, have implications for obesity, which is prevalent among youth in parts of Appalachia.[23] Type 2 diabetes is also widespread in parts of the region, and dietary factors are key to both its prevention and its management.[23] Oral health is associated with systemic health issues as well. For instance, maternal periodontal status has been related to premature birth and low birth weight[13]; periodontal disease has been linked to cardiovascular disease and stroke.[14] To the extent that Appalachia or parts of it have higher rates of periodontal disease, this may be related to a greater prevalence of negative birth outcomes,[51] cardiovascular disease, and stroke, all of which may be connected with other factors such as smoking and socioeconomic status.

Oral Self-Care and Professional Dental Services

Preventive oral health behaviors, such as brushing, flossing, and regular dental visits, are affected by myriad factors, including the social environment (e.g., the expectation that one's visible dentition is complete, structurally intact, and without obvious discoloration), the physical environment (e.g., the number of bathrooms in a home and the availability of toothbrushes and sinks), prosperity and well-being, the health care system, and even genetic endowment. Generational issues abound in Appalachia; self-care behaviors are transmitted, in part, within families, as are perceptions of dental care and reactions to it (e.g., fear[52]) and health-seeking behaviors such as keeping dental appointments.

Access to and utilization of dental care are related to the number and distribution of oral health care professionals (e.g., dentists, dental hygienists) in a community, state, or region; the patient loads of these professionals; costs and other financial aspects; availability of transportation; public policy; and psychosocial variables such as socioeconomic status and oral health values.[7] With approximately 60 percent of the counties in the region considered dental health professional shortage areas, the dental workforce is an important issue in Appalachia.[53] Dental practices are unevenly distributed, massed in urban and suburban areas. Data from Ohio indicate that the dentist-to-population ratio in Appalachian Ohio is one-half that in the state's more urban counties.[54]

Public policy about dental care in large part determines access to dental care and profoundly affects utilization. Policies enacted by governments and positions taken by dental professional groups (sometimes in opposition to each other) impact the oral health of the population, for better or worse. For example, in West Virginia, dental hygienists were historically allowed to practice only under the direct supervision of a dentist who was physically present at the office location. This policy contributed to more restricted access and higher costs, but the counterargument was that quality of care demanded direct supervision by dentists. This policy has been changing in West Virginia and across many other states. Now, some services can be offered by hygienists under the "general supervision" of a dentist—that is, the dentist need not be physically present at the hygienist's practice location. As of February 2011, only three of the thirteen Appalachian states still required direct supervision of all dental hygienists' activities.[55]

Public policy has also attempted to meet the oral health needs of children, with variable and less than ideal results. Although Medicaid and the Children's Health Insurance Program provide funding for dental services, availability varies across states. In addition, reimbursement rates for dentists are limited, making the provision of such care less inviting economically, and sometimes even producing a net loss for a dental practice after overhead costs are considered.[56]

There is, nevertheless, a growing awareness of the need to promote oral health early in life, as evidenced by the creation of numerous school-based programs. Seal Kentucky, for example, provides dental services to eastern Kentucky primary schools through a mobile van; this program applies sealants to the children's teeth, as well as providing other dental preventive and treatment services.[57]

To help counteract the access problem, there have been numerous grassroots attempts to meet the immediate oral health needs of low-income individuals.[58] One example is Missions of Mercy through the America's Dentists Care Foundation,[59] which sponsors multiple-day events providing free dental care by volunteer dental professionals to the underserved in various communities across the country, including Appalachia. Though these efforts are laudable and certainly provide humanitarian aid to many people, such events (which are often inundated with large crowds, including many individuals with severe dental problems) address only a very small portion of the need. These individuals may obtain treatment and pain relief, but they still have no "dental home" and no access to ongoing preventive services.

Oral Health Research: Family-Based Cohort in North-Central and Northern Appalachia

The Center for Oral Health Research in Appalachia (COHRA) was established in 2000, with the University of Pittsburgh School of Dental Medicine as the coordinating center and West Virginia University as the organizational center. COHRA's aim is to document the status of oral health and diseases in Appalachia, as well as related biological, psychological, and social factors. COHRA has taken a multifactorial, developmental approach to the study of child-environment interactions that lead to the development of oral disease. Given the focus on children and their caregivers, COHRA's particular goal is to examine how families buffer or impart risk for oral disease among their children. For example, the high incidence of caries in early childhood has led to the study of pregnant women and their offspring in the first two years of life.

COHRA Methods and Findings. There is a lack of population-based data to establish the oral health status of the entire Appalachian region. To address the need for scientific information that transcends stereotypes and anecdotal reports, COHRA conducted a comprehensive family-based study of oral health in four counties in north-central and northern Appalachia. This resulted in the creation of a data source with approximately 650 household-based family groups, including approximately 3,000 individuals.[a]

The COHRA protocol[60] was designed to assess oral health in families or households with one or more children using a multilevel (child, family, community) framework. Included in the evaluation was a dental screening to identify the presence or absence of teeth, suspected caries, lesions that might be indicative of oral cancer, orthodontic status, and possible periodontal problems. Additionally, oral microbiological sampling was performed to assess for pathogens associated with caries and periodontal disease, as well as biological sampling of blood or saliva for eventual DNA extraction. Finally, there was a battery of self-report questionnaires and interviews on oral hygiene behaviors, other preventive health behaviors, dental fear, fear of pain, and health attitudes in general. Although not generalizable to all of Appalachia, the findings from this family-based sample can help guide communities and policy makers in setting goals, establishing priorities, and planning prevention efforts. Some of the findings from the COHRA project are presented here.

Heritability (i.e., the proportion of variability in the development of caries that is likely attributable to genetic factors) was estimated in COHRA families in the primary and permanent dentition and was found to be substantial, indicating the existence of underlying genes for different caries phenotypes.[61] DNA sequence variations, known as single nucleotide polymorphisms (SNPs), were assessed in candidate genes associated with caries. SNPs in the taste receptor pathways were associated with caries risk in the primary and mixed primary and permanent dentitions.[62]

Caries and tooth sealant use were analyzed among COHRA children in comparison to National Health and Nutrition Examination Survey (NHANES) norms.[63] Although the use of tooth sealants on selected permanent teeth in children aged 5 to 17 years exceeded the national rate (44.8 versus 18.5 percent), the rate of caries in the primary teeth of 2- to 10-year-olds and the rate of untreated caries in 6- to 18-year-olds were also higher (136 and 167 percent of the national rate, respectively). In younger children (aged 6 to 11 years), the overall rate of caries in the permanent teeth was 132 percent of the national rate. These findings raise a question: why is the rate of caries so high—particularly untreated caries and at such young ages—when the rate of sealant use is so high? Poor oral hygiene and dietary behaviors are possible explanations. These findings are both hopeful and disturbing. Sealant programs appear to be achieving some success, testimony to the work of social programs that help fund and promote such dental health behaviors. Nevertheless, the high rate of caries despite sealant use is a concern.

Periodontal disease indicative of periodontitis was found to be much greater in the adult COHRA sample (83.9 percent) than in the U.S. population.[64] In the latter, mild to moderate forms of periodontal disease affect 30 to 50 percent of adults, and the severe generalized form affects 5 to 15 percent.[65]

In a preliminary COHRA study of the occlusal (orthodontic) status of parents and their adolescent children,[66] parents had a high rate of full or partial toothlessness, very little history of orthodontic care, a great unmet need for orthodontic care, and less demand for orthodontic care than would be suggested by clinically determined need. Among the adolescents, however, their orthodontic histories and needs were similar to national norms, but with a lower demand for orthodontics. This finding is a concern, given that it may indicate less focus on oral health later in life. The oral health status of the parents suggested that they were considerably worse off than their children and in comparison to national population-based statistics. This finding is consistent with reports from many adults in the COHRA project who indicated that their children's dental care was a high priority, given their own oral health problems and negative dental experiences, which were often related to symptomatic care focused on pain relief.

In a COHRA study assessing dental fear and anxiety in parents and children,[52] parents' dental fear, including avoidant behavior and fear of pain, were positively correlated with dental fear in their children. The possibility of intergenerational transmission of dental fear was suggested in this Appalachian sample, as parents' fears about pain and dentistry, as well as their avoidant behaviors, were associated with their children's dental fear.

Implications of the COHRA Data. So far, the COHRA findings suggest that Appalachians develop caries very early in life, experience dental fear that may be transmitted intergenerationally, have a lower demand for orthodontic care, and, in spite of a high rate of sealant use, have a much higher rate of untreated caries than the national norm. These findings prompt questions regarding maternal oral health during and after pregnancy and its relation to the oral health of the child. These findings also raise several concerns. First, the apparently high rate of periodontal disease in adults may be a step along the road to tooth loss. Second, the lower demand for orthodontics among adolescents in the COHRA cohort relative to national norms may relate to other oral health values and future behaviors. Third, the likely intergenerational transmission of dental fear suggests that the oral health status of parents and their oral health behaviors, values, beliefs, and attitudes are important influences on the oral health of Appalachian children throughout their lifetimes. Finally, the genetic results, though not exclusive to Appalachia, indicate how research about oral health in the region may inform research, practice, and policy outside of Appalachia.

Oral health is a complex interplay of individual behavior rooted in family and broader social influences. Psychological states such as dental fear, beliefs, attitudes, and values; topography and other geographic variables; economics; and public policy are also prominent factors. Although access to professional oral health care is a frequently cited problem and is a valid concern for many consumers, resolving access problems alone is unlikely to turn the tide in addressing the oral health problems in Appalachia. Failure to utilize available services before experiencing symptoms that require more expensive care is a concern; this issue is evident in the lack of enrollment and follow-through in social services programs for children.[67] Other parts of the world that provide greater public funding for comprehensive dental care still have problems with a lack of voluntary utilization of the dental health care system.[68] Influencing oral health values, attitudes, and beliefs among consumers and in public and private institutions may be the greatest challenge, but doing so may ultimately improve oral health in Appalachia.[69] The often invoked concept of "fatalism" is a simplistic, offhand way of associating oral and other health problems with behaviors, beliefs, attitudes, and energy at the individual level. This conceptualization masks the broader influences in Appalachia, which are complex, multilayered, and interactive.

Further Research

There is a dearth of empirical data delineating the scope and extent of oral health problems in Appalachia. Available indicators suggest that oral health problems, like general health issues, are considerable and represent a health disparity that places a disproportionate burden on Appalachians. Nevertheless, broad-based empirical data are needed, including a focus on states and localities in the region.

A population-based, comprehensive study of oral health in Appalachia is needed to provide a benchmark for future efforts. Work should not be confined to state boundaries, because there are many similarities among parts of states (e.g., areas within West Virginia and Kentucky).

Although some adult data are available on a state-by-state basis,[4] biennial assessments of representative portions of the Appalachian population should be implemented, perhaps through telephone surveys, to assess oral self-care behaviors, dental visits, perceived oral health status, and oral health quality. In addition, methods to positively impact individual behaviors, such as increasing the rate and effectiveness of toothbrushing and flossing, should be investigated in a broad-based fashion, including a view of longitudinal changes across developmental stages in life.

Health promotion interventions to address oral health problems in

Appalachia should be sensitive to local conditions and subjected to trials in representative areas of the region before implementing them more broadly.

Genome-wide approaches are necessary to fully understand the genetic etiologies of oral health disparities in Appalachia and, by extension, in similar populations.

Policy Recommendations

Public policy about dental care in large part determines access to such care and profoundly affects utilization in Appalachia and elsewhere. These policies (e.g., Medicaid funding of extractions but not preventive services) often do not support the best oral health practices. As such, more nuanced and contingency-based policies are needed if the oral health of Appalachians is to improve.

Residents of Appalachia, particularly consumers, should be integral partners in—even drivers of—oral health research and health promotion efforts. Work must be community driven—by Appalachian people, for Appalachian people.[70]

Funding should be allocated not only to meet the immediate restorative dental treatment needs of the population but also to invest in research. Greater funding of and focus on prevention activities should be the emphasis. Inculcating preventive behaviors in children and adolescents is vital, but this must be followed through at least into early adulthood.

Oral health should be a concern not only of dental health professionals but also of physical and mental health professionals. Preventive oral health care (e.g., sealants) should be in the purview of a variety of health professionals who are well trained to offer these services in concert with other health care (e.g., primary care visits).

Novel ways to provide and fund oral health services for low- and middle-income consumers should be explored, as well as methods of rewarding consumers for engaging in preventive behaviors such as regular toothbrushing and flossing. Due to the links between periodontal disease and pregnancy outcome, diabetes, hypertension, heart attack, stroke, and cognitive function, reducing health care costs for the treatment of these comorbid conditions may help offset the costs of such programs.

A public-private infrastructure should be developed—perhaps one for each state, with a regional superstructure—to initiate and support ongoing efforts to improve oral health. One possible model comes from West Virginia, which recently promulgated a statewide oral health plan for 2010–2015.[71]

Acknowledgments

The authors express their appreciation to the families participating in the COHRA project, as well as to Hilda Heady, Robert Blake, Bill Moughamer, Linda Brown, Stella Chapman, Dr. Leroy Utt, the late Kim Clayton, the collaborating health centers and hospitals, the GORGE Connection Rural Health Board, the Rural Health Education Partnerships program in West Virginia, and the Anxiety, Psychophysiology, and Pain Research Laboratory at West Virginia University. Preparation of this chapter was supported in part by grants (R01 DE014899) from the National Institutes of Health/ National Institute of Dental and Craniofacial Research (Marazita) and by a Fulbright senior scholar fellowship (McNeil).

Note

a. COHRA first operated in concert with the Webster-Nicholas Rural Health Education Partnerships (RHEP) program in West Virginia, which later evolved into the GORGE Connection RHEP.

References

1. U.S. Department of Health and Human Services. Oral health in America: a report of the surgeon general. Rockville, MD: U.S. Department of Health and Human Services, National Institute of Dental and Craniofacial Research, National Institutes of Health; 2000.

2. Lauren S. *A Covered Smile: A True Story.* Richmond, VA: Brandylane Publishers; 2003.

3. Garreau J. A moment of tooth: advances to regrow decaying choppers offer more to chew on than you'd think. *Washington Post,* January 4, 2009.

4. Centers for Disease Control and Prevention. Behavioral Risk Factor Surveillance System survey data. Atlanta, GA: U.S. Department of Health and Human Services; 2008.

5. Eyre E. The state of decay. Four-part series. *Charleston Gazette,* April 29, 2007. Available at: http://www.oralhealthwv.org/newsarticles/cg042907.htm. Accessed June 1, 2010.

6. Heaton LJ, Smith TA, Raybould TP. Factors influencing use of dental

services in rural and urban communities: considerations for practitioners in underserved areas. *J Dent Educ.* 2004;68:1081–1089.

7. McNeil DW, Crout RJ, Lawrence SM, Shah P, Rupert N. Oral health values in Appalachia: specific dental-related fatalism? *J Dent Res (Abst).* 2004;83:A-203.

8. McCord JF, Grant AA, Youngson CC, Watson RM, Davis DM. *Missing Teeth: A Guide to Treatment Options.* Edinburgh: Churchill Livingstone; 2003.

9. Sorrell JT, McNeil DW, Gochenour LL, Jackson CR. Evidence-based patient education: knowledge transfer to endodontic patients. *J Dent Educ.* 2009; 73:1293–1305.

10. Joshipura KJ, Willett WC, Douglass CW. The impact of edentulousness on food and nutrient intake. *J Am Dent Assoc.* 1996;127:459–467.

11. Hung HC, Willett W, Ascherio A, Rosner BA, Rimm E, Joshipura KJ. Tooth loss and dietary intake. *J Am Dent Assoc.* 2003;134:1185–1192.

12. Jeffcoat MK. Bone loss in the oral cavity. *J Bone Miner Res.* 1993;8 (Suppl):S467–S473.

13. Bobetsis YA, Barros SP, Offenbacker S. Exploring the relationship between periodontal disease and pregnancy complications. *J Am Dent Assoc.* 2006; 137(Suppl):7S–13S.

14. Demmer RT, Desvarieux M. Periodontal infections and cardiovascular disease: the heart of the matter. *J Am Dent Assoc.* 2006;137(Suppl):14S–20S.

15. Genco RJ. Clinical innovations in managing inflammation and periodontal diseases: the workshop on inflammation and periodontal diseases. *J Periodontol.* 2008;79:1609–1611.

16. Wu B, Plassman BL, Crout RJ, Liang J. Cognitive function and oral health among community-dwelling older adults. *J Gerontol A Biol Sci Med Sci.* 2008; 63:495–500.

17. Halverson JA, Ma L, Harner EJ. An analysis of disparities in health status and access to health care in the Appalachian region. Washington, DC: Appalachian Regional Commission; 2004.

18. Friedewald VE, Kornman KS, Beck JD, Genco R, Goldfine A, Libby P, Offenbacher S, Ridker PM, Van Dyke TE, Roberts WC. The *American Journal of Cardiology* and *Journal of Periodontology* editors' consensus: periodontitis and atherosclerotic cardiovascular disease. *J Periodontol.* 2009;80:1021–1032.

19. Bergstrom J, Preber H. Tobacco use as a risk factor. *J Periodontol.* 1994;65:545–550.

20. Grossi SG, Genco RJ, Machtei EE, Ho AW, Koch G, Dunford R, Zambon JJ, Hausmann E. Assessment of risk for periodontal disease. II. Risk indicators for alveolar bone loss. *J Periodontol.* 1995;66:23–29.

21. Tomar SL, Asma S. Smoking-attributable periodontitis in the United States: findings from NHANES III. National Health and Nutrition Examination Survey. *J Periodontol.* 2000;71:743–751.

22. Taylor GW, Borgnakke WS. Periodontal disease: associations with diabetes, glycemic control and complications. *Oral Dis.* 2008;14:191–203.

23. Centers for Disease Control and Prevention. Estimated county-level prevalence of diabetes and obesity—United States, 2007. *MMWR Morb Mortal Wkly Rep.* 2009;58:1259–1263.

24. Taylor GW, Burt BA, Becker MP, Genco RJ, Shlossman M, Knowler WC, Pettitt DJ. Non-insulin dependent diabetes mellitus and alveolar bone loss progression over 2 years. *J Periodontol.* 1998;69:76–83.

25. Edelstein BL. The dental caries pandemic and disparities problem. *BMC Oral Health.* 2006;6(Suppl 1):S2.

26. Wilson JH. Report about the status of dental health—West Virginia. *WV Dent J.* 1985;59:20–21.

27. Selwitz RH, Ismail AI, Pitts NB. Dental caries. *Lancet.* 2007;369:51–59.

28. Thorne D, Tickamyer A, Thorne M. Poverty and income in Appalachia. *Journal of Appalachian Studies.* 2005;10:341–357.

29. Hughes J, Whisnant R, Weller L, Eskaf S, Richardson M, Morrissey S, Altz-Stamm B. Drinking water and wastewater infrastructure in Appalachia: an analysis of capital funding and funding gaps. Washington, DC: Appalachian Regional Commission; 2005.

30. Lalumandier JA, Ayers LW. Fluoride and bacterial content of bottled water vs tap water. *Arch Fam Med.* 2000;9:246–250.

31. Moynihan PJ. The role of diet and nutrition in the etiology and prevention of oral diseases. *Bull World Health Organ* [online]. 2005;83:694–699.

32. Wu T, Stoots JM, Florence JE, Floyd MR, Snider JB, Ward RD. Eating habits among adolescents in rural southern Appalachia. *J Adolesc Health.* 2007;40:577–580.

33. Harris PN. Undoing the damage of the Dew. *Appalachian Journal of Law.* 2009;9:53.

34. Mendenhall D. What do you Dew! Dentists sounding the alarm about heavy soft-drink consumption among teens. *Post-Gazette,* September 4, 2001.

35. Sawyer D. A hidden America: children of the mountains. ABC News, *20/20,* February 13, 2009.

36. Casto BC, Sharma S, Fisher JL, Knobloch TJ, Agrawal A, Weghorst CM. Oral cancer in Appalachia. *J Health Care Poor Underserved.* 2009;20:274–285.

37. Wewers ME, Ahijevych KL, Chen MS, Dresbach S, Kihm KE, Kuun PA. Tobacco use characteristics among rural Ohio Appalachians. *J Community Health.* 2000;25:377–388.

38. Bouquot JE, Meckstroth RL. Oral cancer in a tobacco-chewing U.S. population—no apparent increased incidence or mortality. *Oral Surg Oral Med Oral Pathol Oral Radiol Endod.* 1998;86:697–706.

39. Velly AM, Franco EL, Schlecht N, Pintos J, Kowalski LP, Oliveira BV, Curado

MP. Relationship between dental factors and risk of upper aerodigestive tract cancer. *Oral Oncol.* 1998;34:284–291.

40. Weyant RJ, Pandav RS, Plowman JL, Ganguli M. Medical and cognitive correlates of denture wearing in older community-dwelling adults. *J Am Geriatr Soc.* 2004;52:596–600.

41. Bush HM, Dickens NE, Henry RG, Durham L, Sallee N, Skelton J, Stein PS, Cecil JC. Oral health status of older adults in Kentucky: results from the Kentucky elder oral health survey. *Spec Care Dentist.* 2010;30:185–192.

42. Booth BM, Leukefeld C, Falck R, Wang J, Carlson R. Correlates of rural methamphetamine and cocaine users: results from a multistate community study. *J Stud Alcohol.* 2006;67:493–501.

43. National Center on Addiction and Substance Abuse. No place to hide: substance abuse in mid-size cities and rural America. New York, NY: National Center on Addiction and Substance Abuse; 2000. Available at: http://www.casacolumbia .org/Absolutenm/articlefiles/No_Place_to_Hide_1_28_00.pdf. Accessed February 10, 2008.

44. Goodchild JH, Donaldson M, Mangini DJ. Methamphetamine abuse and the impact on dental health. *Dent Today.* 2007;26:124, 126, 128–131.

45. Goodchild JH, Donaldson M. Methamphetamine abuse and dentistry: a review of the literature and presentation of a clinical case. *Quintessence Int.* 2007;38:583–590.

46. Saini T, Edwards PC, Kimmes NS, Carroll LR, Shaner JW, Dowd FJ. Etiology of xerostomia and dental caries among methamphetamine abusers. *Oral Health Prev Dent.* 2005;3:189–195.

47. Jones KD. Viewpoint: spotting meth mouth. Available at: http://www.ada .org/prof/resources/pubs/adanews/adanewsarticle.asp?articleid=1517. Accessed February 10, 2008.

48. McGrath C, Chan B. Oral health sensations associated with illicit drug abuse. *Br Dent J.* 2005;198:159–162.

49. Behringer G, Friedell GH. Appalachia: where place matters in health. *Prev Chronic Dis.* 2006;3:A113.

50. Holben DH, Pheley AM. Diabetes risk and obesity in food-insecure households in rural Appalachian Ohio. *Prev Chronic Dis.* 2006;3:A82.

51. Bailey BA, Cole LKJ. Rurality and birth outcomes: findings from southern Appalachia and the potential role of pregnancy smoking. *J Rural Health.* 2009;25:141–149.

52. Davis B, McNeil DW, Crout RJ, Cohen LL, Casto GT, Weyant RJ. Fear of pain relates to patient comfort, satisfaction, and desire for information among Appalachia youth and their parents. *J Dent Res (Abst).* 2002;81:A-269.

53. Health Resources and Services Administration. Shortage designation: HPSAs, MUAs and MUPs. Available at: http://bhpr.hrsa.gov/shortage/. Accessed February 28, 2011.

54. Susi L, Mascarenhas AK. Using a geographical information system to map the distribution of dentists in Ohio. *J Am Dent Assoc.* 2002;133:636–642.

55. American Dental Hygienists' Association. Dental hygienist practice act overview: permitted functions and supervision levels by state. Available at: http://www.adha.org/. Accessed February 28, 2011.

56. Higgins S. Medicaid recipients search for dental care. West Virginia Public Broadcasting, October 18, 2009. Available at: http://www.wvpubcast.org/newsarticle .aspx?id=11696. Accessed June 1, 2010.

57. University of Kentucky. Seal Kentucky and East Kentucky Mobile Dental Program. Available at: http://www.mc.uky.edu/dentistry/service/outreach.html. Accessed February 28, 2011.

58. Sonja Lauren Foundation. Available at: http://www.sonjalaurenfoundation .org/. Accessed September 2, 2010.

59. America's Dentists Care Foundation, Missions of Mercy. Available at: http://www.adcfmom.org/. Accessed September 23, 2011.

60. Polk DE, Weyant RJ, Crout RJ, et al. Study protocol of the Center for Oral Health Research in Appalachia (COHRA) etiology study. *BioMed Centra, Oral Health.* 2008;8:18.

61. Wang X, Shaffer JR, Weyant RJ, et al. Genes and their effects on dental caries may differ between primary and permanent dentitions. *Caries Res.* 2010; 44:277–284.

62. Wendell S, Wang X, Brown M, et al. Taste genes associated with dental caries. *J Dent Res.* 2010,89:1198–1202.

63. Polk DE, Weyant RJ, Crout RJ, et al. What is the dental caries experience of children in northern Appalachia? University of Pittsburgh; 2008.

64. Crout R, McNeil DW, Thomas J, Weyant R, Marazita M. Oral health disparities in rural Appalachian families. Poster presentation. Nashville, TN: National Primary Oral Health meeting; November 2009.

65. Research, Science and Therapy Committee of the American Academy of Periodontology. Position paper: epidemiology of periodontal diseases. *J Periodontol.* 2005;76:1406–1419.

66. Martin CA, McNeil DW, Crout RJ, Ngan PW, Weyant RJ, Heady HR, Marazita ML. Oral health disparities in Appalachia: orthodontic treatment need and demand. *J Am Dent Assoc.* 2008;139:598–604.

67. Pew Center on the States. The cost of delay: state dental policies fail 1 in 5 children. Washington, DC: Pew Charitable Trusts; 2010.

68. Skaret E, Raadal M, Berg E, Kvale G. Dental anxiety and dental avoidance among 12 to 18 year olds in Norway. *Eur J Oral Sci.* 1999;107:422–428.

69. Coyne CA, Demian-Popescu C, Friend D. Social and cultural factors influencing health in southern West Virginia: a qualitative study. *Prev Chronic Dis.* 2006;3:A124.

70. Cram F, Smith L, Johnstone W. Mapping the themes of Maori talk about health. *NZ Med J.* 2003;116:1170.

71. Oral Health Advisory Committee. West Virginia's oral health plan 2010–2015: addressing the crisis of oral health in West Virginia. Charleston, WV: West Virginia Department of Health and Human Resources; 2010.

Part III

Urban Appalachian Health

There is little information about the health of the millions of Appalachians who have migrated to urban areas outside the region. Many of these migrants and their descendants may be experiencing health disparities similar to those of their counterparts in the region. Given the genetic, social, and socioeconomic similarities between the migrant and nonmigrant populations, a greater understanding of Appalachian health can be had by examining what is known about the health of all Appalachians, regardless of their geographic location.

This part presents techniques for identifying Appalachians who reside outside the region, a task that becomes more complicated after the first and second generations of migrants. Of particular interest is an analysis of the health status of Appalachians in the Greater Cincinnati area, which may serve as a reference point for studying similar health issues among migrant families in other metropolitan areas. The concluding chapter discusses the techniques and outcomes of community-based participatory research projects focused on the health status of women and children in an urban Appalachian neighborhood.

14

Identifying Appalachians Outside the Region

Robert L. Ludke, Phillip J. Obermiller,
Eric W. Rademacher, and Shiloh K. Turner

Since the time of the Great Migration, when millions of Appalachians moved to urban centers outside the Appalachian region, questions have been raised about the status of those migrants and their descendants. How are these people faring in the cities? How do they compare with other urban groups on key social indicators? Do they show signs of economic and social assimilation? What are their social, economic, educational, and health needs, if any, and what programs and services might be required to meet those needs?

It has been difficult to answer these questions definitively, in large part because urban Appalachians are an "invisible minority." That is, there is no broadly accepted definition of who is an Appalachian and who is not. This issue is central to understanding and addressing the health and well-being of Appalachians residing outside of as well as within Appalachia. Health professionals interested in providing effective and efficient health care services that meet specific Appalachian needs must be able to identify this population to do so. Identifying clusters of Appalachians in larger populations is key to conducting health needs assessments, designing suitable intervention programs, training practitioners, attracting Appalachian patients, devising patient education methods, and evaluating service outcomes.

This chapter explores the practical aspects of Appalachian identity, discusses various approaches used to identify persons of Appalachian heritage, and illustrates the difficulty of selecting a best method for identifying

Appalachians. It also examines the consequences of applying these different approaches by analyzing the concordance among them and using them to describe the demographic characteristics and health status of urban Appalachians. The chapter concludes with a discussion of further research needs and policy recommendations.

Appalachian Identity

Not until the early twentieth century did place become a critical element of defining human populations in modern social theory. The growing awareness that social groups live in "communities defined territorially" led to an emphasis on an identity derived from location.[1] Thus, the idea of place joined that of culture in developing a contemporary notion of ethnicity, which, in many cases, lies at the heart of group and individual identity.[1]

Sociologists Richard Alba and Mitchell Chamblin have shown that "ethnic differentiation remains a prominent axis of social life" (p. 246).[2] In the areas of applied medical and health research in particular, race and ethnicity remain key constructs.[3] But the possibility of a group identity invites the question of how to elicit that identity. The cognitive aspects of ethnic identification have several components: the felt significance of group membership, the various labels by which members identify themselves to others, the group's reaction to various labels by which nonmembers identify group members, and the availability of alternative identities in the wider society. Hence, identity is not an either-or option referencing specific and exclusive cultural content but a multidimensional personal option exercised for a variety of reasons.[4] A person's identity is a shifting social construct rather than a fixed social determinant, which makes it particularly difficult to determine.

Place is an implicit part of the concept of Appalachia. Since the late 1800s, the region has been physically "placed" along varying historical, cultural, economic, and political lines.[5–9] Well over a century later, the region's boundaries remain quite fluid, and the same is true of Appalachian identity.

However, the question "Where is Appalachia?" is subtly different from the question "Who is Appalachian?" Latino immigrants in Pittsburgh's Shadyside neighborhood live in the Appalachian region. The grandchildren of eastern Kentucky coal miners who migrated to Detroit are now two generations or more removed from the coalfields. Both examples point to the subtleties involved in ascertaining Appalachian identity.[10]

The distinct nature of a mountain identity was explored by a two-year National Science Foundation–sponsored study conducted in western North Carolina.[11–13] Study participants expressed "a strong sense of cultural identity as mountain people" that persisted across social classes.[12] However, the participants also indicated a growing degree of ambiguity or cultural "disorientation" due to the rapid pace of social change in the mountains.[13]

The salience of Appalachian identity among the region's out-migrants, as well as its persistence among their offspring, has led some social scientists to entertain the possibility of ethnic group formation among urban Appalachians.[14–18] However, the migration experience may be contributing geographic "dislocation" to the social "disorientation" already felt by some rural Appalachians. A changing social environment as well as a change of place makes the task of determining urban Appalachian identity even more difficult. Yet Appalachian migrants and their descendants have been identified by researchers for well over half a century.

Identifying Appalachians: Three Standard Techniques

In every case, the operational issue is how to identify people of Appalachian heritage who live in urban areas both inside and outside the region. To date, three broad methodological strategies have emerged: place-based, self-identification, and attribute-based. Each has its advantages and disadvantages, which makes it difficult to arrive at a single definitional approach.

Place-Based Approach. The place-based strategy is straightforward and consistent with the common definition of an Appalachian: if a person has roots in the federally defined region, the person is considered an Appalachian. Several methods have been used to operationalize the concept of having roots in Appalachia. One is direct inquiry—that is, asking a person whether he or she was born in a designated Appalachian county (first-generation Appalachian), has at least one parent born in a designated county (second generation), has grandparents born in a designated county (third generation), and so forth.[14] A less frequently used alternative is to examine public records, such as birth and marriage certificates, or genealogical records, such as family Bibles or other documents, and relate them to states and counties of origin.[19]

The inherent strength of this place-based technique is that people generally know where they were born and often where their parents and even their grandparents were born.[a] Its weakness involves the fundamental issue of determining what constitutes the Appalachian region. Moreover, as noted earlier, not everyone born in Appalachia—however it is defined—is of Appalachian heritage. There are also limitations when identifying multigenerational descendants of Appalachian migrants whose family roots may be in Appalachia but who are no longer associated by birth to Appalachia—for example, fourth-generation migrants who were born and reside in non-Appalachian cities such as Cincinnati, Chicago, or Detroit.

Large national data sets are available to track Appalachian migrants using a place-based methodology. Gross migration data compiled by the Bureau of the Census from Internal Revenue Service (IRS) sample files allow county-to-county tracking of tax return filers by Social Security number.[20] Public Use Microdata Samples (PUMS) have also been employed to document historical migration flows into and out of Appalachia.[21, 22] The decennial census has, until recently, provided the best overview of not only Appalachian in- and out-migration but also the socioeconomic characteristics of the migrants.[23]

Again, there are drawbacks to these techniques. IRS data, though useful for tracking intercensal migration trends, are available only for tax return filers and do not include socioeconomic variables. PUMS data are based on samples and can have high probabilities of error, especially when applied to small areas. Census data are heavily reliant on how researchers specify the region. For instance, a nuclear physicist of East Indian origin transferring from the Oak Ridge National Laboratory near Knoxville, Tennessee, to the Fermi National Accelerator Laboratory near Chicago, Illinois, could be counted as an Appalachian migrant.

Another place-based method that is useful for research in local communities and neighborhoods assumes that if an individual lives in an identified urban Appalachian neighborhood, that person is very likely to be Appalachian. For example, in each of the past four decades, social planner Michael E. Maloney and his colleagues have published *The Social Areas of Cincinnati,* a report that identifies predominantly Appalachian neighborhoods based on selected census indicators such as race and poverty status, along with levels of employment and education.[24] Software for translating census tract data into readily recognizable neighborhood areas is available in many urban planning departments. This technique is often used when seeking opportunities to serve minorities in neighborhood settings. Its primary weakness is that not everyone who lives in a predominantly Appalachian neighborhood, however defined, is necessarily of Appalachian heritage. For example, Orthodox Jews in downtown Pittsburgh live in the designated Appalachian region, and recent Latino immigrants in Cincinnati's Lower Price Hill reside in a heavily Appalachian neighborhood, but few would maintain that either group is of Appalachian heritage. Although the danger of the ecological fallacy haunts all place-based research, this method of identifying Appalachians has proved reasonably reliable and useful when it is carefully employed.

For health studies, the place-based approach of identifying urban Appalachian migrants and their descendants by neighborhood allows the use of other techniques, such as overlaying postal ZIP codes onto known urban Appalachian enclaves. For example, patient ZIP code data are neither scarce nor sensitive, and they can readily be used to identify disease clusters or treatment needs in known Appalachian neighborhoods.[25] The environmental justice movement in Cincinnati has shown how health status is affected by proximity to sources of pollutants using the ZIP code–based toxic release inventory published by the Environmental Protection Agency. Although environmental pollution is spread over wide areas, living near a point source with a heavy toxic load has been associated with negative health outcomes for urban Appalachian children.[25] Small-area research also allows for community-based participatory research, a procedure that has proved effective in both urban and rural Appalachian settings (see chapter 16).[26–28]

Self-Identification Approach. A second major strategy for ascertaining Appalachian identity is simply to ask people whether they think of themselves as Appalachian.[29] Historians J. Trent Alexander and Chad Berry, for instance, used this strategy to examine self-reported Appalachian ancestry in the 2000 census.[30] An obvious strength of this approach is that it allows people to select their own social identities. Its major weakness is that persons of Appalachian heritage may choose not to be identified as such or may not want to be associated with the Appalachian region for a variety of reasons, the primary one being negative stereotyping.[31] Also, there is the issue of whether *Appalachian* is a concept that is recognizable by persons of

Appalachian heritage. In the words of Theresa Myadze, "some Appalachian migrants may not have a uniform understanding or acceptance of the term 'Appalachian'" (p. 185).[17] The way the respondent is asked and the vocabulary used to phrase the question are crucial to the effectiveness of this technique. In some cases, persons of Appalachian heritage may associate more strongly with the derogatory term *hillbilly,* as pointed out by John Hartigan Jr. in his study of migrants in Detroit.[32]

Attribute-Based Approach. The third major strategy for identifying Appalachians is to use cultural attributes. Over time, certain characteristics have become associated with Appalachians. For example, Jones[33] lists ten values common to Appalachians, including individualism, familism, love of place, neighborliness, and religion. Out of fear or ignorance, others have characterized Appalachians in negative terms such as uneducated, poor, lacking intelligence, and slovenly. Either way, the assumption is that persons who share the same characteristics or values are of the same heritage. This method makes intuitive sense, but the inherent weaknesses quickly become obvious. In addition to a lack of agreement regarding the specific attributes of Appalachians, the issue is confounded by different groups sharing identical cultural characteristics. For instance, characterizations such as individualistic, family oriented, place loving, neighborly, and religious may be equally apt for Appalachians in eastern Kentucky, Old Order Amish in Indiana, Swedish Americans in Minnesota, and Native Americans in New Mexico.

Selecting the Best Identification Method

Although several cognitive and place-based methodologies for identifying rural and urban Appalachian populations have been developed in the past forty years, evidence is lacking on which method is best for identifying Appalachians, particularly those who have migrated to urban areas and their descendants. The elusiveness of a single best method is illustrated by an empirical study conducted in the Cincinnati metropolitan area,[b] using health surveys to examine several different types of Appalachian identifiers.[34] The identifiers were based on the approaches described in the previous section and included the following questions:

1. "In what state were you born?" "In which county were you born?" These questions identified only first-generation Appalachians.[c]

2. "In what state was your father born?" "In what county was your father born?" "In what state was your mother born?" "In what county was your mother born?" These questions identified second-generation Appalachians.[d]

3. "Were you, or any of your people,[e] born in southeastern Ohio, eastern Kentucky, eastern Tennessee, or West Virginia?" The vast majority of post–World War II migrants to Greater Cincinnati came from these four areas of Appalachia. This family roots question overcame the difficulties of precisely identifying state and county of birth and identified Appalachians of any generation.

4. "Do you consider yourself to be Appalachian or of Appalachian ancestry?" This question allowed persons to self-identify as Appalachian.

Respondents were subsequently classified as Appalachian if they met the definition of either first- or second-generation Appalachian, had Appalachian family roots, and/or self-identified as Appalachian.

As illustrated in table 14.1, there was a lack of concordance across these questions in identifying persons of Appalachian heritage.[f] Some of the differences can reasonably be attributed to fourth and subsequent generations showing up in some questions and not others. Also, some respondents may have migrated from places other than the Appalachian portions

Table 14.1. Percentage Agreement among Identification Methods

Identifier Type	1st and 2nd Generation (Yes)	Self-Identified (Yes)	Family Roots (Yes)
1st and 2nd Generation			
Yes	—	40.4	55.6
No	—	9.0	24.6
Kappa	—	0.35	0.27
Self-identified			
Yes	56.8	—	60.7
No	16.2	—	26.0
Kappa	0.35	—	0.25
Family roots			
Yes	40.0	31.0	—
No	14.8	9.3	—
Kappa	0.27	0.25	—

Source: Greater Cincinnati Community Health Status Survey, 2005.

of the specified states. The fundamental finding persists, however: there was little or no overlap among the various cohorts identified as Appalachian. The term *Appalachian*, if understood and accepted, may consist of multiple identities, depending on the criteria used, and convergence to a single identity may be difficult if it is possible at all.

Lack of concordance among identifiers may have several pragmatic consequences. First, the estimated size of the Appalachian population may vary dramatically by the type of identifier. For example, the above study found that slightly less than 11 percent of the Cincinnati area population were first-generation Appalachian, based on respondents' state and county of birth (table 14.2); about 25 percent were determined to be first or second generation, based on their own or their parents' state and county of birth (11 percent first generation, and 14 percent second generation). Approximately 16 percent of the population self-identified as Appalachian, and 32 percent claimed Appalachian family roots in southeastern Ohio, eastern Kentucky, eastern Tennessee, or West Virginia. Based on all identifiers combined, about 47 percent of the population of Greater Cincinnati is estimated to be of Appalachian heritage.

Second, different identification methods may result in different demographic characterizations of the Appalachian population. For example, the above study found that the identifier of one's own county of birth (first generation) portrays an Appalachian population that tends to be older; have a lower income; be attending school or keeping house and not working full- or part-time; be widowed, divorced, separated, or never married; be living in smaller households; and be living in Greater Cincinnati's urban fringe (table 14.3). Self-identification tends to characterize the adult Appalachian population with a slightly different gender composition (i.e.,

Table 14.2. Estimated Number of Appalachians by Identification Method	
Identifier Type	**Number (%)**
State/county of birth (1st generation)	223 (10.7)
State/county of father's/mother's birth (1st or 2nd generation)	509 (24.5)
Self-identification	331 (16.0)
Family roots	671 (32.3)
Any type	970 (46.7)
Source: Greater Cincinnati Community Health Status Survey, 2005.	

Table 14.3. Demographic Characteristics of Respondents by Identification Method

Demographic Characteristic	1st Generation (%)	1st and 2nd Generation (%)	Self-Identified (%)	Family Roots (%)	Total (%)
Age (years)					
18–29	8.9	10.3	12.2	12.6	14.0
30–39	15.5	23.8	21.6	26.8	24.6
40–49	19.6	27.6	32.3	24.8	25.3
50–59	16.0	15.0	16.8	14.8	16.0
60–69	18.6	11.7	11.2	10.7	10.2
70+	20.5	11.2	5.2	9.4	9.3
Female gender	58.3	56.4	42.7	54.1	52.9
White race	94.4	91.8	96.6	88.9	90.4
Education					
< High school	28.6	27.8	25.6	24.6	21.7
High school graduate	29.8	31.2	34.4	33.0	33.8
Some college	25.8	25.6	23.4	26.1	26.8
College graduate	15.9	15.5	16.4	16.0	17.6
Income					
< $34,750	42.4	33.8	29.5	30.2	29.6
$34,751–$69,500	26.9	33.3	35.3	36.4	34.2
> $69,500	20.3	25.2	27.1	22.6	26.1
Unknown	10.3	7.6	8.1	10.9	10.1
Employment status					
Working full-time	43.6	48.3	50.5	49.6	52.0
Working part-time	12.1	15.8	18.3	17.7	15.0
Not working	21.7	17.2	17.8	16.4	16.1
Attending school/ keeping house	22.7	18.8	13.4	16.4	16.9
Marital status					
Married	55.6	60.4	66.0	65.4	62.6
Widowed	16.0	8.7	6.4	7.2	7.1
Divorced/separated	20.0	18.1	10.6	14.0	15.1
Never married	8.4	12.8	17.0	13.3	15.2
Household size					
1	15.1	11.6	10.4	10.8	11.3
2	39.0	29.6	27.8	27.8	28.3
3	20.1	21.6	20.5	19.8	19.6
4	16.5	20.7	26.4	24.3	22.3
≥ 5	9.2	16.5	14.9	17.1	18.3
Residence					
City of Cincinnati	6.5	8.3	9.0	11.8	11.6
Suburbs	52.8	55.3	56.1	60.8	61.0
Urban fringe	39.9	29.5	24.6	21.5	22.7

Source: Greater Cincinnati Community Health Status Survey, 2005.

a higher percentage of males and a lower percentage of females), while the family roots identifier results in a slightly greater percentage of nonwhite (predominantly black) Appalachian adults. Additional demographic data might be able to distinguish among these identification methods. For instance, respondents' length of residence in their current locations (often referred to as "years lived") could be a telling factor. The fact that most Appalachian migrants and their descendants are like their neighbors may be a function of assimilation over decades, whereas Appalachian newcomers to Greater Cincinnati may have a heightened sense of regional identity.

Third, different identification methods may result in different assessments of the health status and health disparities of the adult Appalachian population. For example, the results of the above study suggest that the identifier of one's own county of birth (first generation) portrays an Appalachian population with a poorer overall health status, greater risk for heart trouble, and lower risk for severe allergies and migraine headaches (table 14.4). Inclusion of mother's or father's county of birth (second generation) changes this characterization and suggests that the Appalachian population is at relatively greater risk for migraine headaches. Use of the self-identification approach portrays a population that is at higher risk for diabetes and possibly severe allergies but at relatively less risk for chronic lung disease. Identifying the Appalachian population using the family roots question or a combination of methods suggests a lower prevalence of high blood pressure, high cholesterol, and stroke. It is uncertain whether these differences are related to differences in demographics or other potential risk factors among the various identification approaches or to other explanations. Although the characterization of their health status appears to be relatively insensitive to the approach used to identify Appalachians, there are subtle differences in diabetes, heart disease, hypertension, high cholesterol, and allergies that warrant further investigation. Accurate identification of the health disparities and health risks of the Appalachian population is essential for enhancing the well-being and prosperity of the population and their contribution to society.

This study suggests that establishing Appalachian identity is difficult, and there may be no single best method for identifying Appalachians. However, selecting an appropriate method may be situation specific. For instance, if migration is a substantive issue, the identification of first- and

Health Status Measure	1st Generation (%)	1st and 2nd Generation (%)	Self-Identified (%)	Family Roots (%)	Total (%)
Table 14.4. Health Status of Respondents by Identification Method					
Self-rated overall health					
Excellent	11.8	17.0	18.4	19.1	17.8
Very good	29.6	28.3	26.8	28.7	29.2
Good	34.0	32.8	33.4	33.7	33.7
Fair	15.2	15.1	15.5	13.3	13.2
Poor	9.4	6.9	6.0	5.3	6.1
Self-rated oral health					
Very good	37.7	39.4	37.3	34.2	36.0
Good	30.3	32.0	34.9	37.8	37.7
Fair	25.3	20.6	19.0	19.5	18.3
Poor	6.8	8.0	8.8	8.6	8.0
Chronic health condition					
Present	80.8	81.1	78.4	76.4	76.5
Average number	2.6	2.8	2.6	2.4	2.3
Type of condition					
Asthma	15.2	15.4	15.2	14.7	14.0
Arthritis or rheumatism	38.2	35.0	36.8	31.1	30.1
Cancer	7.8	6.3	6.1	5.5	5.7
Chronic back pain	21.6	26.3	24.8	25.8	25.1
Chronic digestive disease	6.4	8.6	5.5	8.5	7.2
Chronic lung disease	9.4	9.4	3.7	8.0	6.8
Depression	24.9	26.4	23.0	23.0	22.6
Diabetes	9.7	13.0	18.1	13.1	11.3
Heart trouble or angina	22.4	13.8	11.0	12.2	11.6
High blood pressure or hypertension	47.8	44.5	45.9	38.8	38.5
High cholesterol or triglycerides	41.9	41.5	40.2	34.9	33.9
Migraine headaches	19.6	31.3	29.7	23.7	23.8
Osteoporosis	6.2	10.9	5.1	8.3	8.0
Severe allergies	9.9	18.8	20.6	17.3	16.1
Stroke	2.3	2.2	2.0	1.5	1.7

Source: Greater Cincinnati Community Health Status Survey, 2005.

second-generation Appalachians may be most appropriate. Conversely, when the interest includes subsequent generations of Appalachians, self-identification may be more suitable. If rural southerners (of whom many Appalachians are a subset) are of interest, a family roots approach may be best. As historian James C. Cobb[35] points out, regional identity in the United States is an evolving, situational reality that is always changing in response to contemporary political and social conditions. However elusive Appalachian identity may be, it is not necessarily illusory. The challenge for researchers is to find it in its current manifestation.

Further Research

The task of measuring Appalachian identity requires additional investigation to find a preferred definitional approach, whether generic or situation specific. The approaches applied in this study included nominal classifications and subjective self-classifications, as well as a somewhat mixed method that invoked both place and group identification in ascribing Appalachian identity. Each of these approaches has its drawbacks, yet each appears to be effective for a specific purpose. The results indicate that these approaches identify different groups of people as being Appalachian. As such, future research is needed in the following areas.

Studies need to be conducted to determine the level of understanding of and identification with the term *Appalachian,* particularly by persons of Appalachian heritage living outside the Appalachian region. The question is whether identification with the term *Appalachian* has salience for persons outside of Appalachia.

The influence of negative stereotyping on various identification methods needs investigation. In particular, does stereotyping affect the reliability and validity of self-identification and self-reported place-based methods?

Research is required to determine the underlying reasons for the lack of concordance among the different methods for identifying Appalachians. Of particular interest is the reason for the lack of Appalachian self-identification among persons who acknowledge family roots in Appalachia.

The validity of the attribute-based approach to identifying Appalachians needs further investigation, particularly given its widespread application by various advocacy and service organizations and individuals. The concept of cultural competence is based on this approach and is widely promoted as a means of tailoring services to individual clients.

New techniques for identifying multigenerational urban Appalachians residing outside the region should be developed and deployed. Questions other than the ones used in this study should be formulated, field-tested, and evaluated for effectiveness across a variety of situational contexts to determine the applicability of various approaches.

Future research should be based on an awareness that issues of Appalachian identity may be more amenable to qualitative methods such as participant observation, focus groups, structured interviews, or content analysis. Such approaches may provide the necessary insight into the structuring of quantitative identifiers.

Policy Recommendations

The work to date on identifying Appalachians who have moved outside the region has several policy implications.

General policies, including funding guidelines at both the state and national levels, should be developed. The urban Appalachian population residing outside the region should be recognized as a legitimate target group for purposes of data collection as well as health education programs, demonstration projects, and full-scale, long-term health interventions. Proven methods for identifying Appalachians are essential to understanding health disparities and targeting appropriate service delivery.

Appalachian identifiers should be included in administrative forms, registry protocols, and survey instruments so that the health of the Appalachian population outside the region can be ascertained and monitored, allowing comparisons between multigenerational Appalachians and non-Appalachians within and outside the region. Information such as the state and county of both residence and birth would allow classification according to Appalachian Regional Commission counties.

Research funding agencies should establish priority areas that stimulate and support research focusing on the development of valid and reliable methods for identifying Appalachians outside the region, as well as the application of those methods to enhance the understanding of the health needs and potential health disparities of this population subgroup.

Service and educational organizations need to adopt proven methods

of identifying Appalachians to permit the implementation of successful interventions tailored to the needs and contexts of Appalachians living outside the region. This includes training practitioners in the use of
situation-sensitive approaches to ensure the acceptance and effectiveness
of interventions designed for Appalachians outside the region.

Notes

a. Due to memory decay, however, eliciting the birth location of a respondent's grandparents does not provide statistically meaningful information.

b. In fall 2005, random-digit-dialed telephone interviews were conducted with
2,007 randomly selected adults residing in eight Ohio counties, nine Kentucky
counties, and five Indiana counties within the Greater Cincinnati metropolitan
area. Of the twenty-two counties surveyed, four were federally designated Appalachian counties in Ohio. Although the primary purpose of the survey was to assess
the self-reported health status, health behaviors, and health opinions of adults living in the area, a secondary purpose was to examine various ways of identifying
Appalachian adults. In addition to basic demographic questions, survey respondents were asked a series of questions regarding their Appalachian heritage based
on the first two strategies described earlier: place-based and self-identification.[36]

c. Those born in one of the 416 counties designated Appalachian by the Appalachian Regional Commission at the time of the survey were classified as first-
generation Appalachian. Currently, there are 420 federally designated Appalachian
counties.

d. Those whose fathers, mothers, or both were born in one of the 416 federally designated Appalachian counties were classified as Appalachian. This classification included (1) persons who were not born in Appalachia themselves but who
were the offspring of at least one parent who was born in Appalachia (second-
generation Appalachian) and (2) persons who were born in Appalachia and had at
least one parent born in Appalachia (first-generation Appalachian).

e. The phrase "your people" was suggested by local ethnographic research.[37]

f. Two-way cross-tabulations of the data by identification method (Appalachian generation versus Appalachian family roots, Appalachian generation versus
Appalachian self-identification, and Appalachian self-identification versus Appalachian family roots) were performed to assess concordance across the identification methods. Pair-wise concordance between the identification methods was
measured by the kappa statistic. A kappa statistic is always less than or equal to
1. A value of 1 implies perfect agreement; values less than 1 imply less than perfect agreement. In rare situations, kappa can be negative, indicating that the respondents agreed significantly less than would be expected by chance. The general
consensus is that a kappa value greater than 0.75 has a high degree of agreement

beyond chance, whereas a value less than 0.40 has a low degree of agreement.[38] To make these comparisons more meaningful, first- and second-generation Appalachians were combined for the Appalachian generation method. In addition, the demographic characteristics of respondents classified as Appalachian by each of the methods were tabulated and compared descriptively.

References

1. Shapiro HD. The place of culture and the problem of identity. In: Batteau A, ed. *Appalachia and America: Autonomy and Regional Dependence.* Lexington, KY: University Press of Kentucky; 1983:111–141.

2. Alba RD, Chamblin MB. A preliminary examination of ethnic identification among whites. *Am Sociol Rev.* 1983;48:240–247.

3. Kaplan JB, Bennett T. Use of race and ethnicity in biomedical publication. *JAMA.* 2003;289:2709–2716.

4. Nagel J. Constructing ethnicity: creating and recreating ethnic identity and culture. *Soc Probl.* 1994;41:152–176.

5. Walls D. On the naming of Appalachia. In: Williamson JW, ed. *An Appalachian Symposium.* Boone, NC: Appalachian State University Press; 1977:56–76.

6. Raitz KB, Ulack R, Leinbach TR. *Appalachia, a Regional Geography: Land, People, and Development.* Boulder, CO: Westview Press; 1984.

7. Bradshaw MJ. *The Appalachian Regional Commission: Twenty-Five Years of Government Policy.* Lexington, KY: University Press of Kentucky; 1992.

8. Williams JA. *Appalachia: A History.* Chapel Hill, NC: University of North Carolina Press; 2002.

9. Appalachian Regional Commission. The Appalachian region. Available at: http://www.arc.gov/appalachian_region/TheAppalachianRegion.asp. Accessed September 1, 2010.

10. Campbell RM. Appalachian experience and self-concept: toward a critical theory of regional identity [PhD dissertation]. Lexington, KY: University of Kentucky; 1994.

11. Hatch E, Keefe SE. Exploring mountain identity. Paper presented at the annual meeting of the American Anthropological Association, Chicago, IL, November 1999.

12. Keefe SE. Mountain identity and the global society in a rural Appalachian community. Paper presented at the national conference of the Center for Ethnicity and Gender in Appalachia, Huntington, WV, March 2000.

13. Keefe SE. Mountain values and resistance to late capitalism. Paper presented at the annual meeting of the Appalachian Studies Association, Knoxville, TN, March 2000.

14. Philliber WW. *Appalachian Migrants in Urban America: Cultural Conflict or Ethnic Group Formation?* New York, NY: Praeger; 1981.

15. Obermiller PJ. Labeling urban Appalachians: the role of stereotypes in the formation of ethnic group identity [PhD dissertation]. Cincinnati, OH: Union Institute and University; 1982.

16. Marger MN, Obermiller PJ. Urban Appalachians and Canadian maritime migrants: a comparative study of emergent ethnicity. In: Obermiller PJ, Philliber WW, eds. *Too Few Tomorrows: Urban Appalachians in the 1980s.* Boone, NC: Appalachian Consortium Press; 1987:23–34.

17. Myadze T. Revisiting urban Appalachian ethnicity. In: Obermiller PJ, Wagner TE, Tucker B, eds. *Appalachian Odyssey: Historical Perspectives on the Great Migration.* Westport, CT: Praeger; 2000:181–189.

18. Tucker B. Toward a new ethnicity: urban Appalachian ethnic consciousness in Cincinnati, 1950–1987. In: Obermiller PJ, Wagner TE, Tucker B, eds. *Appalachian Odyssey: Historical Perspectives on the Great Migration.* Westport, CT: Praeger; 2000:159–180.

19. Alexander JT. Great migrations: race and community in the southern exodus [PhD dissertation]. Pittsburgh, PA: Carnegie Mellon University; 2001.

20. Obermiller PJ, Oldendick RW. Moving on: recent patterns of Appalachian migration. In: Obermiller PJ, Philliber WW, eds. *Too Few Tomorrows: Urban Appalachians in the 1980s.* Boone, NC: Appalachian Consortium Press; 1987:51–65.

21. Alexander JT. "They're never here more than a year": return migration in the southern exodus, 1940–1970. *J Soc Hist.* 2005;38:653–671.

22. Alexander JT. Defining the diaspora: Appalachians in the Great Migration. *J Interdiscipl Hist.* 2006;37:219–247.

23. Obermiller PJ, Howe S. Moving mountains: Appalachian migration patterns, 1995–2000. *Journal of Appalachian Studies.* 2004;10:359–372.

24. Maloney ME, Auffrey C, eds. *The Social Areas of Cincinnati: An Analysis of Social Needs.* 4th ed. Cincinnati, OH: University of Cincinnati School of Planning and the University of Cincinnati Institute for Community Partnerships; 2004.

25. Hansel P, Brown K, Collins S, et al. Health, education, and pollution in Lower Price Hill. Cincinnati, OH: Urban Appalachian Council; 1990.

26. Couto RA. *Streams of Idealism and Health Care Innovation: An Assessment of Service-Learning and Community Mobilization.* New York, NY: Teachers College Press; 1982.

27. Couto RA, DeBruicker J. Lessons from community-based participatory research in Appalachia. In: Obermiller PJ, Maloney ME, eds. *Appalachia: Social Context Past and Present.* 5th ed. Dubuque, IA: Kendall/Hunt Publishing; 2007:337–343.

28. Obermiller PJ. Crossing the campus-community divide: new trends in research collaboration. *Appalachian Journal.* 2007;34:409–412.

29. Miller TR. Urban Appalachian ethnic identity: the current situation. In: Weiland S, Wagner TE, Obermiller PJ, eds. *Perspectives on Urban Appalachians.*

Cincinnati, OH: Ohio Urban Appalachian Awareness Project, University of Cincinnati; 1978.

30. Alexander JT, Berry C. Who is Appalachian? Self-reported Appalachian ancestry in the 2000 census. *Appalachian Journal.* 2010;38:46–54.

31. Billings DB, Norman G, Ledford K. *Back Talk from Appalachia: Confronting Stereotypes.* Lexington, KY: University Press of Kentucky; 1999.

32. Hartigan J. "Disgrace to the race": hillbillies and the color line in Detroit. In: Obermiller PJ, Wagner TE, Tucker EB, eds. *Appalachian Odyssey: Historical Perspectives on the Great Migration.* Westport, CT: Praeger; 2000:143–158.

33. Jones L. *Appalachian Values.* 1st ed. Ashland, KY: Jesse Stuart Foundation; 1994.

34. Ludke RL, Obermiller PJ, Rademacher EW, Turner SK. Identifying Appalachian adults: an empirical study. *Appalachian Journal.* 2010;38:36–45.

35. Cobb JC. *Away Down South: A History of Southern Identity.* New York, NY: Oxford University Press; 2005.

36. Rademacher EW, Ludke RL, Misner JM. 2005 Greater Cincinnati community health status report. Cincinnati, OH: Institute for Policy Research, University of Cincinnati; 2006.

37. Halperin RH. *Practicing Community: Class Culture and Power in an Urban Neighborhood.* 1st ed. Austin, TX: University of Texas Press; 1998.

38. Green AM. *Kappa Statistic for Multiple Raters Using Categorical Classifications.* Research Triangle Park, NC: Westat; 2006.

15

The Health Status and Health Determinants of Urban Appalachian Adults and Children

*Robert L. Ludke, Phillip J. Obermiller,
and Ronnie D. Horner*

The health status of urban Appalachians—those who have migrated out of the region to urban areas such as Cincinnati, Columbus, Chicago, Baltimore, and Detroit—is largely unknown. What is known is tentative due to a greater emphasis on health care delivery than on health status and due to a heavy focus on Appalachian migrant populations in central and southwestern Ohio.[1-6] Beginning in the early 1990s, a number of studies sought to more fully describe the health status of urban Appalachians, although this literature retained its focus on Appalachians residing in Greater Cincinnati. Several interesting patterns began to emerge from this work. For example, Obermiller and Oldendick[7] found that, similar to urban blacks, white Appalachians' major health concerns included heart attack, stroke, emotional or mental illness, and serious accidental injury. In a follow-up report two years later, Obermiller and Handy[8] added information on black urban Appalachians, whose health concerns were similar to those of white urban Appalachians. Based on interviews and case records obtained in the late 1990s, Halperin and Reiter-Purtill[9] documented that urban Appalachian women who had migrated to Cincinnati experienced more severe symptoms of "nerves" than did rural Appalachian women.

As health issues among Appalachians became more urgent, the Appalachian community responded by initiating research and advocacy groups to address its health problems. Foremost among these groups was the task force formed by Cincinnati's Urban Appalachian Council to study the health status of children in one of the city's Appalachian neighborhoods.[10] The work of this task force and of two community-based groups is discussed in chapter 16.

The dearth of health status information on Appalachians in Cincinnati proved to be a formidable barrier to designing interventions to address the health problems of the community. Local data gathered by the urban Appalachian groups, though important in documenting health problems among Appalachian residents of the city, did not permit the large-scale assessment required to devise effective interventions.[a] Subsequently, the Health Improvement Collaborative of Greater Cincinnati and the Health Foundation of Greater Cincinnati initiated the Greater Cincinnati Community Health Status Survey in 1996.[b] This survey was complemented by the Child Well-Being Survey conducted by the Child Health Policy Research Center at Cincinnati Children's Hospital Medical Center in partnership with the Health Foundation of Greater Cincinnati and the United Way of Greater Cincinnati.[c] These community surveys are the data sources used in this chapter to illustrate the health status of Appalachian migrants and their descendants residing in the Greater Cincinnati metropolitan area and to examine some of the potential determinants of their health.[d]

Appalachian migrants pose some interesting challenges, in that they are a dynamic population comprising both first-generation migrants (those born in Appalachia) and second-generation migrants (individuals born and raised in Cincinnati). First-generation migrants may have a "health heritage" that is a more important contributor to their current health status than their more immediate surroundings. The health status of second-generation individuals is likely influenced more by the local environment.

The first section of this chapter looks at changes in the health status and health determinants of first-generation white Appalachian adults between 1999 and 2005. The second section examines changes in the health status and health determinants of first- and second-generation Appalachian children between 2000 and 2005. The chapter concludes with recommendations for further research to improve our current understanding of the health of Appalachian migrants and their descendants and the policy initiatives emanating from this work.

First-Generation White Appalachian Adults

The term *first generation* refers to individuals who were born in the Appalachian region and subsequently migrated to the Cincinnati area. In a sense, their health experience is informative in much the same way as that of international immigrants. Unfortunately, this discussion is restricted to white respondents simply because there were insufficient nonwhite respondents in the Greater Cincinnati Community Health Status surveys. Regrettably, it is unknown when during their lives the immigrant Appalachians migrated, because length of time in the new location influences the extent to which the local environment impacts health status. The comparison group consisted of non-Appalachian white survey respondents.

Health Status. Health status was examined in three dimensions: health-related quality of life, self-reported health, and health conditions. Health-related quality of life, or the perceived level of physical and mental health functioning, was based on the SF-12 health assessment.[11] Self-reported health, both overall and oral health, was assessed by asking respondents to rate their health from excellent to poor. The presence of various health conditions was determined by asking respondents to indicate whether they had ever been told by a doctor or other health professional that they had any of fourteen chronic physical health conditions plus depression.

The overall health-related quality of life of Appalachians, though stable over the period 1999–2005, was lower than that of non-Appalachians. Appalachians scored not only significantly lower than non-Appalachians on physical health functioning (45.5 versus 49.7) but also significantly below the national norm of 50. Appalachians and non-Appalachians had identical average scores for mental health functioning (51.5), which was slightly above the national norm of 50.

Appalachians perceived their health to be poorer than did non-Appalachians, with no significant change between 1999 and 2005. A significantly higher percentage of Appalachians than non-Appalachians, on average across the three periods (1999, 2002, and 2005), reported that their overall health was either fair or poor (27 versus 15 percent, respectively). Also, 28 percent of Appalachians, on average, reported having fair or poor oral health, which was higher (but not significantly higher) than the 21 percent of non-Appalachians.

Appalachians were at greater risk for chronic physical health problems compared with non-Appalachians. Although overall risk and risk for some specific health conditions did not change between 1999 and 2005, there was some evidence that the risk for hypertension, high cholesterol, and depression may be increasing among Appalachians. In particular, the surveys found the following:

- Approximately 80 percent of Appalachians, on average across the three periods, reported having at least one chronic physical health condition; this was higher than the 69 percent of non-Appalachians, but not significantly so.
- Appalachians averaged almost three chronic physical health conditions, compared with two for non-Appalachians.
- With the exception of migraine headaches, Appalachians had higher average prevalence rates than non-Appalachians for all the chronic physical health conditions assessed (figure 15.1). In particular, Appalachians had significantly higher rates of arthritis/rheumatism, hypertension, chronic digestive diseases, and osteoporosis.
- Although the prevalence of asthma, chronic lung disease, diabetes, chronic digestive disease, arthritis/rheumatism, stroke, and migraine headaches among Appalachians remained relatively constant between 1999 and 2005, there were significant increases in hypertension (from 40 to 49 percent) and high cholesterol (from 28 to 45 percent) and significant decreases in cancer (from 19 to 9 percent) and severe allergies (from 23 to 9 percent).
- The average rate of self-reported depression among Appalachians (18 percent) was comparable to that among non-Appalachians, but the rate increased significantly between 2002 and 2005, going from 15 to 25 percent. This rate of increase was significantly greater than that for non-Appalachians.

What might explain these differences in health between Appalachians and non-Appalachians? According to the Evans and Stoddart framework of health,[12] the determinants of health can be divided into five categories: genetic endowment, physical environment, social environment, health care system, and individual response. Data from the three community health

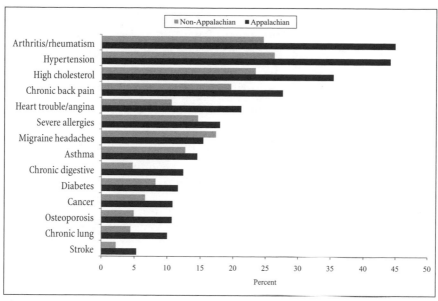

Figure 15.1. Average prevalence of chronic physical health conditions for white, first-generation Appalachians and white non-Appalachians, 1999–2005. *Source:* Greater Cincinnati Community Health Status Surveys, 1999, 2002, and 2005.

status surveys were analyzed to determine the relative importance of each category as an explanation of the observed differences in health status.

Genetic Endowment. The only two genetic endowment indicators available in the data were age and gender. Although no clear-cut conclusions could be drawn with regard to differences in the genetic endowment between Appalachians and non-Appalachians or the influence of these indicators on the health of Appalachians, there were two notable findings.

First, Appalachians were significantly older than non-Appalachians, but the age difference between them decreased during the study period: there was an average age difference of 13.7 years in 1999, 9.2 years in 2002, and 8.0 years in 2005. This decline was attributable to both the increasing average age of non-Appalachians between 1999 and 2005 and the decreasing average age of Appalachians—from 56.5 years in 1999 to 53.7 years in 2002 to 52.8 years in 2005. A possible explanation for this trend is that Appalachians experienced higher rates of mortality, particularly among the older cohort, as a consequence of the higher prevalence of chronic conditions.

Second, there was a significantly higher average percentage of women in the Appalachian population than in the non-Appalachian population (57 versus 52 percent). Since men are generally more vulnerable to health problems and have shorter life spans than women, the greater proportion of women in the Appalachian population may suggest a lower future risk of poor health and mortality compared with non-Appalachians.

Physical Environment. The survey data provided limited insight into the specific nature of the physical environments in which Appalachians and non-Appalachians reside. However, the physical environment of Appalachians appears to be changing as they migrate toward a less urban environment. The importance of this migration trend is difficult to assess because both urban and rural environments pose risks and benefits.

Specifically, the surveys found that Appalachians migrated from the city of Cincinnati to the surrounding suburbs between 1999 and 2002. This was followed by a further migration from the suburbs to the more rural fringe areas of the Cincinnati region between 2002 and 2005. During these same periods, there was only a slight migration of non-Appalachians from the city and suburbs to the rural fringe areas. As a result, in 2005, 55 percent of Appalachians lived in the suburbs, 42 percent lived in the rural fringe areas, and only 3 percent lived in the city. The percentages for non-Appalachians were 71 percent, 17 percent, and 12 percent, respectively.

Social Environment. Appalachians' comparatively lower socioeconomic status may place them at greater risk for poor health. In addition, Appalachians' social support networks—which, research suggests, are positively related to health—may be undergoing changes. These conclusions are based on findings related to education, employment, marital status, and household size.

Appalachians had less formal education than non-Appalachians, although there was a shift toward greater educational parity between 1999 and 2005. In 1999, 52 percent of Appalachians had less than a high school education, compared with 24 percent of non-Appalachians; 21 percent of Appalachians had a post–high school education, compared with 43 percent of non-Appalachians. By 2005, 27 percent of Appalachians had less than a high school education and 42 percent had a post–high school education, compared with 16 percent and 50 percent, respectively, for non-Appalachians.

Appalachian employment rates increased significantly between 1999 and 2002 and remained steady, at 57 percent, in 2005. This was lower (but not significantly lower) than the 69 percent for non-Appalachians. On average across the three periods, approximately 41 percent of Appalachians had low family incomes (less than $30,000 in 1999, less than $32,750 in 2002, and less than $34,750 in 2005), compared with 28 percent of non-Appalachians. Despite their lower socioeconomic status, Appalachians were significantly more likely than non-Appalachians to own their homes (86 versus 76 percent), with no significant changes between 1999 and 2005.

In 1999 significantly more Appalachians than non-Appalachians were married, and significantly fewer were never married; also, significantly more Appalachians were divorced or separated. However, between 1999 and 2005, the proportion of married Appalachians decreased significantly to 54 percent, while the proportion of widowed Appalachians increased significantly to 20 percent; the proportion of divorced or separated and never married Appalachians remained constant at about 17 percent and 9 percent, respectively. This implies that spousal-based social support among Appalachians may be declining.

Appalachians resided in significantly smaller households (fewer children and adults) than non-Appalachians, with no significant change in household size over time. However, Appalachians perceived stronger community support than non-Appalachians, with little change over time.

Health Care System. A willingness to use the health care system for preventive, diagnostic, and treatment services depends on how the system is perceived and how accessible it is. In this regard, Appalachians appeared to be as well positioned as non-Appalachians to use the health care system, a situation that did not change significantly across the three periods. This conclusion is supported by the fact that approximately 36 percent of Appalachians had positive attitudes toward the health care system, 21 percent had negative views, and 42 percent were neutral. Although significantly fewer Appalachians than non-Appalachians were dissatisfied with the quality of care, more Appalachians than non-Appalachians perceived the cost of care to be unreasonable. For both groups, the percentage who perceived the cost of care to be unreasonable increased over time. The cost of care may be a greater barrier to Appalachians' use of the health care system, particularly if they are paying more out of pocket for health care services.

The availability of a usual source of medical care appeared to be similar for Appalachians and non-Appalachians, but this may be declining for both groups. Approximately one-fifth of both Appalachians and non-Appalachians had no usual source of medical care in 2005—a proportion higher than that reported in 1999.

Despite having poorer dental health than non-Appalachians, Appalachians appeared to have comparable access to dental services. Fewer than two-thirds of Appalachians had a usual source of dental care; this proportion did not change over time and was lower (but not significantly lower) than the proportion of non-Appalachians.

There was no significant difference between Appalachians and non-Appalachians in the percentage of uninsured, although the percentage increased for both groups over time. For Appalachians, the percentage of uninsured doubled from 4 to 8 percent between 1999 and 2005. Likewise, Appalachians and non-Appalachians appeared to be similar in terms of those whose access to the health care system was constrained by a lack of resources. Among Appalachians, 4 percent had a household member who had to forgo a doctor's care and 7 percent had a household member who had to forgo prescription medications because the household needed the money to buy food or clothing or pay for housing.

Individual Response. Appalachians and non-Appalachians had different lifestyle behaviors that might negatively impact their health. In particular, tobacco use, weight status, level of physical activity, and diet were potential risk factors for Appalachians, whereas alcohol consumption was less of a concern. With a few exceptions, neither group significantly changed their health risk behaviors over the study period.

Even though cigarette smoking among Appalachians decreased significantly between 2002 and 2005 (from 39 to 26 percent), Appalachians were significantly more likely than non-Appalachians to be cigarette smokers. Appalachians also had a higher prevalence of smokeless tobacco use than non-Appalachians. The rate of smokeless tobacco use decreased among non-Appalachians between 1999 and 2002 (no data were available for 2005), while the rate increased among Appalachians (from 4 to 6 percent).

In 1999 there was no significant difference in weight status between Appalachians and non-Appalachians. However, the body mass index (BMI) of both groups increased between 1999 and 2005, with Appalachians gaining more weight than non-Appalachians. As a result, Appalachians were significantly heavier than non-Appalachians in 2005, with 1 percent of Appalachians being underweight, 39 percent normal weight, 35 percent overweight, 21 percent obese, and 3 percent morbidly obese.

Appalachians were significantly less likely than non-Appalachians to engage in physical activity (69 versus 82 percent), with no significant change between 1999 and 2002. Between 1999 and 2002 there was a decline in the frequency of physical activity for both Appalachians and non-Appalachians. The percentage of Appalachians engaging in physical activity three to five times a week decreased, and the percentage engaging in activity one to two times a week increased. Of those Appalachians who were physically active in 2002, 34 percent engaged in physical activity one to two times a week, 31 percent three to five times a week, and 34 percent six to seven times a week; levels for non-Appalachians were comparable. In 2005 half of Appalachians failed to engage in the recommended level of physical activity—that is, at least thirty minutes of moderate physical activity five days a week or at least twenty minutes of vigorous activity three days a week. Non-Appalachians had a similar level of inactivity.

The percentage of Appalachians eating high-cholesterol or high-fat foods every day, such as fatty meat, cheese, fried foods, or eggs, remained at about 30 percent between 1999 and 2002 (no data were available for 2005); the percent of non-Appalachians decreased. Approximately 30 percent of both Appalachians and non-Appalachians perceived their diets to be very or extremely healthy; however, significantly more Appalachians than non-Appalachians considered their diets to be not too healthy or not at all healthy (18 versus 13 percent), with no significant change between 1999 and 2002. In 2005 Appalachians were significantly less likely than non-Appalachians to eat the recommended five servings of fruits and vegetables per day six to seven times a week.

Appalachians were significantly less likely than non-Appalachians to consume alcohol (37 versus 56 percent), with little change in the rates between 1999 and 2005. Among those who consumed alcohol, the average daily amount consumed was not significantly different between Appalachians and non-Appalachians and did not change between 1999 and 2005. Approximately 12 percent of Appalachians who consumed alcohol were heavy drinkers (two or more drinks per day for men, one or more drinks per day for women), with the rates decreasing from 13 percent in 2002 to 10 percent in 2005 (no data were available for 1999). Although Appalachians and non-Appalachians were similar in terms of heavy drinking, Appalachians were significantly less likely than non-Appalachians (20 versus 37 percent) to be binge drinkers (consume five or more drinks at one time) in both 2002 and 2005 (no data were available for 1999). Also, Appalachians were significantly less likely than non-Appalachians to engage in alcohol-related risky behavior, such as driving when they had too much to drink (2 versus 8 percent).

Appalachians and non-Appalachians were relatively similar in terms of individual preventive health behaviors (with the exception of dental health), with little change in these behaviors across the three periods. For example:

- Approximately 97 percent of Appalachians had their blood pressure checked in the past two years and 86 percent had their blood cholesterol checked in the past five years, rates comparable to those for non-Appalachians.
- Appalachian women were just as likely as non-Appalachian women to be compliant with mammogram and Pap smear screening guidelines, but Appalachian men were significantly less likely than non-Appalachian men to be compliant with rectal exam screening guidelines (72 versus 81 percent).
- Appalachians and non-Appalachians were equally compliant with routine medical checkup guidelines, but Appalachians were significantly less likely to have had a dental checkup in the past two years (57 versus 74 percent) or to have had their teeth cleaned within the past year (55 versus 68 percent).
- Significantly more Appalachians than non-Appalachians received a flu shot in 1999 (48 versus 30 percent), but these rates decreased significantly to 33 and 26 percent, respectively, in 2002 (no data were available for 2005).
- Between 1999 and 2002 (no data were available for 2005), the percentage of Appalachians who reported always wearing a seat belt increased from 58 to 77 percent, a level comparable to that for non-Appalachians.

• Appalachians were significantly less likely than non-Appalachians to have a loaded firearm in the home (6 versus 10 percent), with no significant change between 1999 and 2002 (no data were available for 2005). The majority of Appalachian gun owners in 2002 (69 percent) reported storing the gun in a locked place or having a trigger lock, as did non-Appalachian gun owners.

Summary for Appalachian Adults. In the Greater Cincinnati area, first-generation white Appalachian adults appear to have a poorer quality of life and poorer oral health status than white non-Appalachian adults, with little change since 1999. Although both groups have a comparable mental health status, depression is a growing problem in the Appalachian population. Appalachians may also be at greater risk for chronic physical health problems than their non-Appalachian counterparts. Most troubling is the increase over time in the prevalence of high blood pressure and high cholesterol or triglycerides—conditions that often contribute to the onset of other health problems, such as heart disease.

Although not examined directly, some of the disparities in health status may be a result of differences in health determinants. Compared with white non-Appalachians, first-generation white Appalachian adults reside in less urbanized physical environments and have a lower socioeconomic status. Though comparable in terms of their perceptions of and access to the health care system, as well as preventive health care behaviors, Appalachians are more likely to have lifestyle behaviors, such as tobacco use, overweight, physical inactivity, and diet, that may contribute to a poorer health status.

First- and Second-Generation White Appalachian Children

The focus of this section is the health of urban Appalachian children younger than 18 years. Unlike the case for urban Appalachian adults, data were available on second-generation Appalachian children—that is, those born outside the Appalachian region to first-generation Appalachian parents—as well as first-generation Appalachian children. Again, because of sample sizes, the focus is on whites as opposed to other racial groups. The comparison group was composed of non-Appalachian white children younger than 18 years, which might include unidentifiable Appalachian children of third or higher generations.

Health Status. The health status of urban Appalachian children relative to non-Appalachian children can be examined over the two periods covered by the Child Well-Being Surveys (2000 and 2005), based on four dimensions of health: perceived health status, health conditions, behavioral or emotional problems, and health care utilization.

Based on the perceptions of primary caregivers, the overall health status of Appalachian children was comparable to that of non-Appalachian children and remained constant between 2000 and 2005. Approximately 86 percent of caregivers of Appalachian children considered them to be in excellent or very good health, while 4 percent reported that their children were in fair or poor health.

With few exceptions, the prevalence rates of various health conditions affecting Appalachian children did not change significantly between 2000 and 2005 and were similar to those for non-Appalachian children. In particular, the surveys found the following:

- Approximately 15 percent of Appalachian children had asthma, and 7 percent of children without asthma had a recurrent cough, wheezing, or shortness of breath.
- Although the proportion of Appalachian children with learning disabilities remained relatively constant at about 7 percent between 2000 and 2005, the proportion with attention-deficit disorder increased from 5 percent in 2000 to 11 percent in 2005.
- A greater percentage of Appalachian than non-Appalachian children had hearing problems in 2000 (10 versus 6 percent), with no significant difference in their likelihood of receiving treatment for the problem.
- Among Appalachian children, rates of speech problems (11 percent), mental retardation (2 percent), and other developmental delays (5 percent) were comparable to those among non-Appalachian children.

Based on the perceptions of their caregivers, Appalachian children were at greater risk for poor behavioral and emotional health than were non-Appalachian children, and the disparity widened between 2000 and 2005. In 2000, 8 percent of Appalachian children aged 6 to 17 years were perceived to have a high level of behavioral and emotional problems—slightly higher than, but not significantly different from, the 6 percent for non-Appalachian children. By 2005, the percentage of Appalachian children with behavioral and emotional problems had increased significantly to 22 percent; the percentage of non-Appalachian children with these issues also increased significantly, but to only 10 percent.

In 2005 Appalachian children aged 6 to 17 years were less likely than their non-Appalachian peers to be perceived by their caregivers as usually or always showing respect for teachers or neighbors (90 versus 95 percent) and trying to resolve conflicts with classmates, family, or friends (64 versus 75 percent). They were also significantly less likely to try to understand other people's feelings (70 versus 83 percent). When subdivided by age into those 6 to 11 years and those 12 to 17 years, Appalachian children in both age groups experienced significant increases in behavioral and emotional problems between 2000 and 2005 (table 15.1).

In 2000 Appalachian children aged 6 to 11 were significantly more likely than their non-Appalachian peers to be unable to concentrate or pay attention and to be high-strung or tense. Because these problems increased significantly among non-Appalachian children between 2000 and 2005, the differences between the two groups of preteen children were not significant in 2005. However, the percentage of Appalachian preteen children who acted too young for their age increased significantly between 2000 and 2005; as a result, this was more of a problem for Appalachian than non-Appalachian children in 2005. With the exception of feeling worthless or inferior, more than 40 percent of Appalachian preteen children experienced one or more of these behavioral and emotional problems in 2005, with more than 50 percent having difficulty concentrating or paying attention.

Appalachian and non-Appalachian children aged 12 to 17 had similar prevalence rates of behavioral and emotional problems in 2000. However, between 2000 and 2005, these older Appalachian children experienced significantly increased rates of difficulty concentrating or paying attention, trouble sleeping, lying or cheating, and doing poorly in school. Thus, in 2005, Appalachian teenagers were significantly more likely than their non-Appalachian peers to have problems concentrating or paying attention, lying or cheating, and doing poorly in school. With the exception of having trouble sleeping, more than 40 percent of the older Appalachian children

Table 15.1. Percentage of Appalachian and Non-Appalachian Children with Behavioral and Emotional Problems by Age and Year

Problem	2000		2005	
	Non-Appalachian	Appalachian	Non-Appalachian	Appalachian
Ages 6–11				
Doesn't get along with other kids	36.2	35.0	46.5	46.1
Can't concentrate or pay attention for long	43.0	50.0	47.4	55.7
Has been unhappy, sad, or depressed	41.2	37.2	50.4	44.8
Feels worthless or inferior	15.6	12.6	19.3	25.4
Has been nervous, high-strung, or tense	30.7	43.7	43.8	46.1
Acts too young for his/her age	21.6	28.1	24.2	43.1
High problem level	4.7	8.8	10.2	22.8
Ages 12–17				
Doesn't get along with other kids	30.4	33.3	39.2	46.0
Can't concentrate or pay attention for long	38.2	36.6	41.2	66.8
Has been unhappy, sad, or depressed	49.5	40.1	53.5	53.4
Has trouble sleeping	19.6	17.8	28.3	34.9
Lies or cheats	23.5	27.4	27.8	45.5
Does poorly at schoolwork	32.2	35.0	30.9	48.1
High problem level	8.2	7.0	10.5	22.1

Source: Child Well-Being Surveys, 2000 and 2005.

experienced one or more of these problems in 2005, with two-thirds having difficulty concentrating or paying attention and more than half being unhappy, sad, or depressed.

Appalachian children appear to use the health care system for preventive care, including well-child checkups, routine physical exams, immunizations, or health screening tests, at about the same level as non-Appalachian children. Appalachian and non-Appalachian children were equally likely to have had an injury requiring medical attention (21 percent), but Appalachian children were significantly more likely to have had at least one emergency room visit (33 versus 26 percent). It is worth noting that there was no difference in the frequency of emergency room use between Appalachian and non-Appalachian children with at least one emergency room visit.

Similar to the discussion of the health status determinants for first-generation Appalachian adults, the health determinants that can be drawn from the Child Well-Being Surveys are examined according to the same five categories: genetic endowment, physical environment, social environment, health care system, and individual response.[12]

Genetic Endowment. Based on the only two genetic indicators available in the data—age and gender—Appalachian and non-Appalachian children were similar and exhibited no differences between 2000 and 2005. The ages of the Appalachian children ranged from less than 1 year to 17 years, with an average age of 9.0 years. Approximately 58 percent of the Appalachian children were boys.

Physical Environment. Appalachian children lived in a more rural environment than non-Appalachian children, with little change between 2000 and 2005. In 2005, 36 percent of Appalachian children lived in the rural fringe counties of Greater Cincinnati, compared with 15 percent of non-Appalachian children; 19 percent of Appalachian children lived in the urban county that includes the city of Cincinnati, compared with 32 percent of non-Appalachian children.

Substantial percentages of both Appalachian and non-Appalachian children were exposed to the hazards of secondhand smoke. In 2005 (no data were available for 2000), 32 percent of Appalachian children were living in households where the primary caregiver was a current smoker, versus 26 percent of non-Appalachian children; these rates were not significantly different when adjusted for socioeconomic status.

Social Environment. More Appalachian than non-Appalachian children were living in single-parent households of lower socioeconomic status, which might expose them to greater risks for unfavorable health conditions. However, Appalachian and non-Appalachian children were living in comparable environments in terms of food security, supportive family environments, and outside social involvement. The social environments of Appalachian and non-Appalachian children did not change substantially between 2000 and 2005. Some of the relevant survey findings are examined below.

Compared with non-Appalachian children, Appalachian children were (1) less likely to have a married primary caregiver and more likely to have a primary caregiver who had never been married or was widowed; (2) more likely to have a primary caregiver with less than a high school education or with a high school diploma or its equivalent and less likely to have a college graduate as the primary caregiver; (3) more likely to have a primary caregiver who worked full-time and less likely to have one who worked part-time; (4) more likely to be subject to some type of child-care arrangement during the day, typically with a relative or friend rather than a child-care center, while the primary caregiver worked outside the home or after school; (5) just as likely to spend time caring for themselves, either at home or elsewhere, without an adult or older child responsible for them (children aged 6 to 17 years in 2000); and (6) less likely to have moved in the past year or the past five years, as well as less likely to have moved frequently in the past five years.

Appalachian children were more likely to live in households where the annual family income was low (less than $35,000) and were less likely to live in households where the income was high (more than $70,000). For both Appalachian and non-Appalachian children, there was a significant shift toward higher-income households between 2000 and 2005, which might simply be due to inflation. In 2005, 18 percent of Appalachian children were living in households with incomes below 100 percent of the federal poverty level, 27 percent had household incomes between 100 and 200 percent of the federal poverty level, and 55 percent had household incomes above 200 percent of the federal poverty level. The rates were 10, 15, and 75 percent, respectively, for non-Appalachian children.

Appalachian children were just as likely as non-Appalachian children to live in food-secure households in 2005 (no data were available for 2000). Approximately 17 percent of primary caregivers of Appalachian children bought food that did not last and lacked the money to get more, 18 percent could not afford to eat balanced meals, and 13 percent had to cut the size of their meals or skip meals because there was not enough money for food. In 2000 (no data were available for 2005) Appalachian children were significantly more likely to live in households where the family received food stamps (9 versus 6 percent).

In 2000 there was no significant difference between Appalachian and non-Appalachian children in terms of how much time the primary caregiver or other adults in the household spent at home playing with the child, reading to the child, participating in leisure activities or outings away from home, working on projects together at home, having private talks, and helping with schoolwork. However, Appalachian children younger than 6 years were significantly less likely to be read to compared with their non-Appalachian peers in 2000; this improved to the same level as non-Appalachian children by 2005.

Household members of Appalachian children aged 5 years and older were significantly less likely to participate in school activities than were non-Appalachian household members. Adults in Appalachian households were significantly less likely to attend an open house or back-to-school night; attend a meeting of a PTA, PTO, parent-teacher student organization, parent advisory group, or policy council; go to a regularly scheduled parent-teacher conference; act as a volunteer at the school; or serve on a committee. However, they were equally likely to attend a school or class event such as a play, sports competition, or science fair.

Caregivers of Appalachian children aged 6 years and older were similar to caregivers of non-Appalachian children in terms of talking with children about alcohol and other drugs, setting clear rules, and punishing children when they broke the rules. Approximately 73 percent of caregivers of Appalachian children had talked to their children about alcohol and other drugs in the past month, 95 percent set clear rules for their children often or a lot, and 61 percent punished their children often or a lot when they broke the rules.

In 2005, 82 percent of Appalachian households had cable television, and 77 percent of the caregivers of Appalachian children used the Internet at home; approximately 20 percent used the Internet frequently to find information about recreational activities for their children, and 13 percent used it to find health information related to children. These percentages were similar among caregivers of non-Appalachian children.

Fifty-eight percent of both Appalachian and non-Appalachian children aged 6 to 17 years were involved in some type of community service or volunteer work at school, at church, or in the community in 2000 (no data were available for 2005). Also, 61 percent of Appalachian children aged 6 to 17 years were involved with a club or organization (e.g., Scouts, a religious group, a boys' or girls' club) after school or on weekends during the past year, participating an average of 2.2 days per week. This level of participation was similar to that of non-Appalachian children.

Health Care System. Compared with non-Appalachian children, Appalachian children had more primary care services at their disposal and comparable levels of resources to access those services, except for private insurance coverage. Significantly more Appalachian children than non-Appalachian children (95 versus 88 percent) had a medical home—that is, a personal doctor or nurse (generalist, pediatrician, specialist, nurse practitioner, or physician assistant) who knew the child well and was familiar with the child's health history. However, Appalachian children were significantly less likely than non-Appalachian children to have private insurance coverage (75 versus 85 percent). The percentage of both Appalachian and non-Appalachian children covered by Medicaid or the Child Health Insurance Program increased significantly between 2000 and 2005; the percentage of covered Appalachian children increased from 15 to 19 percent, comparable to the increase among non-Appalachian children. Whereas the percentage of non-Appalachian children without health insurance did not change significantly between 2000 and 2005, the percentage of Appalachian children without health insurance decreased significantly from 8 to 3 percent.

In terms of resources to access the health care system, in 2000 (no data were available for 2005), 2 percent of Appalachian children did not receive a doctor's care because of a lack of transportation, 2 percent did not receive care because the household needed the money to buy food or clothing or pay for housing, and 2 percent did not receive prescription medications because the household needed the money for those other necessities. These percentages were similar for non-Appalachian children.

Individual Response. Childhood obesity is not only a major health determinant for childhood health problems but also a precursor of poor health in adulthood. There were no significant differences between Appalachian and non-Appalachian children in either weight status or physical activity (an underlying obesity determinant). In 2005 approximately 15 percent of caregivers of Appalachian children considered their children to be overweight, which was higher (but not significantly higher) than that for non-Appalachian children. In addition, similar percentages of caregivers of Appalachian and non-Appalachian children were likely to consider their children to be underweight (5 versus 8 percent). There was no significant difference between Appalachian and non-Appalachian children aged 6 to 17 years in the average number of days they exercised or participated in physical activity for at least twenty minutes that made them sweat and breathe hard. Appalachian children engaged in physical activity an average of 3.9 days per week.

Summary for Appalachian Children. In the Greater Cincinnati area, it appears that first- and second-generation white Appalachian children are largely comparable to white non-Appalachian children in terms of health status and health utilization. However, these Appalachian children may be at greater risk for poor behavioral and emotional health, with the disparity between Appalachian and non-Appalachian children potentially increasing over time. It is uncertain, however, whether the risk is actually greater or whether the caregivers simply have different standards for judging behavioral and emotional health. If the caregivers' perceptions are correct, the prevalence of these problems among Appalachian children may be contributing to the above-average high school dropout rate among the urban Appalachian population of Cincinnati.

It is uncertain to what extent this disparity in behavioral and emotional health is related to the health determinants collected in the Child Well-Being Surveys. Although the Appalachian children appear to reside in more rural areas and in more single-parent, lower socioeconomic households than their non-Appalachian counterparts, they have comparable exposure to second-hand smoke and to social support environments, both inside and outside the household. Also, the availability of health care services appears to be similar, although Appalachians are more likely to be covered by Medicaid than by private insurance. The two groups also have similar lifestyle behaviors.

Further Research

Clearly, there is a dearth of information about the health status and underlying health determinants of the population of Appalachians who migrated out of the region to urban areas. This sparseness is apparent in both the number of studies and the comprehensiveness of the assessments. Thus, current understanding provides limited guidance as to points of intervention and health improvements for urban Appalachians. The following are some key research areas that would lead to a more informative evidence base.

Improved methods of identifying persons of Appalachian heritage need to be developed, evaluated, and incorporated into national, regional, and local data-collection efforts. These are required to better identify the health status and health determinants of all Appalachians, not just first- or second-generation individuals. Currently, there is high likelihood of misclassifying Appalachians, which likely obfuscates their true state of health and well-being relative to non-Appalachians.

Studies comparing the health status of Appalachians residing in metropolitan areas *outside* the Appalachian region with that of rural Appalachians would improve the understanding of the combined effects of rural predisposition and migration on the health and well-being of this population. In addition, studies comparing the health status of Appalachians residing in metropolitan areas *inside* the region with that of rural Appalachians are needed to assess the impact of urban integration on the health and well-being of Appalachians. Finally, comparing the health determinants and health status of Appalachians residing in the Greater Cincinnati area with those of urban Appalachians living in other metropolitan areas would reveal whether urban Appalachians in general face similar health and well-being challenges and whether there are unique, context-specific challenges.

Urban Appalachians are not officially recognized as a minority population, despite having recognizable socioeconomic and demographic characteristics. Therefore, the health determinants and health status of urban Appalachians should be compared with those of other urban minorities, such as African Americans and Hispanics, to assess the extent to which Appalachians share a level of disadvantage in terms of health and well-being.

The health determinants and health status of Appalachians and non-Appalachians are often similar when controlling for age, gender, and socioeconomic status. Where significant differences exist, the variations are clear, but their causes are not. Focused research is needed to establish and test explanatory hypotheses to fully understand the differences.

Policy Recommendations

The research on Appalachian migrants and their descendants living in urban areas leads to a number of policy recommendations to address their health and well-being. For instance, in light of the health disparities that exist between urban Appalachians and non-Appalachians, policies need to recognize Appalachians as a minority group to facilitate the development, funding, and implementation of programs and services to address those disparities.

Appalachian identifiers need to be incorporated into the health information and surveillance systems of urban health care providers and public health agencies so that the health status of Appalachian adults and children can be monitored. This will help identify interventions to address the needs of those residents and determine the extent to which those needs are being met.

Academic institutions and funding agencies should consider creating educational and research capabilities to focus on the health and well-being of urban Appalachians. These capabilities would be similar to educational and research programs addressing the educational and health needs of residents of Appalachia, but they would adopt an urban rather than a rural Appalachian focus.

Given that urban Appalachian adults are predisposed to chronic disease, potentially due to their socioeconomic status and individual behaviors, community organizations and agencies need to consider policies that address the onset of chronic disease and ameliorate its underlying causes. This would include interventions among children to prevent the adoption of unhealthy lifestyle behaviors that may result in the onset of chronic disease in adulthood.

Given high dropout rates among urban Appalachian children and their predisposition for behavioral and emotional problems that may contribute to these rates, elementary and secondary school systems need to adopt policies to address the underlying problems rather than continuing punishment-based practices such as detention and dismissal.

Notes

a. It is worth noting that the lack of health status information was not unique to the Appalachian community. It was true for other residents as well, impeding efforts to improve the health of Cincinnatians generally.

b. The Greater Cincinnati Community Health Status Survey is a random-digit-dialed telephone survey, conducted every three years through 2005, to examine the health status, lifestyle behaviors, and health opinions and practices of approximately 2,000 adult residents in the multicounty area surrounding Cincinnati.[13–16] There were 251, 236, and 231 first-generation Appalachians in the 1999, 2002, and 2005 surveys, respectively, compared with 1,568, 1,558, and 1,634 non-Appalachians. It is possible that the non-Appalachian comparison groups included unidentifiable Appalachians of second, third, or higher generations. The survey responses were weighted to be representative of the Appalachian and non-Appalachian populations in the Greater Cincinnati area. When assessing differences, statistical adjustments were made for differences in gender and socioeconomic status (education and income).

c. Carried out in 2000 and 2005, the Child Well-Being Survey was a random-digit-dialed telephone survey of approximately 1,500 adult caregivers to assess the health and well-being of children in the multicounty area surrounding Cincinnati.[17, 18] The Child Well-Being Surveys included children and their primary caregivers as respondent dyads; there were 438 Appalachians and 1,513 non-Appalachians in the 2000 survey and 172 Appalachians and 1,069 non-Appalachians in the 2005 survey. These surveys produced information on first- and second-generation white Appalachian children in a twenty-nine-county area surrounding Cincinnati in 2000[17] and in a twenty-two-county area in 2005.[18] The survey responses of the primary caregivers were weighted to be representative of the Appalachian and non-Appalachian populations in the Greater Cincinnati area. Significant differences either between Appalachians and non-Appalachians or between the two survey periods were identified using statistical analyses that adjusted for age, gender, and socioeconomic status (education and income) of the primary caregivers as well as age and gender of the children, where appropriate.

d. Data from the 1999, 2002, and 2005 Greater Cincinnati Community Health Status Surveys and the 2000 and 2005 Child Well-Being Surveys are available at: http://www.oasisdataarchive.org/OASIS_CODE/Templates/Login.cfm.

References

1. Porter ER. From mountain folk to city dwellers. *Nurs Outlook.* 1963; 11:514–515.

2. Porter ER. When cultures meet—mountain and urban. *Nurs Outlook.* 1963;11:418–420.

3. Watkins VM. Consideration of factors relevant to the development of adequate health support systems for Appalachian migrants [master's thesis]. Cincinnati, OH: University of Cincinnati; 1973.

4. Friedl J. *Health Care Services and the Appalachian Migrant.* Vol. 42. Columbus, OH: The Ohio State University; 1978.

5. Friedl J. Health care: the city versus the migrant. In: Batteau A, ed. *Appalachia and America: Autonomy and Regional Dependence.* Lexington, KY: University Press of Kentucky; 1983:189–209.

6. Helton LR. Urban Appalachian health care: attitudes and practices. *Mountain Life and Work.* 1988;64:13–26.

7. Obermiller PJ, Oldendick RW. Urban Appalachian health concerns. In: Borman KM, Obermiller PJ, eds. *From Mountains to Metropolis: Appalachian Migrants in American Cities.* Westport, CT: Bergin and Garvey; 1994:51–60.

8. Obermiller PJ, Handy WS. Health education strategies for urban blacks and Appalachians. In: Borman KM, Obermiller PJ, eds. *From Mountains to Metropolis: Appalachian Migrants in American Cities.* Westport, CT: Bergin and Garvey; 1994:61–70.

9. Halperin RH, Reiter-Purtill J. "Nerves" in rural and urban Appalachia. In: Keefe SE, ed. *Appalachian Cultural Competency: A Guide for Medical, Mental Health, and Social Service Professionals.* Knoxville, TN: University of Tennessee Press; 2005:265–284.

10. Hansel P, Brown K, Collins S, et al. Health, education, and pollution in Lower Price Hill. Cincinnati, OH: Urban Appalachian Council; 1990.

11. Ware JE, Kosinski M, Keller SD, eds. *SF-12: How to Score the SF-12 Physical and Mental Health Summary Scales.* Boston, MA: The Health Institute, New England Medical Center; 1996.

12. Evans RG, Stoddart GL. Producing health, consuming health care. In: Evans RG, Barer ML, Marmor TR, eds. *Why Are Some People Healthy and Not Others: The Determinants of Health of Populations.* New York, NY: Aldine de Gruyter; 1994:27–64.

13. Downing K, Tuchfarber AJ. The Greater Cincinnati Community Health Foundation Survey. Cincinnati, OH: Institute for Policy Research, University of Cincinnati; 1996.

14. Ludke RL, Rademacher EW, Tuchfarber AJ. The Greater Cincinnati Community Health Status Survey. Cincinnati, OH: Institute for Health Policy and Health Services Research, University of Cincinnati; 2000.

15. Ludke RL, Rademacher EW, Tuchfarber AJ. The Greater Cincinnati Community Health Status Survey 2002. Cincinnati, OH: Institute for Health Policy and Health Services Research and Institute for Policy Research, University of Cincinnati; 2002.

16. Rademacher EW, Ludke RL, Misner JM. 2005 Greater Cincinnati community health status report. Cincinnati, OH: Institute for Policy Research, University of Cincinnati; 2006.

17. Donovan EP, Rose B. The state of our children: report on the well-being of children in the tristate region. Vol. 2. Cincinnati, OH: Child Policy Research Center, Cincinnati Children's Hospital Medical Center; 2001.

18. Rademacher EW. 2005 Child Well-Being Survey. Cincinnati, OH: Institute for Policy Research, University of Cincinnati; 2006.

16

Community-Based Participatory Health Research in an Urban Appalachian Neighborhood

M. Kathryn Brown

Community-based participatory research (CBPR) is an appropriate and effective research methodology for areas that are underserved or completely missed by health data-collection protocols that typically operate at the federal, state, county, or metropolitan level.[1] In this research paradigm, communities identify their health issues of concern and then systematically collect local data to better understand those issues so that practical intervention and prevention strategies can be developed and implemented. CBPR is no less scientific or accurate than conventional investigator-initiated research models. When done right, CBPR is a rigorous research methodology that builds capacity and generates reliable data for improving health.

This chapter discusses CBPR and its applicability to understanding and addressing the health issues of urban Appalachians from a neighborhood perspective. This is accomplished by describing the development, implementation, and outcomes of two CBPR projects—one focused on children and the other on women—carried out in Lower Price Hill, a predominantly Appalachian neighborhood in Cincinnati, Ohio. The significance of these collaborative health research projects stemmed from the direction and control exerted by community residents over the projects and the usefulness and quality of the data collected. Often overlooked by local health researchers, service providers, and environmental regulators, specific information about women and children in the neighborhood became an essential part of the community's efforts to impact health determinants. Outcomes of these efforts included changes in the behaviors of parents vis-à-vis themselves and their children, as well as in the behaviors and practices of health care providers vis-à-vis their patients. In addition, residents leveraged the data to promote changes in the attitudes, practices, and policies of health care providers, politicians, and regulators. The availability of detailed information specific to Lower Price Hill, coupled with residents' knowledge of the genesis and significance of the data, was critical in effecting each of these changes.

Before describing the research strategies and findings developed in the community, brief descriptions of CBPR and the Lower Price Hill neighborhood set the background. The chapter concludes with research and policy suggestions.

Community-Based Participatory Research

Much has been written about the roots of CBPR.[2-5] Common themes from seemingly divergent perspectives began to converge, and new directions in public health research began to take shape in the 1990s. Growing interest in health disparities,[6,7] environmental justice,[8] and health as an ecological phenomenon shaped by economic, social, and political factors[9,10] broadened the perspectives of community advocates, researchers, and public health analysts. The push for the democratization of science and collaborative approaches to community issues offered alternative approaches.[11,12] New funding strategies to build capacity and support the conduct of collaborative, community-based research followed. Some of the efforts that helped launch CBPR were the National Institute of Environmental Health Sciences' Environmental Justice Partnerships for Communication (1994)[13] and Community-Based Prevention Intervention Research (1999),[14] the Centers for Disease Control and Prevention's Urban Centers for Applied Research in Public Health (1994),[15] and the W. K. Kellogg Foundation's Community-Based Public Health Initiative (1990).[16]

Community-based and participatory research has a long and substantial track record in Appalachia.[17] Since the 1970s, the Highlander Research and Education Center in New Market, Tennessee, has been a source of instruction and inspiration for generations of community activists seeking justice and community knowledge on local issues, especially environmental health. The techniques of participatory research and popular education programs are taught at retreats and workshops conducted at the Highlander Center and are practiced in communities throughout Appalachia and beyond.[18] The Highlander Center also trained more than 100 community researchers to search rural county tax assessor records for the Appalachian Land Ownership Study. The Appalachian Land Ownership Task Force, founded under the auspices of the Appalachian Alliance, consisted of fifteen members from citizens' groups, along with eight members from local colleges, and received funding from the Appalachian Regional Commission. This grassroots effort to investigate the patterns of landownership and taxation in six Appalachian states concluded that land reform was essential if local communities were to prosper.[19] The study galvanized communities and academics from small colleges in the region to create collaborative approaches to address local and regional issues of economic development.[20–22]

Health disparities remain a distressing feature of life in Appalachia.[23] In 1992 the National Cancer Institute (NCI) issued a request for "applications that propose mobilization of community lay and professional leaders to develop and support community cancer control coalitions throughout Appalachia."[24] Concurrently, the NCI issued a comparable request for the formation of the National Hispanic Leadership on Cancer. This onetime solicitation, using a cooperative agreement funding mechanism, replicated the community-coalition approach introduced by the NCI in 1986 with the National Black Leadership Initiative on Cancer. Four centers were funded as part of the Appalachian Leadership Initiative on Cancer, representing the Central Highlands, North-Central Appalachia, Southern Appalachia, and Northern Appalachia. The strategies and challenges of these community coalitions are presented in *Sowing Seeds in the Mountains: Community-Based Coalitions for Cancer Prevention and Control.*[25]

CBPR employs a variety of study designs and methods. Although there are no strict rules defining this process, CBPR is an integration of the following elements: recognition of the community as the unit of identity; building on strengths and resources within the community; facilitation of the collaborative, equitable involvement of all partners in all phases of the research; integration of knowledge and intervention for the mutual benefit of all partners; promotion of a colearning and empowering process that attends to social inequalities; application of a cyclical and iterative process; understanding health from both positive and ecological perspectives; dissemination of findings and knowledge gained to all partners; and a long-term commitment by all partners.[26]

Lower Price Hill

Lower Price Hill is a predominantly urban Appalachian neighborhood located on Cincinnati's near west side. Appalachian families began moving into the area after World War II as the mostly German population moved to middle-class neighborhoods in the western suburbs. Unlike some Cincinnati neighborhoods, Lower Price Hill has remained a coherent entity with strong kinship networks. It is common to find several generations of a family living within a single building or within a few blocks of one another. A funeral becomes a community event as neighbors share food and condolences in a local school hall. The annual Appalachian Mini-Festival in the spring and Lower Price Hill Day in the fall have the flavor of reunions as former neighbors return to renew old ties and support those who still reside in the community. The Cincinnati Public Schools has operated a school in the neighborhood since 1931, and the Cincinnati Health Department has operated a primary care health clinic in the neighborhood since 1976.

Lower Price Hill faces many of the problems found in low-income neighborhoods. Census data for 2000[27] reveal that more than half (56 percent) of households in the neighborhood are below the poverty line. Women with children account for 49 percent of heads of households. The median household income is $17,500, compared with the citywide median of $37,500. The mean income for female heads of households with children is $5,242. The unemployment rate is 16 percent, compared with the city's rate of 5 percent; when students and the retired are included, the rate rises to 50 percent. Among adult residents, 62 percent do not have a high school diploma—the highest rate in the city; 46 percent are neither in school nor employed. Less than 8 percent of the neighborhood's population is African American. The neighborhood is also home to a growing population of Hispanic immigrants from rural areas of Mexico and Central America.

The neighborhood has a number of specific health risks due to its geographic location and local land-use patterns. Lower Price Hill is situated in the floodplains of the Ohio River and Mill Creek valleys, which form its boundaries on the south and east sides, respectively. Price Hill, which forms the neighborhood's western boundary, limits airflow when the winds blow from the east or west, allowing air to stagnate and industrial emissions and odors to concentrate. Several railroad lines pass through Lower Price Hill, and major traffic arteries for automobiles, buses, and commercial trucks crisscross the neighborhood. Zoning in Lower Price Hill is a mixture of high-density residential areas with intermediate and heavy manufacturing districts. Nearly every structure in the neighborhood was built between 1850 and 1900, leading to high risks for lead contamination. Over the years, the scraping and painting of highway and railway overpasses have contaminated neighborhood playgrounds and parks. Industrial processes include the fabrication and painting of metal products, application of industrial coatings, use of degreasing solvents, and use of compounding chemicals for foundries. The county's largest sewage processing facility has operated adjacent to the neighborhood since 1959, including on-site operation of a municipal waste dump and hazardous waste incinerator.

Concerned groups and individuals in Lower Price Hill first began to raise questions about the proximity of industrial and municipal processes and their impact on the environment and human health in the late 1970s. Residents successfully advocated for the shutdown and dismantling of a liquid waste incinerator operated at the nearby Metropolitan Sewer District Mill Creek Facility. Odors from this sewage treatment facility, the county's largest, and the on-site storage of chlorine gas have been constant challenges for the neighborhood. Pressure from the community also led to improvements in environmental controls at Queen City Barrel, which recycled fifty-five-gallon drums in the neighborhood until 2004, when several warehouses storing barrels burned out of control and the facility was closed. Prior to 2004, the "empty" barrels (as much as one inch of residue is legally allowed in each drum) were stockpiled in vacant warehouses, empty lots, and trailers parked along side streets in the neighborhood.

Community Responses: A Collaborative Health Research Approach

The Lower Price Hill (LPH) Task Force Report. The LPH Task Force was an independent coalition of individuals and representatives of organizations who were concerned about the environment, the health and learning abilities of the neighborhood's youngest residents, and the nonresponse of health, school, and environmental officials. The task force was organized after an external study conducted in the early 1980s indicated possible neurological damage among Lower Price Hill's children.

The LPH Task Force accessed and summarized public records from the U.S. Environmental Protection Agency, the Ohio Environmental Protection Agency, the Southwestern Ohio Air Pollution Control Agency, and the city of Cincinnati. A chronology of events in the community was compiled, including health hazard evaluations conducted by the National Institute of Occupational Safety and Health, violations of operating and emission permits, and enforcement actions. Achievement scores, the need for special education services, the frequency of learning disabilities, and indicators of neurological impairment among Lower Price Hill children and those living in other Cincinnati ZIP codes of similar socioeconomic status were compiled and compared.

Admission data from Cincinnati Children's Hospital Medical Center, the only regional hospital to admit young children before the mid-1990s, were obtained. Standardized morbidity ratio (SMR) analyses were conducted on hospital admissions (July 1, 1985–June 30, 1989) and emergency room (ER) visits (January 1, 1986–June 30, 1989) of children younger than 18 years from ZIP code 45204, which encompasses all of Lower Price Hill. Hospital admissions and ER visits for Lower Price Hill children were compared with those for children from the city of Cincinnati as a whole, as well as for children from four other ZIP codes with high percentages of white Appalachians of comparable socioeconomic status.[28, 29]

In June 1990 the LPH Task Force issued a report entitled "Health, Education, and Pollution in Lower Price Hill." It found significant differences among different age groups for a number of different disease codes. Among children younger than 5 years, acute respiratory infections were consistently elevated in children from Lower Price Hill compared with children from Cincinnati and other predominantly white Appalachian ZIP codes. Diseases of the ear and mastoid process were also significantly elevated among the Lower Price Hill children compared with children in the city. The statistically significant findings of the SMR analyses provided evidence that the children of Lower Price Hill faced considerably greater health challenges than their counterparts in other urban Appalachian neighborhoods and in the rest of the city. The LPH Task Force report put the onus for the neighborhood's health problems on industrial pollution instead of on the residents themselves.

The Environmental Leadership Coalition: A Partnership for Justice. In 1996 Cincinnati's Urban Appalachian Council was awarded a National Institute of Environmental Health Sciences grant, along with coinvestigators from the University of Cincinnati's Departments of Environmental Health and Communications and administrators from the Cincinnati Health Department. The grant program required a collaborative framework, stipulating that a community organization, a health care provider, and a research university develop a partnership to address community health issues. This community-based effort, called the Environmental Leadership Coalition: A Partnership for Justice, lasted for nine years, two grant cycles, and an intervening year of interrupted funding.

Leadership development was a core objective of all program activities through the two grant periods. Early in the first grant cycle (1996–1999), the Highlander Research and Education Center (and later Appalachian Focus) consulted with the Environmental Leadership Coalition, conducting a series of workshops on trust building, educational barriers, institutional responsiveness, and leadership development. Appalachian Focus guided the summer internships for neighborhood residents in the summers of 1997–1999. During these internships, core community leaders emerged to form the Lower Price Hill Environmental Leadership Group (ELG). The Urban Appalachian Council had already formed a youth program, the Youth Environmental Project, which would be integrated into the coalition's work.

During this first grant period, the idea of a children's health survey emerged from discussions among community-based interns who noticed recurring themes of frequent ear infections and respiratory illnesses, similar to the findings of the SMR analyses conducted for the 1990 LPH Task Force report. The goal of the survey was to identify the health problems of children living in Lower Price Hill, explore the impact of air pollution on the community's health, and share the results with the community. The survey questions were generated by the survey team, which consisted of members of the ELG, the Environmental Leadership Coalition program coordinator, and researchers from the University of Cincinnati's Department of Environmental Health, including an epidemiologist, a research associate, and an epidemiology graduate student. The idea was to describe the health of the neighborhood children without reference to other communities or other statistics.

Although the questionnaire was homegrown, established survey research methods were followed throughout its conduct. Survey team members were trained in survey research, including recruitment and interview techniques, form completion, procedures for maintaining confidentiality and minimizing bias, quality assurance and quality control protocols, data management procedures, and data analysis. University of Cincinnati researchers experienced in population-based epidemiological research conducted the training sessions.

Households with at least one child younger than 18 years living on the premises were eligible to participate. Only the parent, guardian, or primary caregiver (who had to be over 18) could complete the questionnaire for his or her child. The elements of participation were explained to each potential respondent, and he or she was asked to sign a consent form. Once consent was obtained, a face-to-face interview with the respondent was conducted by one of five trained community-based interviewers. The consent form and survey took about thirty minutes to complete.

The questionnaire focused on health conditions among neighborhood children and air quality conditions in the community. The following information was collected: household demographics; site of primary medical care; medical specialists seen in the previous twelve months; and number of children with selected symptoms (e.g., earaches or infections, diagnosis or treatment of asthma) in the past five years (1993–1997), breathing problems more than one time per month (not related to asthma), use of a breathing machine or inhaler, headaches more than two times per month, diagnosis or treatment of attention-deficit disorder (ADD) or attention-deficit hyperactivity disorder (ADHD), diagnosis or treatment of depression by a doctor, diagnosis of cancer or tumor, use of ear tubes for drainage, treatment for delayed speech, and diagnosis or treatment of muscular dystrophy, cerebral palsy, or multiple sclerosis. Two questions probed school absenteeism for health-related reasons in the previous year, and three questions involved blood testing for lead. Respondents were also asked about the frequency of odors in the neighborhood in a usual week, such as chlorine, paints or chemicals, raw sewage, and rotten eggs, and whether selected symptoms (e.g., watery or burning eyes, coughing, metal taste in the mouth, headaches) were associated with any of the smells. Each respondent was asked how many adults and children in the household smoked. Open-ended questions about the parents' concerns for their children's health were also included.

Data entry was completed by one ELG member, with oversight by the program coordinator. Data entry screens were created by a University of Cincinnati graduate student, and data entry and error checking procedures were developed by the university's epidemiologist on the survey team. The graduate student met with the ELG to identify the data analyses to be performed and to review the output. Data analysis was performed using Epi-Info statistical software.

Households were randomly selected to participate in the survey from a listing of housing units with children compiled by ELG members. Recruitment continued until approximately 50 percent of the Lower Price Hill households with children had been surveyed. One hundred twelve parents or guardians completed the survey, providing information on 264 children. No household with age-appropriate children refused to participate in the survey. Sixty-one percent of the children were 10 years of age or younger, and 72 percent of the children had lived their entire lives in the neighborhood. Key findings were presented in a booklet prepared by the ELG and presented at community meetings. Some of those findings included the following:

- There was a high frequency of breathing problems among Lower Price Hill children: 16 percent had been diagnosed with or treated for asthma, 15 percent had bronchitis symptoms more than three times per year, 14 percent had breathing problems (other than asthma) more than once a month, 15 percent used a breathing machine or inhaler, and 11 percent had visited an asthma or lung specialist in the past year.
- Many households were affected by lead poisoning: 72 percent of households had their children checked for lead, 28 percent of the children tested for lead had severe lead poisoning (greater than 20 micrograms), and 8 percent of the children had visited a lead poisoning specialist in the past year.

- There was a high frequency of children treated with ear tubes: 22 percent of the children had ear tubes inserted (approximately 50 percent of households), and 13 percent of the children had visited a hearing specialist in the past year.
- Many households were affected by tobacco smoke: 80 percent of households had one or more adult smoker, and 10 percent of households had one or more children who smoked.
- Parents were concerned about learning and developmental problems: 18 percent of respondents believed at least one of their children had an undiagnosed learning disability, 15 percent of the children had been treated for delayed speech development, and 10 percent of the children had been diagnosed with or treated for ADD or ADHD.
- Many respondents considered some of their children's health symptoms (e.g., headaches, coughing, burning eyes, shortness of breath, metal taste in the mouth) to be associated with odors they attributed to nearby industries. Between 42 and 77 percent of the respondents indicated that their children experienced each of the symptoms, and more than 85 percent associated each symptom's occurrence with at least one odor.

ELG members designed and produced a comic book entitled "LPH Our Kids' Health Survey, 'Justice or Just Us,'" telling the story of the children's health survey and its results. The story line and illustrations were created by community residents, including some who were not involved in conducting the survey. A two-page booklet of bulleted survey results was also developed and circulated. ELG members presented the survey findings to community residents and community-based agency personnel, who then evaluated these presentations: 68 percent of the residents and agency personnel found the results helpful, and among just the residents, 85 percent found the results helpful. Residents were particularly enthusiastic about the comic book as a meaningful way to communicate the survey findings, with more than 80 percent of presentation attendees approving of the comic book format. The findings about learning disabilities and respiratory problems raised the most concern, with cancer and allergies identified as issues to be addressed in the future.

Based on the survey findings, the ELG focused its attention on developing peer education programs in four health priority areas: asthma, lead poisoning prevention, ear infections and ear tubes, and smoking cessation. Community-specific training on asthma and lead was developed and presented in neighborhood settings, reaching more than 200 residents in the first two years. These peer education sessions were conducted in community centers and homeless shelters, as well as in the kitchens of community residents. Age-appropriate materials for young children and adults were developed. For example, an Old Maid asthma prevention card game was created.

ELG members also researched lead poisoning prevention and lead abatement techniques, creating an education module similar to the one for asthma prevention and management. ELG members shared the lead poisoning prevention measures with the Youth Environmental Project, which incorporated the best practices into a puppet show targeted at young people who babysit for young children and siblings. Both the ELG and the Youth Environmental Project developed smoking cessation and tobacco prevention modules to reach adults in their homes and young children in neighborhood after-school programs.

The program coordinator and assistant director of the Urban Appalachian Council summarized the survey's impact on the community in the following manner: "The health survey was very important to the neighborhood in a number of ways. First, just the act of developing and then conducting the survey got people talking to each other about their children's health and considering the trends and patterns of the illnesses. The most direct result has been the peer health education programs on asthma and lead, which have reached hundreds of neighbors and have raised knowledge and awareness even among those not directly involved."[30]

ELG members were proud of the 100 percent survey participation rate, which they attributed to the fact that community residents conducted the survey, rather than outside professionals. This was an enviable response rate for any survey research project, especially one conducted in a low-income urban community that mistrusts researchers and institutions. Neighbor interviewing neighbor (using a standardized research protocol) generated data that would otherwise not be available for Lower Price Hill. The familiarity among friends and neighbors and the trust that they would use the data responsibly were implicit and were not lost on ELG members—they understood that even the smallest breach of confidentiality could derail the survey and preclude any future survey research in the neighborhood.

The Lower Price Hill health survey gave the community useful information about the health status of children in the neighborhood. Even though the survey was not designed to collect data that could be compared with city, county, state, or national statistics, ELG members and parents began asking about additional issues as the survey progressed. For instance, cancer needed to be studied in more detail, and residents began to wonder how their health compared with that in other neighborhoods. Even before the children's health survey was completed, the ELG and the Environmental Leadership Coalition agreed that a women's health survey was the next priority and that the ability to compare results with other communities was an important factor.

The Women's Health Survey. In anticipation of doing a women's health survey, ELG members began organizing small-group discussions with neighborhood women, young and old, to identify health issues of concern for inclusion in the survey. Over several months, three small-group discussions were conducted in a storefront meeting space in the neighborhood. The atmosphere was nonjudgmental; the women were encouraged to discuss intimate health problems without identifying the persons experiencing those problems. ELG members probed, asking questions about sensitive topics such as abuse, depression, reproductive outcomes, family history, and gynecologic health.

The purpose of the Lower Price Hill women's health survey was to describe the health problems and concerns of women living in the neighborhood, compare the results with other communities, identify needed medical services, identify potential health problems based on family medical histories, identify barriers to health care, and advocate for necessary changes. In addition to demographic data, the following information was collected: work history, diagnosed medical conditions, treatment of medical conditions, screening tests, reproductive history, family history of diagnosed cancers and selected conditions, female health problems, cause of death of blood relatives, domestic abuse, and general well-being. Two final questions asked whether either parent or any grandparent had been born in the Appalachian region. County maps of the federally designated

Appalachian region were available at each interview station to assist respondents in answering these questions. The women's survey ran nineteen pages, compared with the eleven-page children's health survey.

To allow the comparison of Lower Price Hill survey results with results in other communities (something the children's survey was not designed to address), a University of Cincinnati graduate student combed the literature to identify questionnaires that elicited the same types of data that would be collected in the survey. The intent was to use questions from surveys with published results so that the findings could be compared. Questions from four survey instruments were used verbatim or with slight modification in the women's health survey. The instrument used most frequently was the 2000 Greater Cincinnati Community Health Status Survey (GCCHSS).[a] Thirteen questions from the GCCHSS pertaining to the frequency of health screenings, general sense of well-being, satisfaction with health care, personal health concerns, and community health concerns were included in the women's health survey. Three questions adopted from the National Health and Nutrition Examination Survey II pertained to the availability of emotional and financial support from friends and family. Questions about physical, sexual, and emotional abuse were taken from the Abuse Assessment Screen on the Centers for Disease Control and Prevention website and the Women's Health Initiative.

Early in the design process, the survey team and ELG members decided to include Latina women living in the neighborhood. Community members considered the inclusion of Spanish-speaking women important if the survey was to reflect the health of all women living in Lower Price Hill. The survey thus had no length of residency or language restrictions. This decision required that the questionnaire, consent form, and supplemental materials be translated into Spanish; that recruiters and interviewers (potentially from outside the community) be identified and trained; and that awareness sessions be conducted to ensure that the survey team members and interview locations were welcoming and that the Spanish-speaking interviewers and respondents felt comfortable and safe. One bilingual white woman and two women from Central America were hired to conduct the Spanish version of the survey, including recruitment, scheduling, survey interviews, and processing, under the close supervision of the lead researcher.

In all aspects, the women's health survey was larger and more complicated than the children's health survey. As noted, the questionnaire was almost double the length, and many of the health-related issues were addressed in greater detail. The questionnaire was estimated to take up to two hours to complete. Given the length of the questionnaire and the sensitivity of some of the topics covered, the interviews were conducted at a health resource center established in the neighborhood by a group of local women to minimize interruptions by children and intrusions by spouses or male companions. The surveys were conducted in small, intimate spaces where the responses would be confidential and distractions were minimized. Child care was available in a separate area of the health resource center, and men's access was restricted during interview sessions. A University of Cincinnati researcher was on site during each interview to assist with questions.

Female ELG members, members of the local Women's Wellness Group, Urban Appalachian Council personnel, and female community members volunteered to help conduct the survey. Only one male ELG member participated in the survey, assisting with the processing of forms. Women were trained to be recruiters, interviewers, hostess-greeters, child-care supervisors, and processors. Depending on the job, individuals completed between two and ten hours of training. The training topics included the same ones covered in the children's health survey: recruitment and interview techniques, form completion and processing, procedures for maintaining confidentiality and minimizing bias, quality assurance and quality control protocols, and error checking.

Because of the time required to conduct the survey and complete the questionnaire, vouchers were available for the participants and the persons staffing the survey. Each person who completed a questionnaire received a $10 voucher to a grocery store chain. A $20 voucher to the same grocery store chain was given to each interviewer for each successfully completed survey. Successful completion meant that all the questions were answered, the survey was readable, and the answers were consistent and logical.

A detailed door-to-door census of the neighborhood was conducted to identify all inhabited housing units. The definition of the neighborhood was expanded from the customary ZIP code delineation to include all the street blocks considered to be in Lower Price Hill by neighborhood residents. A database of inhabited housing units was used to identify households for recruitment. Two-person recruitment teams went to each randomly selected housing unit to determine whether an eligible woman (i.e., at least 18 years of age) lived at the address. If the woman living in the home was eligible and willing to participate, an interview appointment was scheduled.

A team consisting of three ELG members, two Women's Wellness Group members, and two University of Cincinnati researchers was created to direct the data analysis. The team conducted data management tasks such as categorizing responses to open-ended questions, reviewing output for consistency and logic, identifying data analysis questions for the programmer to perform, and summarizing the findings for dissemination to the community and presentation to professional organizations.

A total of 144 women, approximately 32 percent of the women in Lower Price Hill, completed the survey. Eighty-two percent were white, 11 percent were black, and 5 percent were Latina. The average age was 43 years; 30 percent were aged 50 years or older. Health findings included the following:

- Family medical history: the most common causes of death were cardiovascular disease (23 percent) and cancer (20 percent) among the respondents' fathers and cardiovascular disease (31 percent) and cancer (29 percent) among their mothers.
- Family history of common chronic diseases (depression, diabetes, drug or alcohol problems, heart disease, stomach problems, and stroke): 24 percent of respondents reported their fathers had drug or alcohol problems, 15 percent reported their fathers had heart disease, 28 percent reported their mothers had depression, and 23 percent reported their mothers had diabetes.
- Family history of cancer: 78 percent of respondents had a family history of cancer (cancer diagnosed in a grandparent, parent, aunt or uncle, sister or brother, or daughter or son), 41 percent had a family history of cancer in more than one generation, and the most commonly reported cancers were breast, colon/bowel, lung, and cervix.

The next set of findings compares the Lower Price Hill women's survey responses to those of female respondents in the 2000 GCCHSS (given in parentheses):

- Time since last screening: 23 percent (versus 35 percent) of respondents reported their last mammogram was within the past year, 51 percent (versus 40 percent) reported they had never had a mammogram, 23 percent (versus 52 percent) reported their last cholesterol test was within the past year, and 44 percent (versus 18 percent) reported they had never had a cholesterol test.
- General health and well-being: 6 percent (versus 19 percent) of respondents described their health as excellent, 39 percent (versus 20 percent) described their health as fair or poor, and 40 percent (versus 61 percent) reported that health problems never interfered with their social activities.
- Health care: 72 percent (versus 87 percent) of respondents were very or fairly well satisfied with the quality of their health care, 64 percent (versus 83 percent) were very or fairly well satisfied with the availability of health care, and 37 percent (versus 15 percent) rated their satisfaction with their overall health care as fair or poor.
- Community health concerns: In the Lower Price Hill survey, 28 percent of respondents cited drug abuse, 10 percent cited air quality, and 7 percent cited prostitution as their greatest health concerns for the community. In contrast, GCCHSS respondents identified cancer (13 percent), available health care (6 percent), and cost of health care (5 percent) most frequently.

Presentations to the community proposed the following next steps to take: work with local experts to plan necessary health services and educational programs, seek funding for health services and programs, work with local health care providers on health services and educational programs, and advocate for new or enhanced services and programs with local government agencies. Community residents were also encouraged to promote their own health by knowing their family history for heart disease, cancer, and diabetes; talking with a doctor about their risks for heart disease, cancer, and diabetes; getting screened for breast cancer, cervical cancer, high cholesterol, high blood pressure, and diabetes; and knowing the signs of depression and alcohol or drug dependency and seeking early treatment. In addition, women were encouraged to attend the annual Lower Price Hill Health Fair conducted by the Women's Wellness Group and to join the group.

Conclusions

CBPR methods have been used to identify, document, and characterize environmental and public health issues of concern to Lower Price Hill residents. In a small community such as Lower Price Hill, the funding provided by the National Institute for Environmental Health Sciences, leveraged by a local Appalachian organization, represented a sizable infusion of money and relevant expertise.[b] The two community health surveys afforded community residents, agency personnel, and university-based researchers the opportunity to investigate neighborhood health issues, prioritize the neighborhood's concerns, and develop strategies to improve health. The community's long-standing concerns about environmental pollution provided the incentive to investigate the health impacts of years of exposure. The Women's Wellness Group and the ELG provided critical outlets for residents to use their skills, knowledge, and data to effect change. Prioritizing findings and strategizing approaches to improve the neighborhood's health rested with these groups.

CBPR methods generate data of meaning to the local community. In essence, community residents ask and answer their own research questions—questions that matter to them. Robust data sources are the result when communities have the opportunity to collect information about their neighborhoods using CBPR methods. Residents can then engage one another, health care providers, planners, and policy analysts in meaningful discussions about shared and unique priorities, as well as strategies to leverage resources to better manage if not prevent unhealthy conditions. Healthier and safer communities result when community leaders, residents, providers, analysts, and researchers are informed about local health status and use consensus to build strategies to improve the health of residents and communities.

No research happens in a vacuum, whether it is conducted in a community setting or in a research laboratory. As community residents understand intuitively, many dimensions of health have to do with social, political, environmental, geographic, and other dimensions of human lives. Unlike the traditional course of research that slowly builds a body of knowledge, the origins of CBPR are rooted in change; it is conducted precisely to effect change. Although CBPR can be used to evaluate interventions and investigate the etiologies of diseases, its connection to communities of people necessitates a more immediate link to outcomes. Too often, the response to CBPR and community-driven research by government agencies, health care providers, and researchers is to dismiss the data as nonscientific or inconclusive. Casting doubt on the rigor of the research, the soundness of the findings, or the relevance to hypothesis-driven research data delays meaningful response. When health care providers as well as researchers, planners, and analysts at universities, nonprofit organizations, and government agencies embrace CBPR methods, public health agendas can be formulated from the ground up rather than from the top down. Effective collaborative strategies will result.

Further Research

Greater utilization of CBPR methods is needed to understand and address the health issues facing Appalachians, whether in urban neighborhoods or rural communities. Agencies and organizations that fund research need to engage nonscientists, community residents, patients, survivors, and advocates when setting future research agendas and reviewing grant applications so that all stakeholders have an opportunity to contribute to an understanding of health and disease and the development of effective strategies to improve health.

Federal funding agencies and private foundations need to fund more CBPR projects. These grant programs should be ongoing and adequately funded to support the essential research, education, and health improvement objectives of CBPR. Grant management and reporting requirements need to be streamlined so community-oriented agencies and organizations can serve as the lead institutions.

Institutional review boards need to be better informed about CBPR methods and give community-based coinvestigators access to data so that analyses, interpretations, communications of findings, and publications reflect the input of all the project collaborators. Likewise, published findings need to be readily available to the public at large. Pay-for-view access to study results undermines the ability of individuals not affiliated with academic institutions or government agencies to meaningfully participate in all phases of public health research, priority and policy setting, and practice.

Policy Recommendations

CBPR is a two-way street, with professional researchers and neighborhood residents learning from each other. Flexibility without loss of rigor is important so that good methodological practices are maintained and the immediate concerns of the community are addressed. The following policy recommendations speak to these important aspects of CBPR.

The threshold for public health action needs to be reset so that prevention and intervention strategies are developed and implemented with the best available information. In all likelihood, this will happen based on the precautionary principle: that is, if an action or policy involves a suspected risk of harm to the public or the environment, the burden of proving a lack of harm falls on those taking the action. This principle is often invoked before causation has been proved.

Regulators, public health officials, and community planners need to become knowledgeable about CBPR. They must recognize that no single research discipline or methodology is sufficient to capture all the complexities of public health issues or to creatively design effective strategies to address the multiple aspects of those issues.

Collaborative education and training opportunities need to be expanded. Community residents, patients, survivors, and advocates should be educated in health research concepts, standards, and methods so that they can meaningfully participate in all phases of public health research and practice. Researchers need to be educated about the social context of knowledge production and should be trained in CBPR methods.[31]

Notes

a. The 2000 GCCHSS was a random-digit-dialed telephone survey, consisting of 100+ questions, conducted with more than 2,000 adults in twenty-two counties in southeastern Indiana, southwestern Ohio, and northern Kentucky.

b. The funding partially supported the lead agency's administration and management of the grant, supplies and rental space, salaries for university-based researchers and agency staff members, honoraria for community residents serving as survey workers, and gift cards for survey participants. Given the scope and hands-on participation of community residents who were initially unfamiliar with research principles and methods, it would not have been possible to conduct the community health surveys without multiyear funding. The sense of purpose the surveys engendered and the commitment to the betterment of the neighborhood encouraged all those involved to stay engaged, complete the surveys, and report the findings. Residents, staff, and researchers demonstrated enduring commitments to one another, the process, and the community.

References

1. Couto RA. Failing health and new prescriptions: community-based approaches to environmental risks. In: Hill CE, ed. *Current Health Policy Issues and Alternatives: An Applied Social Science Perspective.* Athens, GA: University of Georgia Press; 1986:53–70.

2. O'Fallon L, Tyson F, Dearry A, eds. Successful models of community-based participatory research: final report of meeting hosted by the NIEHS in Washington, D.C., March 29–31, 2000. Washington, DC: National Institute of Environmental Health Science; 2000.

3. Minkler M, Wallerstein N. *Community Based Participatory Research for Health.* San Francisco, CA: Jossey-Bass; 2003.

4. Israel BA. *Methods in Community-Based Participatory Research for Health.* 1st ed. San Francisco, CA: Jossey-Bass; 2005.

5. Cargo M, Mercer SL. The value and challenges of participatory research: strengthening its practice. *Annu Rev Public Health.* 2008;29:325–350.

6. Krieger N, Rowley DL, Herman AA, Avery B, Phillips MT. Racism, sexism, and social class: implications for studies of health, disease, and well-being. *Am J Prev Med.* 1993;9:82–122.

7. Williams DR, Collins C. U.S. socioeconomic and racial differences in health: patterns and explanations. *Annual Review of Sociology.* 1995;21:349–386.

8. Bullard RD. *Unequal Protection: Environmental Justice and Communities of Color.* San Francisco, CA: Sierra Club Books; 1994.

9. McKinlay JB. The promotion of health through planned sociopolitical change: challenges for research and policy. *Soc Sci Med.* 1993;36:109–117.

10. Brown ER. Community action for health promotion: a strategy to empower individuals and communities. *Int J Health Serv.* 1991;21:441–456.

11. Gaventa J. Toward a knowledge democracy: viewpoints on participatory research in North America. In: Fals-Borda O, Rahman MA, eds. *Action and Knowledge: Breaking the Monopoly with Participatory Action Research.* New York, NY: Apex Press; 1991.

12. Brown P, Kroll-Smith S, Gunter VJ. Knowledge, citizens, and organizations: an overview of environments, diseases, and social conflict. In: Kroll-Smith S, Brown P, Gunter VJ, eds. *Illness and the Environment: A Reader in Contested Medicine.* New York, NY: New York University Press; 2000:9–28.

13. National Institute of Environmental Health Sciences. Environmental justice and community-based participatory research. Available at: http://www.niehs.nih.gov/research/supported/programs/justice/. Accessed May 30, 2011.

14. National Institute of Environmental Health Sciences. Community-based prevention and intervention research. Available at: http://grants.nih.gov/grants/guide/rfa-files/RFA-ES-99–012.html. Accessed May 30, 2011.

15. Community-Institutional Partnerships for Prevention Research Group. Appendix A: selected organizations and websites. Available at: http://depts .washington.edu/ccph/cbpr/append/a_append.php. Accessed May 30, 2011.

16. Community-Campus Partnerships for Health. Community-based participatory research. Available at: http://depts.washington.edu/ccph/commbas.html. Accessed May 30, 2011.

17. Couto RA, DeBruicker J. Lessons from community-based participatory research in Appalachia. In: Obermiller PJ, Maloney ME, eds. *Appalachia: Social Context Past and Present.* 5th ed. Dubuque, IA: Kendall/Hunt Publishing; 2007:337–343.

18. Lewis HM. Participatory research and education for social change: Highlander Research and Education Center. In: Reason P, Bradbury H, eds. *Handbook of Action Research: Participative Inquiry and Practice.* Thousand Oaks, CA: Sage; 2001.

19. Appalachian Land Ownership Task Force. Land ownership patterns and their impacts on Appalachian communities: a survey of 80 counties. ERIC Document No. ED325280. Washington, DC: Appalachian Regional Commission; 1981. Available at: http://www.eric.ed.gov/. Accessed September 11, 2011.

20. Beaver PD. Participatory research on land ownership in Appalachia. In: Bateau A, ed. *Appalachia and America: Autonomy and Regional Dependence.* Lexington, KY: University Press of Kentucky; 1983.

21. Horton BD. The Appalachian land ownership study: research and citizen action in Appalachia. In: Park P, Brydon-Miller M, Hall B, Jackson T, eds. *Voices of Change: Participatory Research in the United States and Canada.* Toronto, Canada: Ontario Institute for Studies in Education; 1993.

22. Scott SL. Discovering what the people knew: the 1979 land ownership study. *Action Research.* 2009;7(2):207–227.

23. Halverson JA, Ma L, Harner EJ. An analysis of disparities in health status and access to health care in the Appalachian region. Washington, DC: Appalachian Regional Commission; 2004.

24. National Cancer Institute. Appalachia leadership initiative on cancer. Available at: http://grants.nih.gov/guide/rfa-files/RFA-CA-92–011.html. Accessed March 1, 2011.

25. Couto RA, Simpson NK, Harris G, National Cancer Institute, Division of Resources Centers and Community Activities. *Sowing Seeds in the Mountains: Community-Based Coalitions for Cancer Prevention and Control.* Washington, DC: Appalachia Leadership Initiative on Cancer, Division of Cancer Prevention and Control, National Cancer Institute; 1995.

26. Israel BA, Schulz AJ, Parker EA, Becker AB. Review of community-based research: assessing partnership approaches to improve public health. *Annu Rev Public Health.* 1998;19:173–202.

27. Maloney ME, Auffrey C, eds. *The Social Areas of Cincinnati: An Analysis of Social Needs.* 4th ed. Cincinnati, OH: University of Cincinnati School of Planning and the University of Cincinnati Institute for Community Partnerships; 2004.

28. Maloney ME. *The Social Areas of Cincinnati: An Analysis of Social Needs.* 2nd ed. Cincinnati, OH: Cincinnati Human Relations Commission; 1985.

29. Brown MK, Obermiller PJ. The health status of children living in urban Appalachian neighborhoods. In: Borman KM, Obermiller PJ, eds. *From Mountains to Metropolis: Appalachian Migrants in American Cities.* Westport, CT: Bergin and Garvey; 1994:71–82.

30. Sonnenberg E. Are the kids all right? Available at: http://www.NeighborhoodAmerica.com. Accessed February 22, 2000.

31. Gibbons M, Limoges C, Nowotny H, Schwartzman S, Scott P, Trow M. *The New Production of Knowledge: The Dynamics of Science and Research in Contemporary Societies.* Los Angeles, CA: Sage; 2007.

Acknowledgments

We deeply appreciate the patience and trust of the contributors to this volume. They persevered through multiple revisions of their chapters over a period of nearly four years, trusting that we would one day shepherd their essays into print.

Barbara Ludke not only provided emotional support for this project but also improved the manuscript by her editorial and substantive insights. Keith Witt at the Appalachian Regional Commission helped us acquire regional maps. Richard P. Mulcahy, coeditor of the health section of the *Encyclopedia of Appalachia,* is a fellow editor whose insight and collegiality we greatly value. We thank each of them most sincerely.

Colleagues in the Appalachian Studies Association, staff at the Urban Appalachian Council, and fellow members of the council's Research Committee supplied the encouragement and criticism necessary to keep us grounded throughout the multiyear process of developing the manuscript. They are our touchstones.

We are also grateful for the work of the peer reviewers who made this volume possible and whose suggestions made it better. Steve Wrinn, Allison Webster, and the staff at the University Press of Kentucky have been unfailingly professional and supportive throughout the publication process.

Both of us enjoyed the support of our respective institutions: the University of Cincinnati Department of Family and Community Medicine, the university's School of Planning, and the University of Kentucky Appalachian Center. We are especially grateful to Ronnie Horner, professor, University of Cincinnati Department of Internal Medicine, for his support and commitment to this venture.

Clearly we were not alone in this endeavor and are deeply indebted to all who had a hand in it. Nevertheless, we alone hold responsibility for any of its defects.

Selected Bibliography

Abramson R, Haskell J. *Encyclopedia of Appalachia*. Knoxville, TN: University of Tennessee Press; 2006.

Ahijevych K, Kuun P, Christman S, Wood T, Browning K, Wewers ME. Beliefs about tobacco among Appalachian current and former users. *Appl Nurs Res*. 2003;16:93–102.

Barnett E, Halverson JA, Elmes GA, Braham VE. Metropolitan and non-metropolitan trends in coronary heart disease mortality within Appalachia, 1980–1997. *Ann Epidemiol*. 2000;10:370–379.

Behringer B, Friedell GH. Appalachia: where place matters in health. *Prev Chronic Dis*. 2006;3:A113.

Bell JL, Helmkamp JC. Non-fatal injuries in the West Virginia logging industry: using workers' compensation claims to assess risk from 1995 through 2001. *Am J Ind Med*. 2003;44:502–509.

Borman KM, Obermiller PJ, eds. *From Mountains to Metropolis: Appalachian Migrants in American Cities*. Westport, CT: Bergin and Garvey; 1994.

Casto BC, Sharma S, Fisher JL, Knobloch TJ, Agrawal A, Weghorst CM. Oral cancer in Appalachia. *J Health Care Poor Underserved*. 2009;20:274–285.

Couto RA, DeBruicker J. Lessons from community-based participatory research in Appalachia. In: Obermiller PJ, Maloney ME, eds. *Appalachia: Social Context Past and Present*. 5th ed. Dubuque, IA: Kendall/Hunt Publishing; 2007:337–343.

Couto RA, Simpson NK, Harris G, National Cancer Institute, Division of Resources Centers and Community Activities. *Sowing Seeds in the Mountains: Community-Based Coalitions for Cancer Prevention and Control*. Washington, DC: Appalachia Leadership Initiative on Cancer, Division of Cancer Prevention and Control, National Cancer Institute; 1994.

Coyne CA, Demian-Popescu C, Friend D. Social and cultural factors influencing health in southern West Virginia: a qualitative study. *Prev Chronic Dis*. 2006;3:A124.

Denham SA. Family health in a rural Appalachian Ohio county. *Journal of Appalachian Studies*. 1996;2(2):299–310.

Denham SA, Meyer MG, Toborg MA, Mande MJ. Providing health education to Appalachia populations. *Holist Nurs Pract*. 2004;18:293–301.

Evans RG, Barer ML, Marmor TR, eds. *Why Are Some People Healthy and Not Others: The Determinants of Health of Populations*. New York, NY: Aldine de Gruyter; 1994.

Hall HI, Rogers JD, Weir HK, Miller DS, Uhler RJ. Breast and cervical carcinoma mortality among women in the Appalachian region of the U.S., 1976–1996. *Cancer.* 2000;89:1593–1602.

Halperin RH, Reiter-Purtill J. "Nerves" in rural and urban Appalachia. In: Keefe SE, ed. *Appalachian Cultural Competency: A Guide for Medical, Mental Health, and Social Service Professionals.* Knoxville, TN: University of Tennessee Press; 2005:265–284.

Halverson JA, Bischak G. Underlying socioeconomic factors influencing health disparities in the Appalachian region. Washington, DC: Appalachian Regional Commission; 2008.

Halverson JA, Ma L, Harner EJ. An analysis of disparities in health status and access to health care in the Appalachian region. Washington, DC: Appalachian Regional Commission; 2004.

Hansel P, Brown K, Collins S, et al. Health, education, and pollution in Lower Price Hill. Cincinnati, OH: Urban Appalachian Council; 1990.

Hendryx M. Mortality from heart, respiratory, and kidney disease in coal mining areas of Appalachia. *Int Arch Occup Environ Health.* 2009;82:243–249.

Hendryx M, Ahern MM. Relations between health indicators and residential proximity to coal mining in West Virginia. *Am J Public Health.* 2008;98:669–671.

Hendryx M, Ahern MM. Mortality in Appalachian coal mining regions: the value of statistical life lost. *Public Health Rep.* 2009;124:541–550.

Holben DH, Pheley AM. Diabetes risk and obesity in food-insecure households in rural Appalachian Ohio. *Prev Chronic Dis.* 2006;3:A82.

Hopenhayn C, Bush H, Christian A, Shelton BJ. Comparative analysis of invasive cervical cancer incidence rates in three Appalachian states. *Prev Med.* 2005;41:859–864.

Huang B, Wyatt SW, Tucker TC, Bottorff D, Lengerich E, Hall HI. Cancer death rates—Appalachia, 1994–1998. *MMWR Weekly.* 2002;51:527–529.

Hutson SP, Dorgan KA, Phillips AN, Behringer B. The mountains hold things in: the use of community research review work groups to address cancer disparities in Appalachia. *Oncol Nurs Forum.* 2007;34:1133–1139.

Huttlinger K, Schaller-Ayers J, Lawson T. Health care in Appalachia: a population-based approach. *Public Health Nurs.* 2004;21:103–110.

Kearney PA, Stallones L, Swartz C, Barker DE, Johnson SB. Unintentional injury death rates in rural Appalachia. *J Trauma.* 1990;30:1524–1532.

Keefe SE. *Appalachian Cultural Competency: A Guide for Medical, Mental Health, and Social Service Professionals.* 1st ed. Knoxville, TN: University of Tennessee Press; 2005.

Lyttle NL, Stadelman K. Assessing awareness and knowledge of breast and cervical cancer among Appalachian women. *Prev Chronic Dis.* 2006;3:A125.

Maloney ME, Auffrey C, eds. *The Social Areas of Cincinnati: An Analysis of Social Needs.* 4th ed. Cincinnati, OH: University of Cincinnati School of Planning and the University of Cincinnati Institute for Community Partnerships; 2004.

Marmot MG, Wilkinson RG. *Social Determinants of Health*. 2nd ed. New York, NY: Oxford University Press; 2006.

Mary Babb Randolph Cancer Center/Office for Social Environmental and Health Research. Underlying socioeconomic factors influencing health disparities in the Appalachian region. Final Report Contract No. CO-15198. Morgantown, WV: Department of Community Medicine, Robert C. Byrd Health Sciences Center, West Virginia University; 2008.

Meyer MG, Toborg MA, Denham SA, Mande MJ. Cultural perspectives concerning adolescent use of tobacco and alcohol in the Appalachian Mountain region. *J Rural Health*. 2008;24:67–74.

Nolan RL, Schwartz JL, eds. *Rural and Appalachian Health*. Springfield, IL: Charles C. Thomas; 1973.

Obermiller PJ, Wagner TE, Tucker B, eds. *Appalachian Odyssey: Historical Perspectives on the Great Migration*. New York, NY: Praeger; 2000.

Rademacher EW, Ludke RL, Misner JM. 2005 Greater Cincinnati community health status report. Cincinnati, OH: Institute for Policy Research, University of Cincinnati; 2006.

Schwartz F, Ruhil AV, Denham S, Shubrook J, Simpson C, Boyd SL. High self-reported prevalence of diabetes mellitus, heart disease, and stroke in 11 counties of rural Appalachian Ohio. *J Rural Health*. 2009;25:226–230.

Shackelford L, Weinberg B, Anderson DR. *Our Appalachia: An Oral History*. Lexington, KY: University Press of Kentucky; 1988.

Shell R, Tudiver F. Barriers to cancer screening by rural Appalachian primary care providers. *J Rural Health*. 2004;20:368–373.

Song H, Fish M. Demographic and psychosocial characteristics of smokers and nonsmokers in low-socioeconomic status rural Appalachian 2-parent families in southern West Virginia. *J Rural Health*. 2006;22:83–87.

Stensland J, Mueller C, Sutton J. An analysis of the financial conditions of health care institutions in the Appalachian region and their economic impacts. Washington, DC: Appalachian Regional Commission; 2002.

Tessaro I, Mangone C, Parkar I, Pawar V. Knowledge, barriers, and predictors of colorectal cancer screening in an Appalachian church population. *Prev Chronic Dis*. 2006;3:A123.

Thoenen E. *Health Risks: The Appalachian Lifestyle*. Charleston, WV: West Virginia Department of Health and Human Resources, Health Statistics Center; 1995.

Tincher RB. Night comes to the chromosomes: inbreeding and population genetics in southern Appalachia. *Central Issues in Anthropology*. 1980;2(1):27–50.

Wallace JP, Baugh C, Cornett S, et al. A family history demonstration project among women in an urban Appalachian community. *Prog Community Health Partnersh*. 2009;3:155–163.

Wewers ME, Ahijevych KL, Chen MS, Dresbach S, Kihm KE, Kuun PA. Tobacco use characteristics among rural Ohio Appalachians. *J Community Health.* 2000;25:377–388.

Williams JA. *Appalachia: A History.* Chapel Hill, NC: University of North Carolina Press; 2002.

Wingo PA, Tucker TC, Jamison PM, et al. Cancer in Appalachia, 2001–2003. *Cancer.* 2008;112:181–192.

Zhang Z, Infante A, Meit M, English N, Dunn M, Bowers KH. An analysis of mental health and substance abuse disparities and access to treatment services in the Appalachian region. Washington, DC: Appalachian Regional Commission; 2008.

Contributors

Carol S. Baugh, PhD, is Coordinator, Appalachian Studies, Sinclair Community College, and Director, Fairborn Education Foundation and Alumni Association.

Bruce A. Behringer, MPH, is Associate Vice President, Division of Health Science, East Tennessee State University.

Andrew C. Bernard, MD, is Associate Professor of Surgery, Acute Care Surgery, Trauma and Surgical Critical Care, College of Medicine, University of Kentucky.

Kristine Harper Bowers, BA, is Research Assistant and Coordinator of Substance Abuse Projects, Office of Rural and Community Health and Community Partnerships, East Tennessee State University.

M. Kathryn Brown, PhD, is an environmental epidemiologist and a community health research consultant based in Cincinnati.

Eleanor Sue Cantrell, MD, is Director, Lenowisco Health District, Virginia Department of Health.

Mark A. Carrozza, MA, is Health Informatics Developer, The Health Foundation of Greater Cincinnati.

Jennifer Chubinski, MSPPM, is Director of Community Research, The Health Foundation of Greater Cincinnati.

Julia F. Costich, MPA, JD, PhD, is Associate Professor and Chair, Department of Health Services Management, College of Public Health, University of Kentucky.

Richard J. Crout, DMD, PhD, is Associate Dean for Research and Professor of Periodontics, School of Dentistry, and Professor of Biochemistry, School of Medicine, West Virginia University.

Lisa Curtin, PhD, is Professor, Department of Psychology, Appalachian State University.

Sharon A. Denham, DSN, RN, is Professor Emerita, School of Nursing, Ohio University.

Mark B. Dignan, PhD, MPH, is Director, Prevention Research Center, University of Kentucky.

Michael S. Dunn, PhD, is Associate Professor of Health Promotion, Coastal Carolina University.

E. Kelly Firesheets, PsyD, is Director of Evaluation, The Health Foundation of Greater Cincinnati.

James L. Fisher, PhD, is Research Scientist, Ohio Cancer Registry, The Ohio State University Medical Center, and Adjunct Assistant Professor, College of Public Health, The Ohio State University.

Gilbert H. Friedell, MD, is Director Emeritus, Markey Cancer Center, University of Kentucky.

Joel A. Halverson, PhD, is Research Assistant Professor, Pharmaceutical Systems and Policy, School of Pharmacy, West Virginia University.

Michael S. Hendryx, PhD, is Director, West Virginia Rural Health Research Center, and Associate Professor, Department of Community Medicine, West Virginia University.

Ronnie D. Horner, PhD, is Professor, Department of Internal Medicine, College of Medicine, University of Cincinnati.

Mira L. Katz, PhD, is Associate Professor, Division of Health Behavior and Health Promotion, College of Public Health, The Ohio State University.

Paul A. Kearney, MD, is Professor of Surgery and Section Head, Acute Care Surgery, Trauma and Surgical Critical Care, College of Medicine, University of Kentucky.

Susan E. Keefe, PhD, is Professor, Department of Anthropology, Appalachian State University.

Evelyn A. Knight, PhD, is Associate Professor, Department of Health Behavior, College of Public Health, University of Kentucky.

Robert L. Ludke, PhD, is Professor, Department of Family and Community Medicine, College of Medicine, University of Cincinnati.

Mary L. Marazita, PhD, is Associate Dean of Research and Director, Center for Craniofacial and Dental Genetics; Professor and Vice Chair, Department of Oral Biology, School of Dental Medicine; Director and Professor of Human Genetics, Graduate School of Public Health; Professor, Clinical and Translational Science Institute; and Professor of Psychiatry, School of Medicine, University of Pittsburgh.

Ann L. McCracken, PhD, is former Director of Evaluation, The Health Foundation of Greater Cincinnati.

John M. McLaughlin, PhD, is Regional Medical Research Scientist and Director of Outcomes Research, Specialty Medicines Development Group, Pfizer, Inc.

Daniel W. McNeil, PhD, is Professor of Psychology and Eberly Professor of Public Service, Eberly College of Arts and Sciences, and Clinical Professor, Department of Dental Practice and Rural Health, School of Dentistry, West Virginia University.

Melanie F. Myers, PhD, MS, CGC, is Assistant Professor, Division of Human Genetics, Department of Pediatrics, and Director, Genetic Counseling Graduate Program, University of Cincinnati and Cincinnati Children's Hospital Medical Center.

Phillip J. Obermiller, PhD, is Senior Visiting Scholar, School of Planning, University of Cincinnati, and Fellow, Appalachian Center, University of Kentucky.

Electra D. Paskett, PhD, is Marion N. Rowley Professor of Cancer Research and Director, Division of Cancer Control and Prevention, Department of Internal Medicine, College of Medicine; Professor, Division of Epidemiology, College of Public Health; and Associate Director for Population Sciences, Comprehensive Cancer Center, The Ohio State University.

Levi D. Procter, MD, is with the Division of General Surgery, College of Medicine, University of Kentucky.

Eric W. Rademacher, PhD, is Co-Director, Institute for Policy Research, University of Cincinnati.

Rebecca J. Schmidt, DO, is Section Chief, Section on Nephrology, Department of Medicine, School of Medicine, West Virginia University.

Shiloh K. Turner, MPA, is Vice President for Community Investment, The Greater Cincinnati Foundation.

Barbara B. Weaner, RN, MSN, RNC, FNP, is Nurse Practitioner, Section on Nephrology, Department of Medicine, School of Medicine, West Virginia University.

Mary Ellen Wewers, PhD, is Professor, Division of Health Behavior and Health Promotion, College of Public Health, The Ohio State University.

Index